12 Lead ECG
Interpretation

NOTICE

Medicine is an ever-changing science. As new research and clinical experience broaden our knowledge, changes in treatment and drug therapy are required. The editors and the publisher of this work have checked with sources believed to be reliable in their efforts to provide information that is complete and generally in accord with the standards accepted at the time of publication. However, in view of the possibility of human error or changes in medical sciences, neither the editors nor the publisher nor any other party who has been involved in the preparation or publication of this work warrants that the information contained herein is in every respect accurate or complete, and they are not responsible for any errors or omissions or for the results obtained from use of such information. Readers are encouraged to confirm the information contained herein with other sources. For example and in particular, readers are advised to check the product information sheet included in the package of each drug they plan to administer to be certain that the information contained in this book is accurate and that changes have not been made in the recommended dose or in the contraindications for administration. This recommendation is of particular importance in connection with new or infrequently used drugs.

12 Lead ECG Interpretation
A Self-Teaching Manual

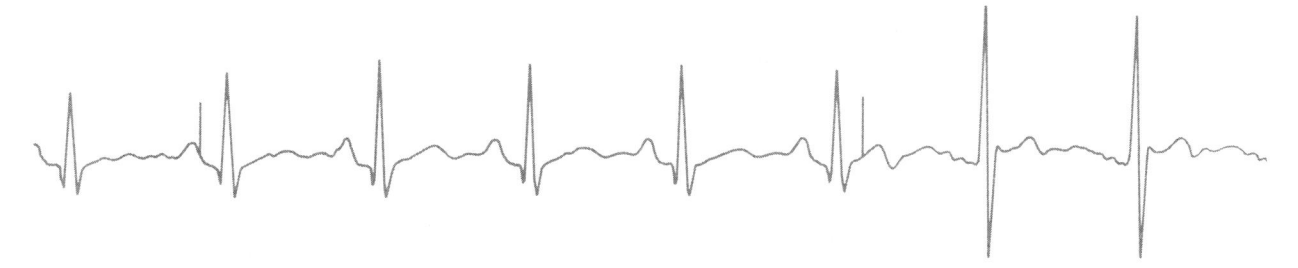

ANN E. NORMAN, R.N., B.A., B.S.N.
Department of Educational and Consulting Services
Los Angeles County + University of Southern California Medical Center

McGraw-Hill, Inc.
New York St. Louis San Francisco Auckland Bogotá
Caracas Lisbon London Madrid Mexico City Milan
Montreal New Delhi San Juan Singapore
Sydney Tokyo Toronto

12 Lead ECG Interpretation: A Self-Teaching Manual

Copyright © 1992 by McGraw-Hill, Inc. All rights reserved. Printed in the United States of America. Except as permitted under the United States Copyright Act of 1976, no part of this publication may be reproduced or distributed in any form or by any means, or stored in a data base or retrieval system, without the prior written permission of the publisher.

34567890 MALMAL 01 00 99

ISBN 0-07-105396-4

This book was prepared camera-ready. The editors were Gail Gavert and Steven Melvin; the production supervisor was Gyl Favours. The cover was designed by José Fonfrias.

Malloy Lithographers, Inc. was printer and binder.

Library of Congress Cataloging-in-Publication data

Norman, Ann E.
　　12 lead ECG interpretation : a self-teaching manual / Ann E.
　Norman.
　　　　p. cm.
　　Includes bibliographical references.
　　ISBN 0-07-105396-4 :
　　1. Electrocardiography—Programmed instruction. I. Twelve lead
　ECG interpretation. II. Title.
　　　[DNLM: 1. Arrhythmia—diagnosis—programmed instruction.
　2. Electrocardiography—programmed instruction. WG 18 N842z]
　RC683.5.E5N65 1992
　6169.1'207547—dc20
　DNLM/DLC
　for Library of Congress　　　　　　　　　　　　　　　　92-6221
　　　　　　　　　　　　　　　　　　　　　　　　　　　　　　CIP

*Dedicated with love
to my husband,
Harry*

Contents

Acknowledgments ix
Objectives xi
Instructions to the Learner xiii

1   INTRODUCTION TO 12 LEAD ECG 1

Assessment of the 12 lead ECG. Principles of 12 lead ECG interpretation.

2   REVIEW OF THE BASICS 8

Conduction system of the heart. qRS complex. T wave. U wave. PR interval (PRI). ST segment. QT interval (QTI). ECG paper: time and voltage. Normal standardization mark. Physiological q waves (septal q waves).

3   LOCATION OF FRONTAL PLANE AXIS 20

Definition of the frontal plane axis. Normal frontal plane axis. The frontal plane leads. Hexaxial reference system. Perpendicular leads. Quadrants. Three principles of electrocardiography: review. Steps to locate the frontal plane axis. The hexaxial quadrants. Frontal plane axis summary. Causes of frontal plane axis deviation.

4   PROGRESSION OF THE R WAVE 46

Location of the precordial V leads. Normal complex morphology in V leads. Practice 12 lead ECGs #1–12. Review of the 12 leads of the ECG.

5   CHAMBER ENLARGEMENTS 64

Review of chambers and valves. Causes of chamber enlargements. Atrial enlargement. Normal P waves. Practice strips #13–20. Ventricular hypertrophy. Left ventricular hypertrophy ECG characteristics. Estes scoring system for LVH. Right ventricular hypertrophy ECG characteristics. Practice 12 lead ECGs #21–35.

6 INTRAVENTRICULAR CONDUCTION DEFECTS (IVCD) 112

Types and causes of IVCD. Normal ventricular depolarization. Right bundle branch block. Left bundle branch block. Axis deviation with bundle branch block. Practice 12 lead ECGs #36–45. Hemiblocks. Bifascicular block. Trifascicular block. Practice 12 lead ECGs #46–70. Correcting the frontal plane axis.

7 MYOCARDIAL ISCHEMIA, INJURY, AND INFARCTION 187

Coronary artery distribution. Review of the leads. Myocardial ischemia, injury, and infarction ECG criteria. Reciprocal changes: acute and posterior. Posterior myocardial infarction V_1 and V_2. Subendocardial infarctions. Practice 12 lead ECGs #71–95.

8 SUPRAVENTRICULAR ABERRANCY VERSUS VENTRICULAR ECTOPY 239

The scope of the problem. ECG characteristics of supraventricular aberrancy. ECG characteristics of ventricular ectopy. Summary. Practice strips.

9 EFFECTS OF DRUGS AND ELECTROLYTES ON THE ECG 261

Changes in waves, intervals, and segments. QT interval. Effects of digitalis on the ECG. Quinidine effects on the ECG: therapeutic and toxic. Other medications. Effects of electrolytes on the ECG. Summary of drug and electrolyte ECG changes. Nonspecific ST segment and T wave changes.

10 WOLFF-PARKINSON-WHITE (WPW) SYNDROME 275

Incidence of WPW. Classification: Types A and B. WPW ECG diagnostic criteria. Clinical significance. Retrograde versus antegrade AV node conduction. Treatment and medication.

11 12 LEAD ECG REVIEW 287

Frontal plane axis. Chamber enlargement. Intraventricular conduction defects. Transmural myocardial ischemia, injury, and infarction. Subendocardial infarction. Supraventricular aberrancy versus ventricular ectopy. Summary of drug and electrolyte ECG changes. Wolff-Parkinson-White (WPW) syndrome.

Glossary 295
Bibliography 299

Acknowledgments

It is my pleasure to express my sincere appreciation to the following people at the Los Angeles County+University of Southern California Medical Center:

Tibor Zempleni, M.D., for his assistance with the manuscript.

Fotine D. O'Connor, R.N., M.N., Director of the Department of Nursing Services and Education, for her support and encouragement in my writing endeavors.

Rosemary J. Free, R.N., B.S.N., M.A., Nurse Education Director, Medical Center, Department of Educational and Consulting Services, for encouraging me to write this book.

Winifred Kataoka, R.N.C., M.A., Nursing Instructor, School of Nursing, for the artwork.

Lorraine Bennett, Word Processor II, Department of Educational and Consulting Services, whose fantastic fingers at the keyboard helped bring this book to fruition.

The nurses, physicians, and technicians who helped me collect the tracings.

I would also like to thank my husband, Harry "buddy," for his patience and contribution to the artwork.

Objectives

Upon completion of this self-teaching manual on the 12 lead ECG, you will be able to

1
Recognize a normal 12 lead ECG.

2
Locate the frontal plane axis.

3
Recognize the normal progression of the R wave in the precordial leads.

4
Identify enlargements of the four chambers of the heart.

5
Identify right and left bundle branch blocks.

6
Identify hemiblocks and bifascicular and trifascicular blocks.

7
Identify areas of myocardial ischemia, injury, and infarction.

8
State the ECG characteristics of supraventricular aberrancy and ventricular ectopy.

9
Recognize ECG changes that occur with certain medications and electrolytes.

10
Identify the Wolff-Parkinson-White (WPW) syndrome.

Instructions to the Learner

This self-instructional text may be used solely on your own or in conjunction with a classroom course. Basic arrhythmia interpretation is not a prerequisite to learning how to interpret 12 lead ECG, but it is helpful to have that background.

To learn 12 lead ECG interpretation, you must learn the principles of and criteria for ECG, and then practice interpretations. Practice 12 lead ECGs are included in this book. The answers to the practice tracings are provided so that you can check yourself as you proceed. Do not just look at the answers. The only way you will really learn 12 lead ECG interpretation is to practice, practice, practice.

12 Lead ECG
Interpretation

CHAPTER 1
INTRODUCTION TO 12 LEAD ECG

Figure I A on the following page is a normal 12 lead ECG. The 12 leads are universal in their placement. Beginning at the top left-hand corner:

Lead I is at the upper lefthand corner

Lead II is below lead I on the middle line

Lead III is below lead II on the lower line

Refer to Figure 1 A on the following page and notice that in the first quarter of the tracing in the upper row is a blip mark and the configuration of the ECG waves change. This alerts you that the lead has changed. Please note the blip marks on Figure 1 A, page 2.

NOTE: Some ECGs do not have blip marks. In this case you know the lead has changed because you are one-fourth of the way across the tracing on the upper row and because the configuration of the ECG waves change.

The augmented vector leads are the second column.

Lead aVR (augmented vector right) is on the upper line
Lead aVL (augmented vector left) is below aVR on the middle line
Lead aVF (augmented vector foot) is below aVL on the lower line

Return to the upper line and notice that halfway across the tracing, the lead changes again. This change is denoted by another blip mark and the changing configuration of the ECG waves. The last six leads are the precordial (chest) leads. These leads are designated V_1, V_2, V_3, V_4, V_5, and V_6. Some 12 leads identify the leads. Some do not. Study Figure 1 A on the following page.

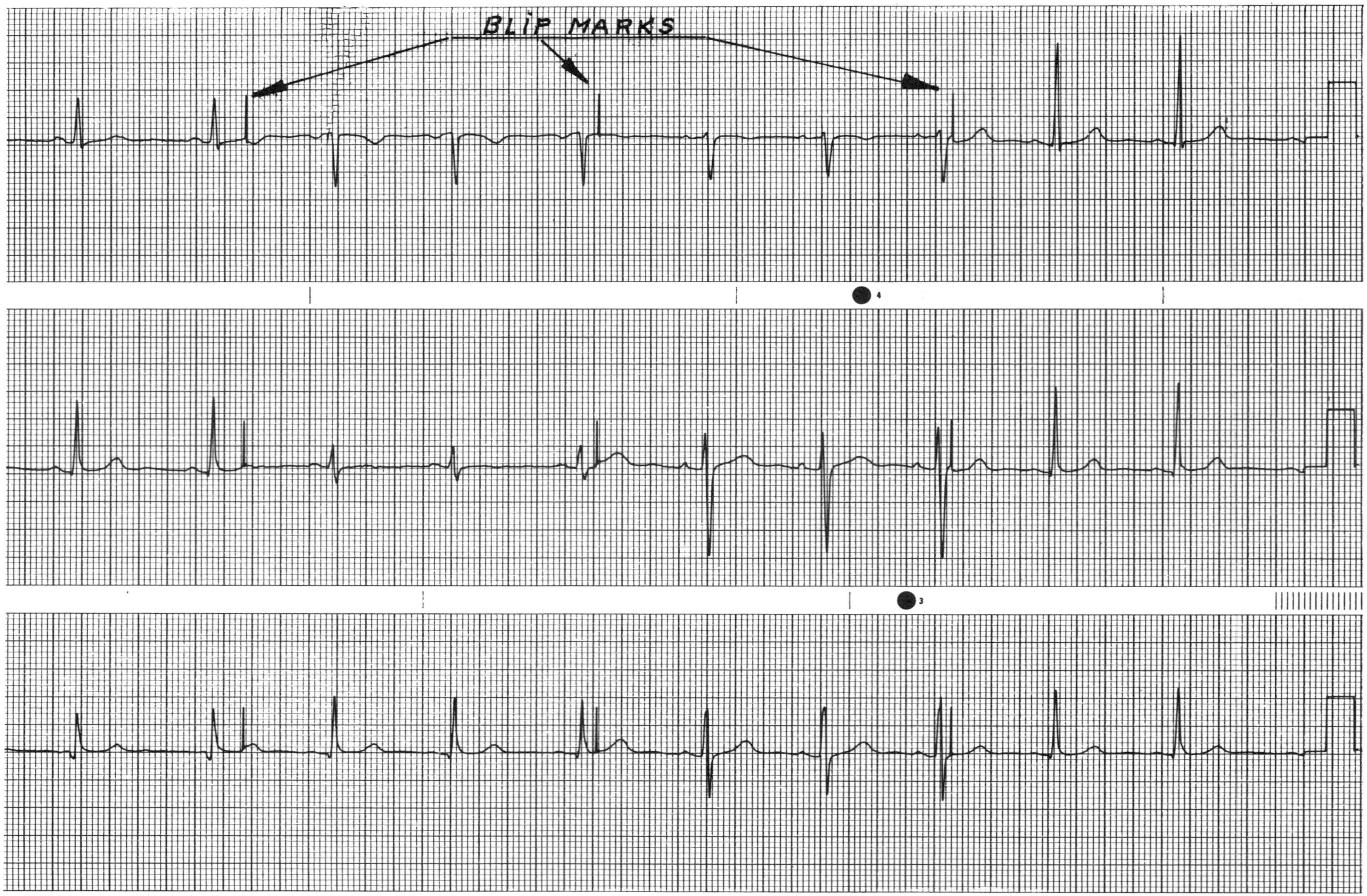

BLIP MARKS

Figure 1 A

Chapter 1 — Introduction to 12 Lead ECG

Figure 1 B on following page is also a normal 12 lead ECG. On this particular tracing, the leads are designated. Study Figure 1 B to familiarize yourself with the location of the 12 leads. Your ECG lab may or may not designate the leads. If not designated, it is universally understood that the leads are arranged as described in Figure 1 A and depicted in Figure 1 B.

ASSESSMENT OF THE 12 LEAD ECG

To interpret the 12 lead ECG you need to assess the following:

1. Basic rhythm
2. Frontal plane axis
3. R wave progression
4. Configuration and duration of the complex
5. Size of the P wave
6. QT interval (to be discussed in Chapter 9)
7. ST segment
8. Size and configuration of the T wave
9. Presence and size of U waves (abnormals will be discussed in Chapter 9)

INTERPRETATION OF FIGURE 1 A (page 2)

Basic rhythm: Normal sinus rhythm
Frontal plane axis: Normal +60° (Chapter 3 will cover this)
R wave progression: Normal (Chapter 4)
Configuration and duration of the complex: Normal
Size of the P wave: Normal (Chapter 2)
QT interval: Normal (discussion will be omitted until Chapter 9)
ST segment: Normal (Chapter 2)
Size and configuration of T wave: Normal (Chapters 2 and 9)
Presence and size of U wave: Normal (Chapter 2)
12 Lead ECG Interpretation: Normal

INTERPRETATION OF FIGURE 1 B (page 4)

Basic rhythm: Normal sinus rhythm
Frontal plane axis: Normal +60°
R wave progression: Normal
Configuration and duration of the complex: Normal
Size of the P wave: Normal
ST segment: Normal
Size and configuration of T wave: Normal
Presence and size of U wave: Normal (seen in V_2 and V_3)
12 Lead ECG Interpretation: Normal

Figure 1 B

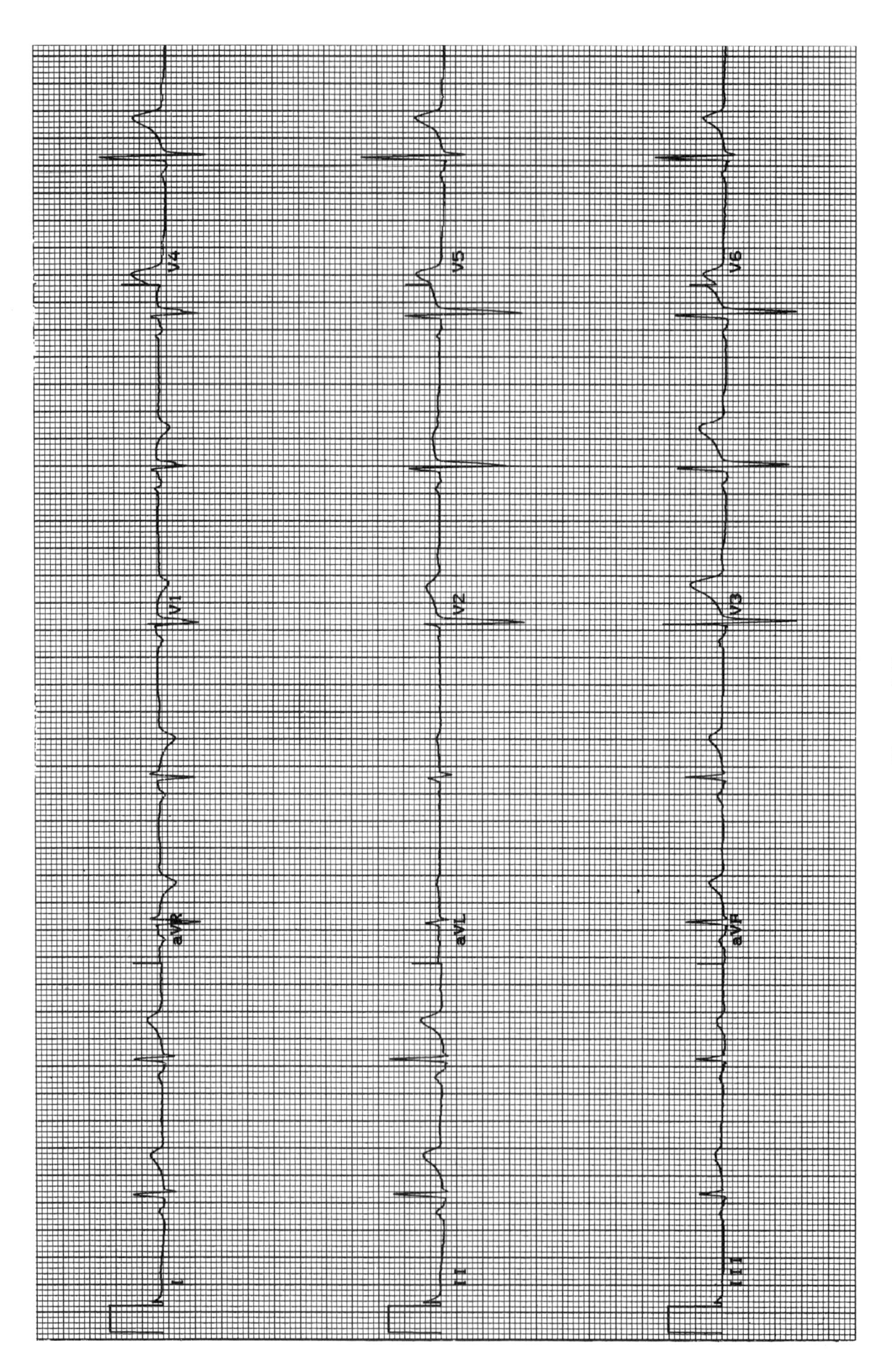

Chapter 1 — Introduction to 12 Lead ECG

PRINCIPLES OF 12 LEAD ECG INTERPRETATION

To interpret the 12 lead ECG, please recall the following three principles:

1.   ⟶ + = ⋀

   When the wave of depolarization moves towards the positive (+) electrode of any lead, an upright wave is inscribed.

2.   ⟵ + = ⋁

   When the wave of depolarization moves away from the positive electrode of any lead, a negative wave is inscribed.

3.   ↑↓ + = ⋀⋁ or —

   When depolarization moves perpendicular to the positive electrode of any lead, either a biphasic complex ⋀⋁ or a straight line _____ will be inscribed.

YOU WILL USE THE ABOVE PRINCIPLES THROUGHOUT THIS BOOK.

Pretend that the positive (+) electrode is an eye looking at the heart.

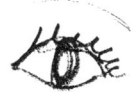

This eye is looking at the electrical activity of the heart. The positive electrode "sees" depolarization moving towards it, or away from it, or at an angle to it.

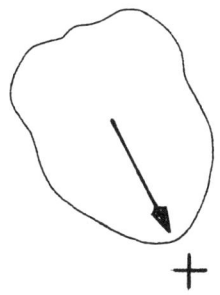

The positive electrode of the above lead sees the wave of depolarization moving towards it. Therefore, according to **principle #1**, an upright complex will be inscribed in this lead.

Chapter 1 — Introduction to 12 Lead ECG

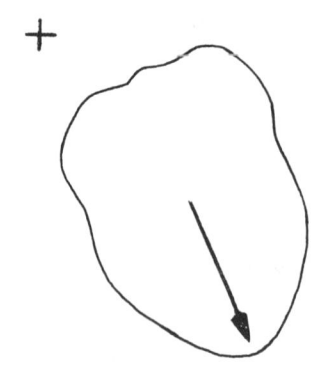

The positive electrode of the above lead sees the wave of depolarization moving away from it. Therefore, according to **principle #2**, a negative complex will be inscribed in this lead.

Refer to Figure 1 B.

QUESTION: What kind of a complex is inscribed in lead II?

A. Positive
B. Negative
C. Biphasic

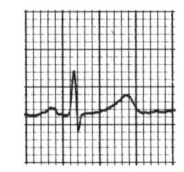

Figure I B lead II

ANSWER: A. The complex in lead II is primarily positive (above the isoelectric line). Therefore, the wave of depolarization is moving towards the positive electrode of lead II.

QUESTION: In Figure 1 B, what kind of a complex do you see in lead aVR?

A. Positive
B. Negative
C. Biphasic

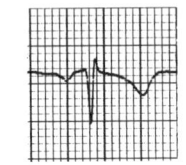

Figure I B aVR

ANSWER: B. The complex in aVR is primarily negative, below the isoelectric line. The wave of depolarization is moving away from the positive electrode of aVR.

QUESTION: In Figure 1 B what kind of a complex is inscribed in aVL?

A. Positive
B. Negative
C. Biphasic

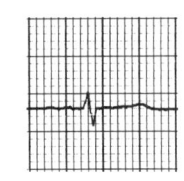

Figure I B aVL

ANSWER: C. A biphasic complex is inscribed in aVL. The wave of depolarization is moving perpendicular to the positive electrode of aVL according to **principle #3**.

Chapter 1 — Introduction to 12 Lead ECG

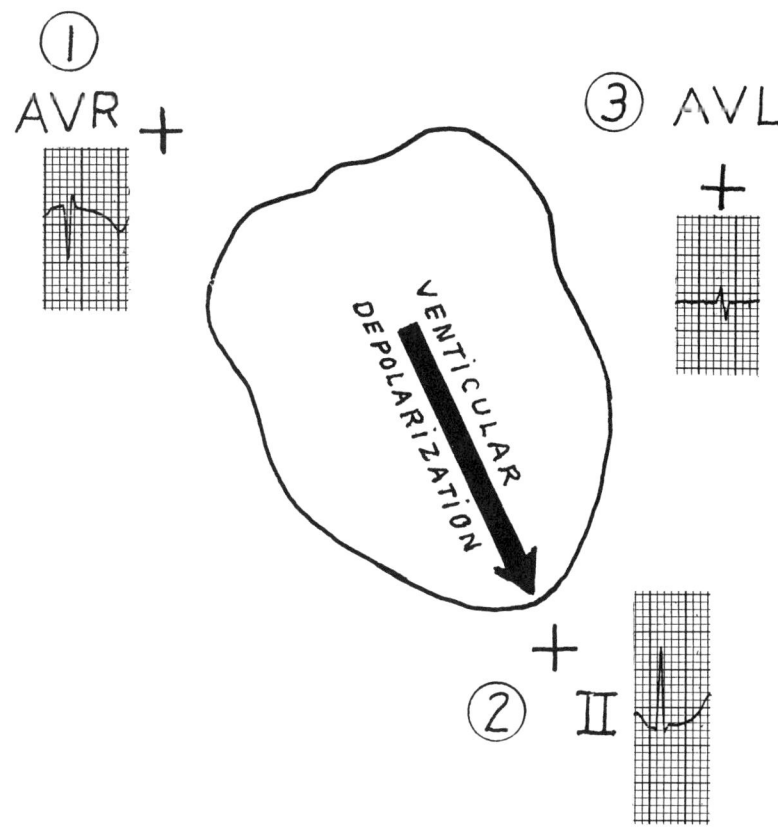

In the above picture you can see what happened in Figure 1 B. The wave of ventricular depolarization: **1, 2, 3**

1. moved away from the positive electrode of lead aVR

2. moved towards the positive electrode of lead II

3. moved perpendicular to the positive electrode of lead aVL

Take a few minutes to relate the above picture and the explanation to Figure 1 B. This concept is crucial to understanding the 12 lead ECG.

CHAPTER 2
REVIEW OF THE BASICS

CONDUCTION SYSTEM OF THE HEART

The conduction system of the heart is composed of specialized fibers that initiate the electrical events and conduct these impulses through the heart.

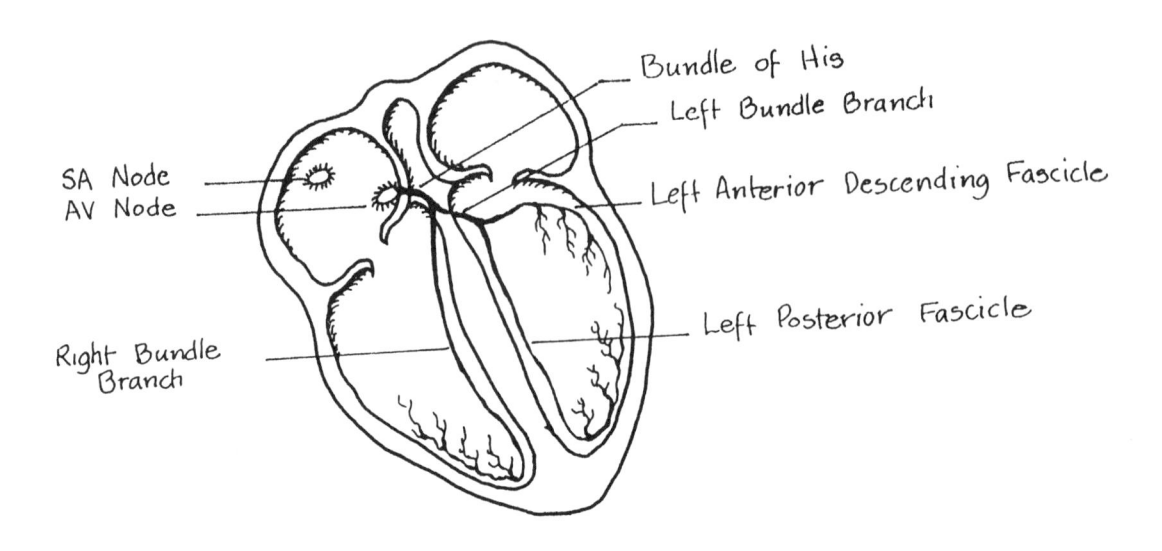

NOTE: Review the anatomy of the conduction system of the heart with the above picture.

- The **S-A node** initiates the normal rhythmic electrical impulse. The S-A node rhythmically depolarizes and this wave of *depolarization* spreads through the atria. The S-A node is very small and you do not see its electrical activity on the ECG. You do see the atria depolarize; depolarization of the atria inscribes the P wave on the ECG. P waves are normally small and round. Normal P waves are no more than 2½ millimeters tall and no more than 2½ millimeters wide.

- The **A-V node** delays the electrical impulse before it proceeds into the ventricles. This normal delay at the A-V node allows time for the atria to depolarize and contract while the ventricles are still in their diastole. Thus, the atria can empty their contents into the ventricles before ventricular contraction begins. This synchronization between the atria and the ventricles accounts for approximately 15% of the cardiac output.

- The **junctional bundle** conducts the impulse from the atria to the **ventricles**. The electrical impulse travels into the ventricular conduction system via the junctional bundle and down the bundle branches. There are two main bundle branches: the **left and the right bundle branches** conduct the electrical impulse into the right and left ventricle respectively. The left bundle branch further divides into two main branches called **fascicles**: an **anterior fascicle** and a **posterior fascicle**. The right bundle branch does not divide into fascicles.

Chapter 2 — Review of the Basics

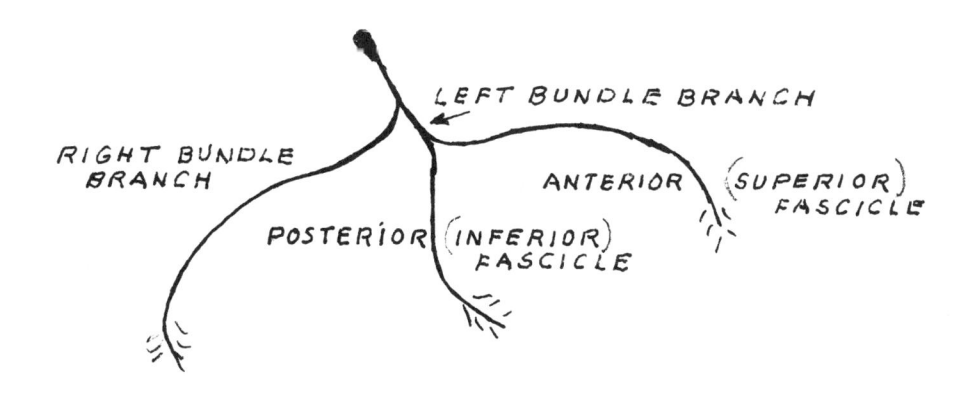

The anterior fascicle is also called the superior fascicle.

The posterior fascicle is also called the inferior fascicle.

- The terminal **Purkinje fibers** enter the myocardial cell and conduct the electrical impulse throughout the ventricles. The electrical impulse travels very rapidly through the Purkinje fibers resulting in rapid transmission of the impulse throughout the ventricular system.

QRS COMPLEX

The electrical event of ventricular depolarization is normally followed by the mechanical event of ventricular contraction. When the ventricles depolarize, the waves of the complex are inscribed on the ECG. The waves of the complex are the qRs. These waves are specifically named.

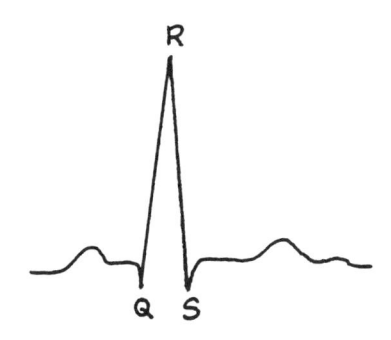

QUESTION: When the first wave of the complex is negative (below the *isoelectric line*) it is called a q wave.

A. True
B. False

ANSWER: A. True. **q Waves must be negative and a q wave must be the first wave of the complex.**

Chapter 2 — Review of the Basics

QUESTION: q Waves normally are very large.

A. True
B. False

ANSWER: B. False. q Waves normally are small and are denoted with a small q. The amplitude of a normal q wave is less than one fourth the height of its R wave.

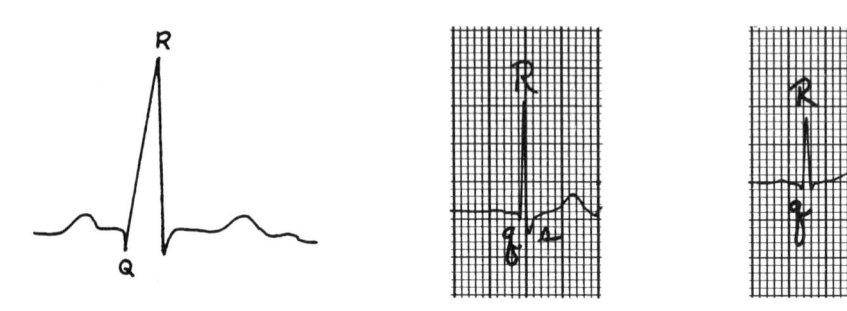

QUESTION: The R wave is the first upward deflection of the complex.

A. True
B. False

ANSWER: A. True. R waves are <u>always</u> positive (above the isoelectric line). There is no such thing as a "negative R wave."

QUESTION: When there are two positive deflections, the second one is called R prime (R').

A. True
B. False

ANSWER: True.

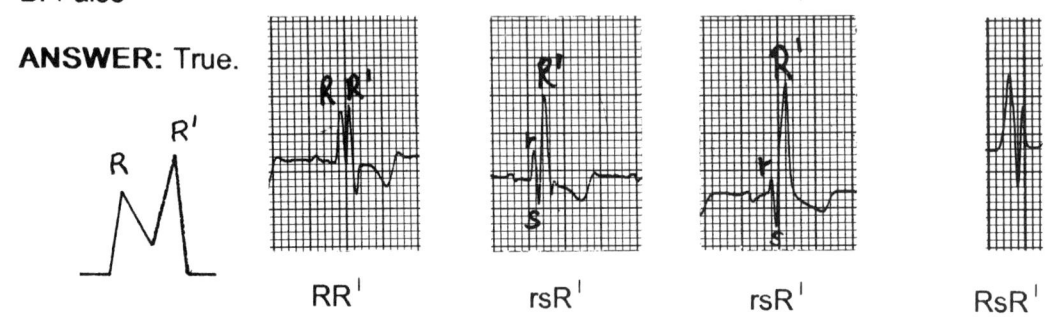

RR'   rsR'   rsR'   RsR'

QUESTION: The S wave is the negative deflection following the R wave.

A. True
B. False

ANSWER: A. True. S waves are always negative, and like the alphabet, S follows R.

NOTE: If the wave of the complex is less than 5 millimeters (5 small boxes) tall or deep it is denoted with a small letter. If the height or depth of the wave is 5 millimeters or more, it is denoted with a capital letter.

Chapter 2 -- Review of the Basics

QUESTION: Name the waves of the complexes in the following:

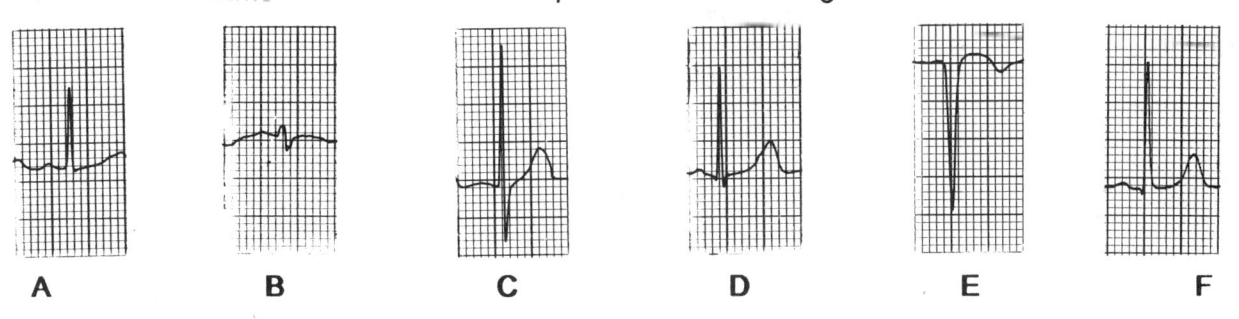

| A | B | C | D | E | F |

ANSWERS:

A. rs
B. R
C. RS
D. qRs
E. QS
F. qR

NOTE: As you can see, complexes do not always have a q, R, and s wave.

QUESTION: The duration of the complex normally is less than 0.12 seconds.

A. True
B. False

ANSWER: True. The normal duration of the complex varies between 0.06 and 0.10 seconds but occasionally a duration of 0.11 seconds is seen in healthy adults.

T WAVE

QUESTION: T waves represent ventricular repolarization.

A. True
B. False

ANSWER: A. True.

Ventricular depolarization occurs from endocardium to epicardium but **repolarization** occurs from epicardium to endocardium. Normally, the last cell to depolarize is the first one to repolarize. Normal T waves are in the same direction as their complex.

Refer back to Figure I A on page 2 and note the T waves in the frontal plane leads. Leads I, II, III, and aVF have tall R waves with upright T waves. Lead aVR has a negative complex with an inverted T wave. Lead aVL is biphasic and the T wave is almost non-existent. These are normal T waves with respect to their complex.

Chapter 2 — Review of the Basics

Normally, **the T wave in V$_1$** is inverted, biphasic, flat, or upright. In other words, the T wave in V$_1$ can pretty much be what it wants to be. An inverted, biphasic, or flat T wave in V$_1$ usually is upright by V$_2$. T waves in V$_3$ through V$_6$ normally are upright. Refer back to Figure I A on page 2 and note the T waves in the precordial leads. V$_1$ has an inverted T wave. V$_2$ through V$_6$ have upright T waves. These are normal T waves.

The normal T wave is asymmetrical, i.e., it peaks towards the end of the wave instead of in the middle. Normally, T waves in the frontal plane are no more than 5 millimeters tall (1 large box); T waves in the precordial plane normally are no more than 10 millimeters tall (2 large boxes).

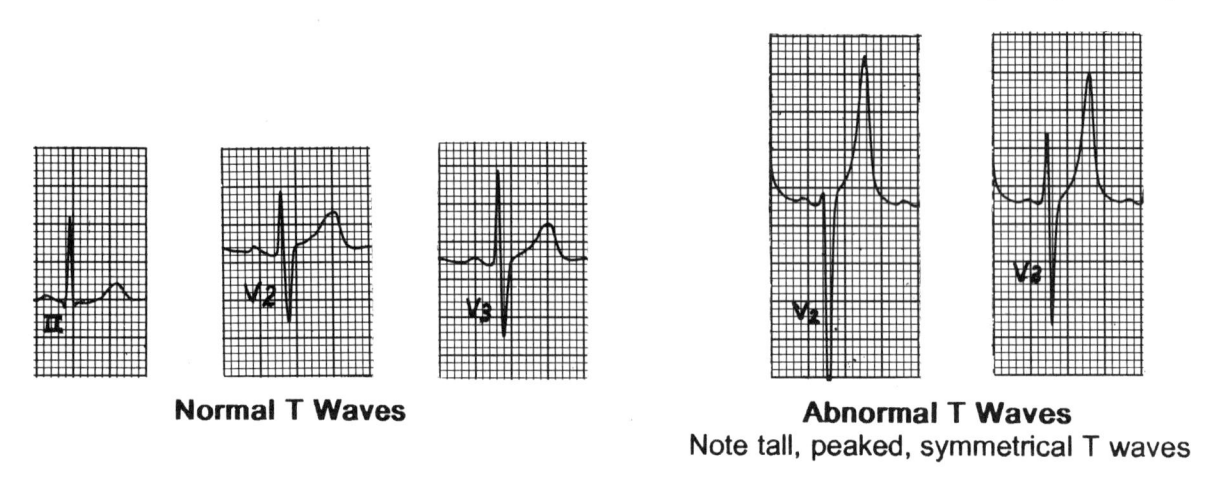

Normal T Waves

Abnormal T Waves
Note tall, peaked, symmetrical T waves

| U WAVE |

QUESTION: Sometimes there is a wave following the T wave, before the next P wave. What is this wave called?

ANSWER: U wave.

Normal U waves represent repolarization of the Purkinje fibers. A normal U wave is no more than one-fourth the height of its T wave and is in the same direction as the T wave. Normal U waves are best seen in V$_2$ and V$_3$ with ventricular rates less than 90 BPM. A U wave with an amplitude greater than 1.5 millimeters is abnormal in any lead.

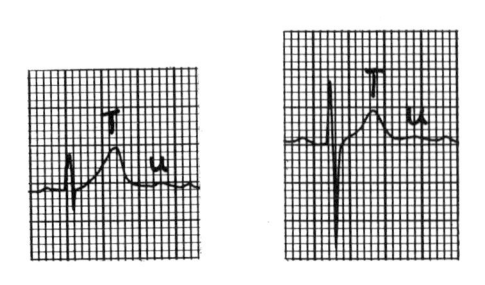

EXAMPLES OF NORMAL U WAVES 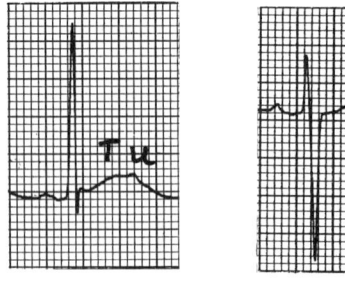 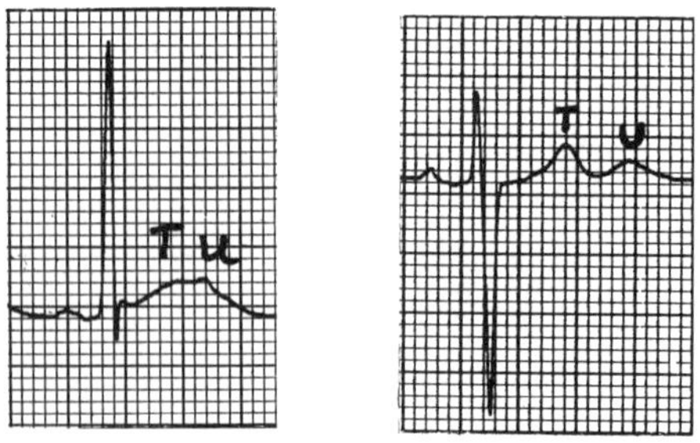   EXAMPLES OF ABNORMAL U WAVES

Chapter 2 -- Review of the Basics

PR INTERVAL (PRI)

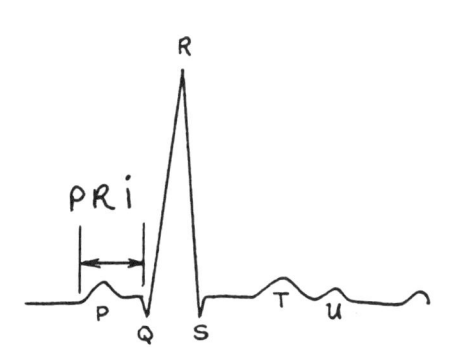

The PRI is measured from the beginning of the P wave to the beginning of the complex. The PRI represents the time it takes the wave of depolarization to spread through the atria, the A-V node, and the A-V junction.

QUESTION: The normal PRI is 0.12 to 0.20 seconds.

A. True
B. False

ANSWER: A. True

ST SEGMENT

The ST segment is measured from the end of the complex to the beginning of the T wave. The ST segment is the beginning of ventricular repolarization.

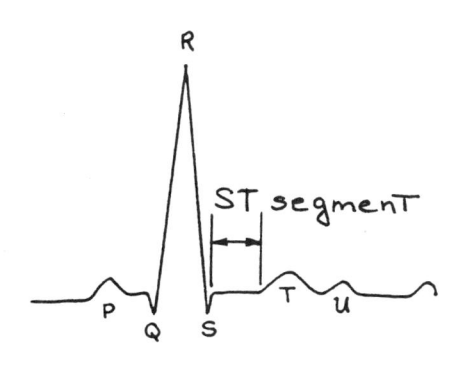

Chapter 2 -- Review of the Basics

QUESTION: The normal ST segment is on the isoelectric line or no more than one millimeter above or below the isoelectric line.

A. True
B. False

ANSWER: A. True. When the ST segment is more than one millimeter above the isoelectric line, it is an *elevated ST segment*. When the ST segment is more than 1 millimeter below the isoelectric line, it is a *depressed ST segment*.

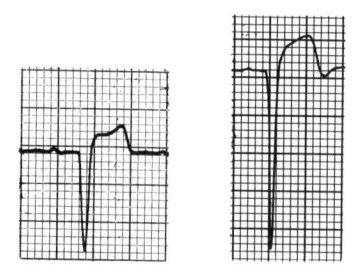

Elevated ST Segment 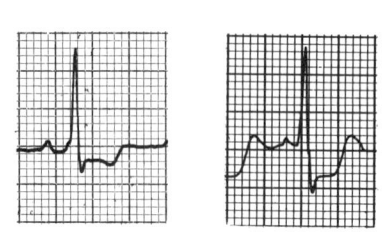   **Depressed ST Segment**

QT INTERVAL (QTI)

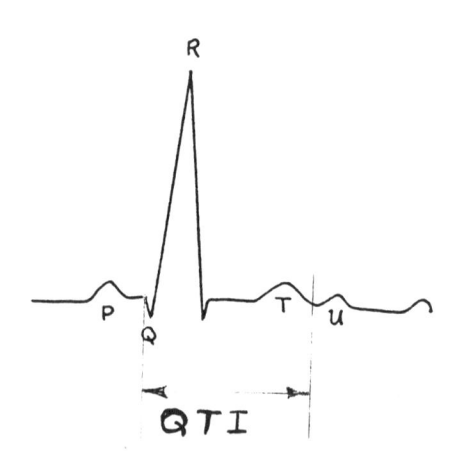

QTI

Chapter 2 -- Review of the Basics

The QTI is measured from the beginning of the complex to the end of the T wave. Generally speaking, a normal QTI is no more than one half the R to R interval.

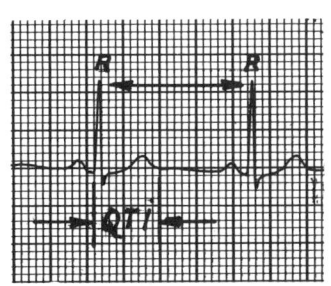

For simplicity's sake, the QT interval will not be discussed further until Chapter 9.

ECG PAPER: TIME AND VOLTAGE

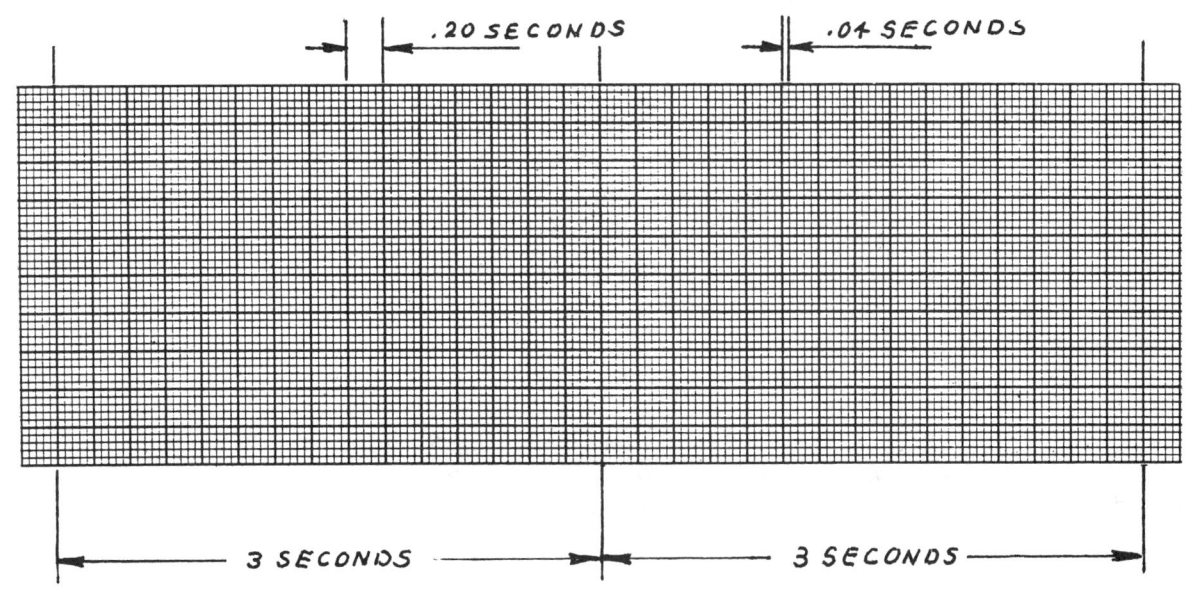

QUESTION: Each **small** box on the **horizontal** line represents 0.04 seconds passage of time when the ECG is recorded at standard time: 25 mm per second.

A. True
B. False

ANSWER: A. True.

QUESTION: Each **large** box on the **horizontal** line represents 0.20 seconds passage of time.

A. True
B. False

ANSWER: A. True. Since there are five small boxes in one large box, each large box on the horizontal line is equal to 0.20 seconds.

Chapter 2 -- Review of the Basics

QUESTION: Each **small** box on the **vertical** line is equal to 0.1 millivolts.

A. True
B. False

ANSWER: A. True.

NORMAL STANDARDIZATION MARK

The normal standardization mark is 10 small boxes (10 millimeters) tall. Therefore, the voltage of the normal standardization mark is 1.0 millivolt (10 X 0.1 = 1.0). ECG voltage is usually expressed in millimeters.

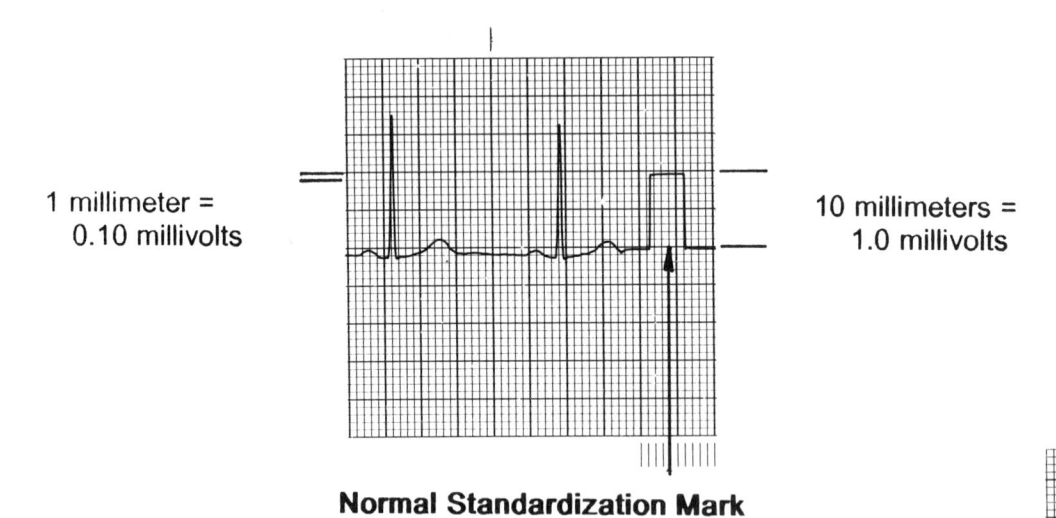

1 millimeter = 0.10 millivolts

10 millimeters = 1.0 millivolts

Normal Standardization Mark

To assess the 12 lead ECG, orient the standardization mark to the upright position: Sometimes it is at the beginning and sometimes at the end of the tracing. If you do not properly orient the standardization mark, you may be looking at the 12 lead ECG upside down.

Chapter 2 — Review of the Basics

PHYSIOLOGICAL q WAVES (SEPTAL q WAVES)

On the left bundle branch, before it bifurcates into the two fascicles, there is a Purkinje-like fiber. In some people, this fiber is large enough to be classified as a third fascicle. In any case, ventricular septum depolarization normally is initiated from this part of the conduction system.

Recall that the intraventricular septum is a wall of the left ventricle. The septum is the first part of the ventricle to depolarize. The left side of the septum depolarizes first and normal septal depolarization spreads from left to right:

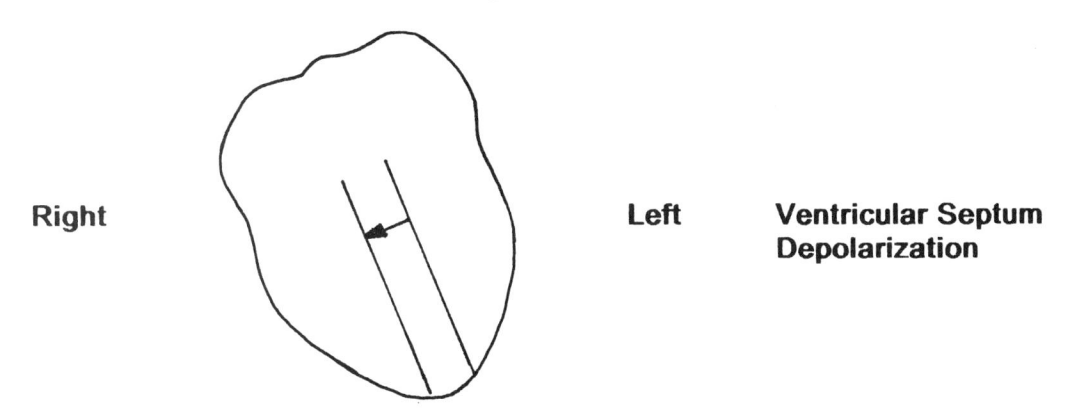

Right   Left   Ventricular Septum
                         Depolarization

QUESTION: The septum is the first part of the ventricle to depolarize and the septum normally depolarizes from left to right.

A. True
B. False

ANSWER: A. True. The septum is the first part of the ventricle to depolarize and septal depolarization normally occurs from left to right. If you missed this question, please refer to the picture of ventricular septum depolarization above.

It is important and bears repeating: The ventricular septum *is the first part of the ventricle to depolarize.* Septal depolarization normally occurs from left to right as depicted in the picture above.

Those leads that have their positive electrode on the left side of the heart will see ventricular septum depolarization moving away from them and inscribe a negative deflection. This negative deflection is the first wave of the complex in the left lateral leads.

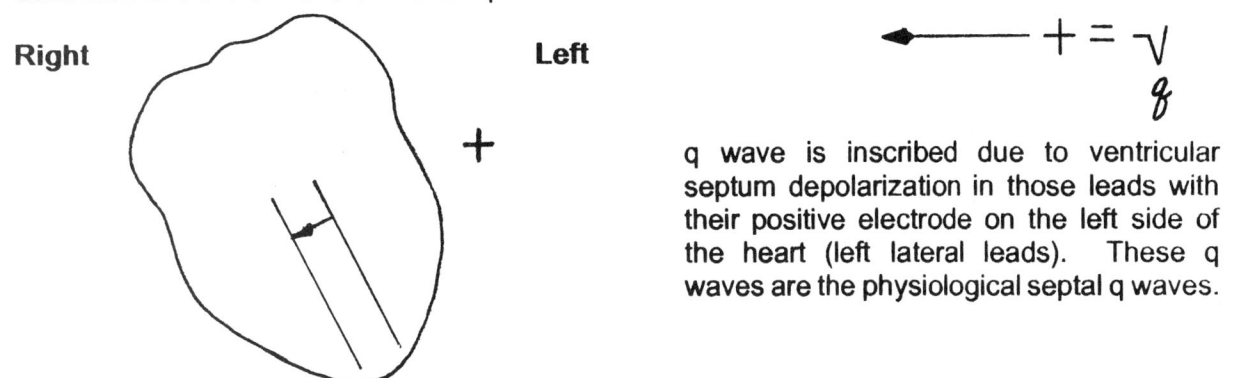

Right   Left

q wave is inscribed due to ventricular septum depolarization in those leads with their positive electrode on the left side of the heart (left lateral leads). These q waves are the physiological septal q waves.

Chapter 2 -- Review of the Basics

QUESTION: What kind of a wave will ventricular septum depolarization inscribe in those leads that have their positive electrode on the left side of the heart?

ANSWER: A q wave will be inscribed in those leads that have their positive electrode left of the heart. If you missed this question please review the last picture on the previous page.

These physiological septal q waves normally are very small. Generally speaking, physiological q waves are less than one millimeter in either direction.

QUESTION: When the wave of the complex is less than 5 millimeters in amplitude it is denoted with a small letter.

A. True
B. False

ANSWER: A. True.

Name the waves of the following complexes and check your answers below.

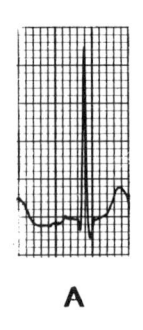

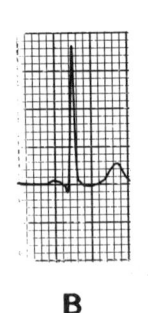

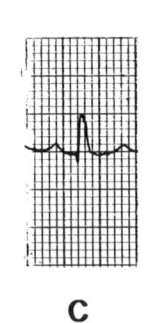

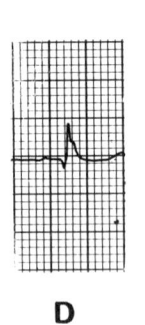

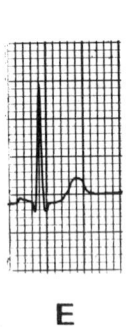

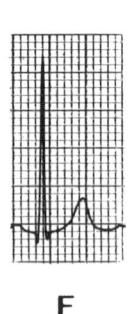

A   **B**   **C**   **D**   **E**   **F**

ANSWERS:

A. qRs   C. qRR^1 E. qRs
B. qR   D. qRr^1 F. qRs

LEFT LATERAL LEADS

All of the above q waves are normal. Please note the size of the normal physiological q waves above.

The leads that have their positive electrode on the left side of the heart are I and aVL in the frontal plane and V_5 and V_6 in the precordial plane. These four leads are called the **left lateral leads: I, aVL, V$_5$, V$_6$.**

Chapter 2 -- Review of the Basics

QUESTION: Physiological q waves normally are seen in leads I, aVL, V_5, and V_6.

A. True
B. False

ANSWER: A. True. Physiological q waves normally are seen in leads I, aVL, V_5, and V_6 as a result of the septum depolarizing away from the positive electrode of these leads.

Recall that physiological q waves are also known as septal q waves. Physiological means that they are normal - they are inscribed as the result of normal depolarization of the ventricular septum.

Normally, ventricular septum depolarization occurs from left to right. In some people, however, septal depolarization occurs somewhat differently. The Purkinje that initiates septal depolarization in some people causes ventricular septum depolarization to occur from inferior to superior.

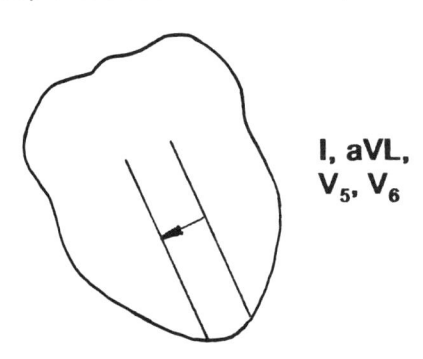

I, aVL, V_5, V_6
Left to right
Ventricular septum depolarization

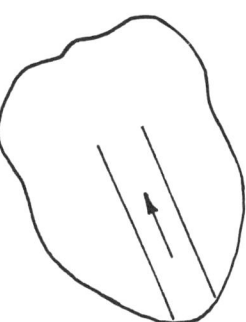

II, III, aVF
Inferior to superior
Ventricular septum depolarization

Inferior to superior ventricular septum depolarization is a normal variant. Those leads that have their positive electrode on the inferior surface of the heart will see septal depolarization moving from inferior to superior and inscribe a negative deflection. This negative deflection is the first wave of the complex - a q wave.
The leads that have their positive electrode inferior to the heart are called the inferior leads. The inferior leads are II, III, and aVF.

QUESTION: As a normal variant, physiological q waves will sometimes be seen in leads II, III, and aVF.

A. True
B. False

ANSWER: True.

In summary, physiological (septal) q waves are the result of ventricular septum depolarization. The septum is the first part of the ventricle to depolarize. In those leads that see ventricular septum depolarization moving away from them, a physiological q wave will be inscribed.

Physiological q waves are normally seen in leads I, aVL, V_5, and V_6. As a normal variant, physiological q waves will be seen in the inferior leads II, III, and aVF.

CHAPTER 3
LOCATION OF FRONTAL PLANE AXIS

DEFINITION OF THE FRONTAL PLANE AXIS

The frontal plane axis is the orientation of the heart's electrical activity in the frontal plane. The frontal plane consists of the right-to-left - left-to-right, and superior to inferior -inferior to superior directions.

SUPERIOR

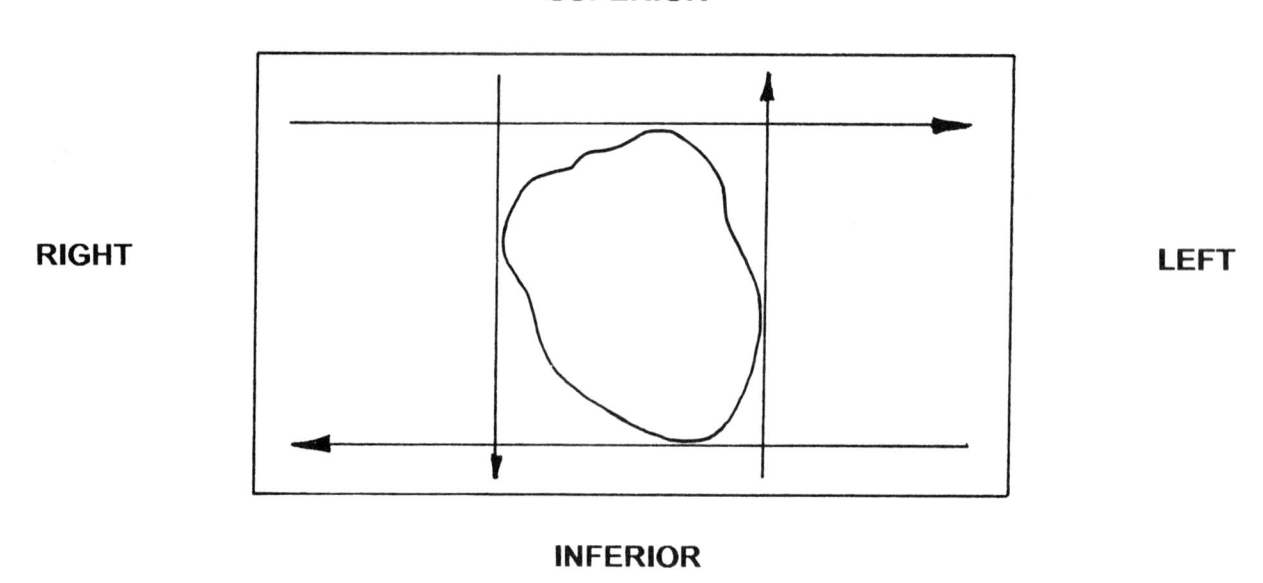

RIGHT **LEFT**

INFERIOR

QUESTION: The frontal plane considers the anterior to posterior orientation of the heart.

A. True
B. False

ANSWER: B. False. The frontal plane is the right-to-left - left-to-right plane; and the vertical (superior to inferior - inferior to superior) plane. See picture above. The frontal plane is a twodimensional surface as depicted above.

The anterior to posterior (forward to backward) plane will be discussed in Chapter 4.

When you locate the frontal plane axis, you determine the direction that the wave of depolarization is traveling.

Review the normal conduction system of the heart: Normally, conduction begins in the S-A node. The wave of depolarization moves across the atria, through the AV node, into the Bundle of His, down the bundle branches, and finally through the Purkinje fibers which conduct the electrical impulse throughout the ventricles.

Chapter 3 -- Location of the Frontal Plane Axis

NORMAL FRONTAL PLANE AXIS

SUPERIOR

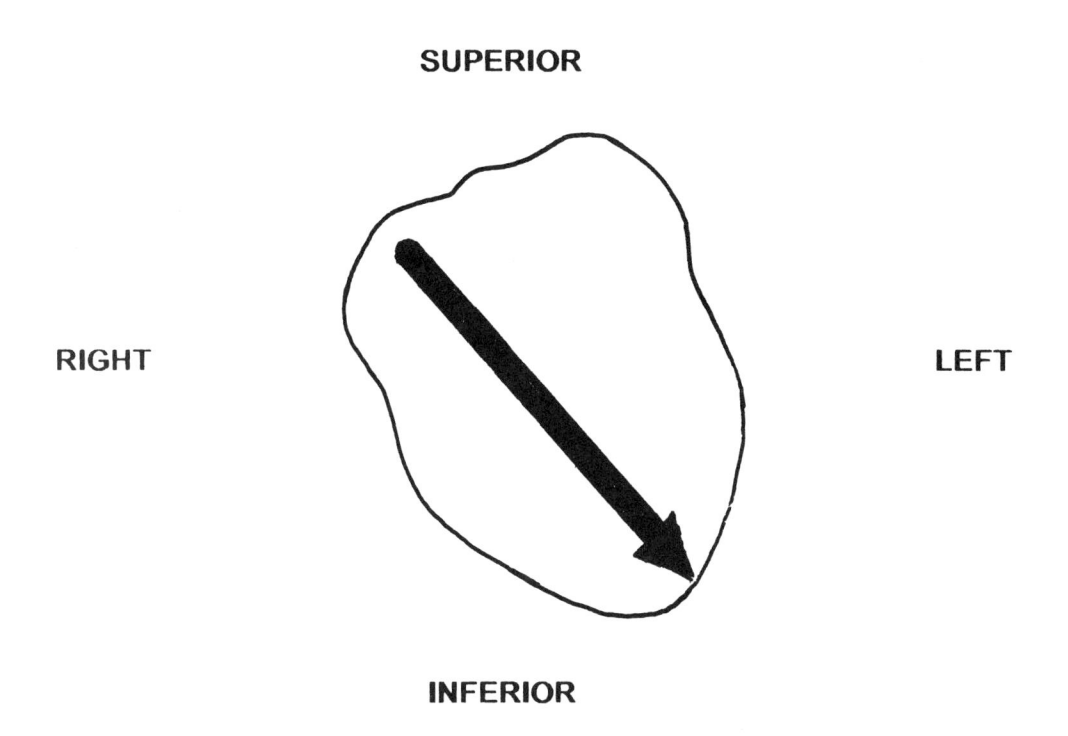

RIGHT   **LEFT**

INFERIOR

QUESTION: Normally, the wave of depolarization travels from right to left.

A. True
B. False

ANSWER: A. True. Depolarization begins in the S-A node which is on the right side of the heart and travels towards the left on its way to the ventricles. Note the direction of the arrow in the picture above is from right-to-left.

QUESTION: Normally, the wave of depolarization travels from superior to inferior.

A. True
B. False

ANSWER: A. True. Depolarization begins in the S-A node which is in the superior aspect of the heart and travels down towards the ventricles. Note the direction of the arrow in the above picture is from superior to inferior.

In summary, frontal plane depolarization normally occurs from right to left and from superior to inferior.

Chapter 3 — Location of the Frontal Plane Axis

THE FRONTAL PLANE LEADS

The activity of the heart produces electrical potentials which can be measured on the surface of the body. Using the galvanometer, differences between electrical potentials at different sites of the body can be recorded.

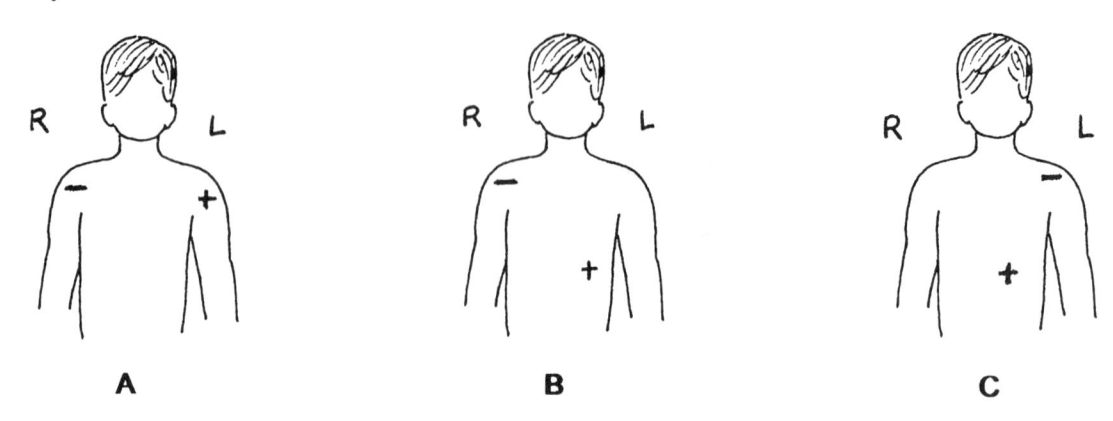

A   **B**   **C**

In picture A above, the negative electrode is on the right arm and the positive electrode is on the left arm. This is lead I. Lead I records electrical differences between the left and right arm electrodes.

In picture B, the negative electrode is on the right arm and the positive electrode is on the left leg (left lower chest). This is lead II. Lead II records electrical differences between the left leg and right arm electrodes.

In picture C, the negative electrode is on the left arm and the positive electrode is on the left leg (left lower chest). Picture C depicts lead III. Lead III records electrical differences between the left leg and the left arm electrodes.

Leads I, II, and III are the limb leads. The limb leads are sometimes referred to as the standard or bipolar leads. These three leads form Einthoven's triangle:

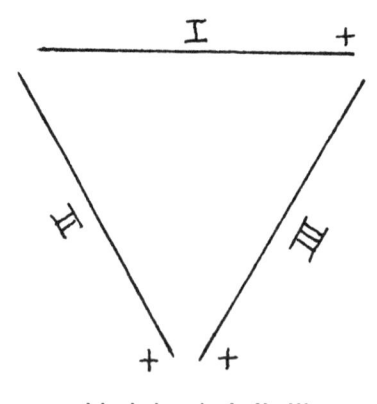

Limb leads I, II, III

Einthoven invented the electrocardiograph in 1903. Einthoven postulated that the right arm, left arm, and left leg formed the apexes of an equilateral triangle. The heart, an electrical source, is the center of this triangle.

Chapter 3 -- Location of the Frontal Plane Axis

The + represents the positive electrode of the lead:

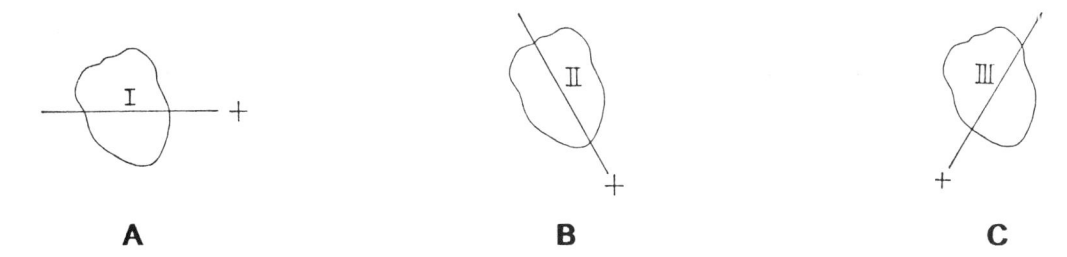

A   **B**   **C**

In picture A above, lead I of Einthovan's triangle is placed across the heart.
In picture B, lead II is placed across the heart.
In picture C, lead III is placed across the heart.

In summary, the three limb leads placed across the heart, pictorially depicted:

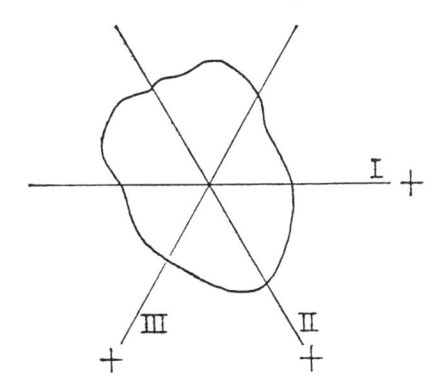

Transposition of the sides of Einthoven's triangle forms the triaxial reference system

Triaxial Reference System

The limb leads have a positive and a negative electrode but we will concentrate only on the positive electrode.

The other three frontal plane leads are the augmented vector leads. The galvanometer records potential differences and, therefore, the technique is bipolar (potential site A minus potential site B). However, if the potential of B is zero, the recorder records the potential of site A. (A - O = A).

Frank Wilson, a pioneer of modern electrocardiography, introduced an electrode which for all practical purposes has a zero potential and does not change during the cardiac cycle. It became known as the central or V electrode and all leads in which it is applied are called V leads or unipolar leads. Leads that reflect the potentials of the right arm, left arm, and left leg are called VR, VL, and VF, respectively. Using this technique the ECG deflections are small compared to the standard limb leads and have to be augmented by 50 percent. These leads are called aVR, aVL, and aVF.

To obtain the augmented vector leads you simply turn the dial on the ECG machine to the desired lead. To obtain lead aVR, turn the dial to aVR; to obtain lead aVL, turn the dial to aVL. To obtain lead aVF, turn the dial to aVF. What does this mean? When you turn the dial, the ECG machine changes it's view of the heart's electrical activity. The heart's electrical activity does not change; the place from which the activity is being viewed changes.

Chapter 3 — Location of the Frontal Plane Axis

aVR means augmented Vector Right,
 the positive electrode is on the right shoulder.

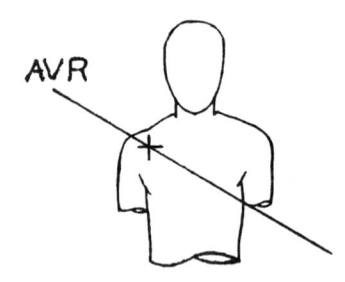

aVL means augmented Vector Left,
 the positive electrode is on the left shoulder.

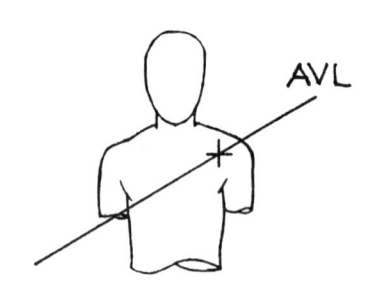

aVF means augmented Vector Foot,
 the positive electrode is on the foot.

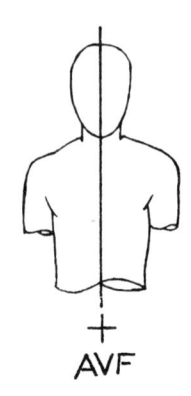

NOTE: Although the F stands for foot, please conceptualize the positive electrode of aVF as being at the umbilicus.

Chapter 3 -- Location of the Frontal Plane Axis

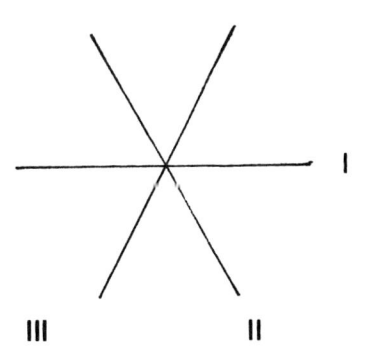

Now combine the three limb leads . . .
    I, II, III

. . . . and the three augmented Vector leads,
    aVR, aVL, aVF

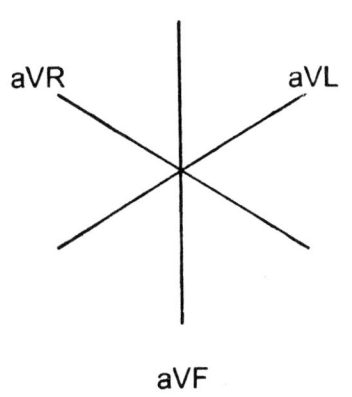

. . . . and this combination creates the Hexaxial Reference System.

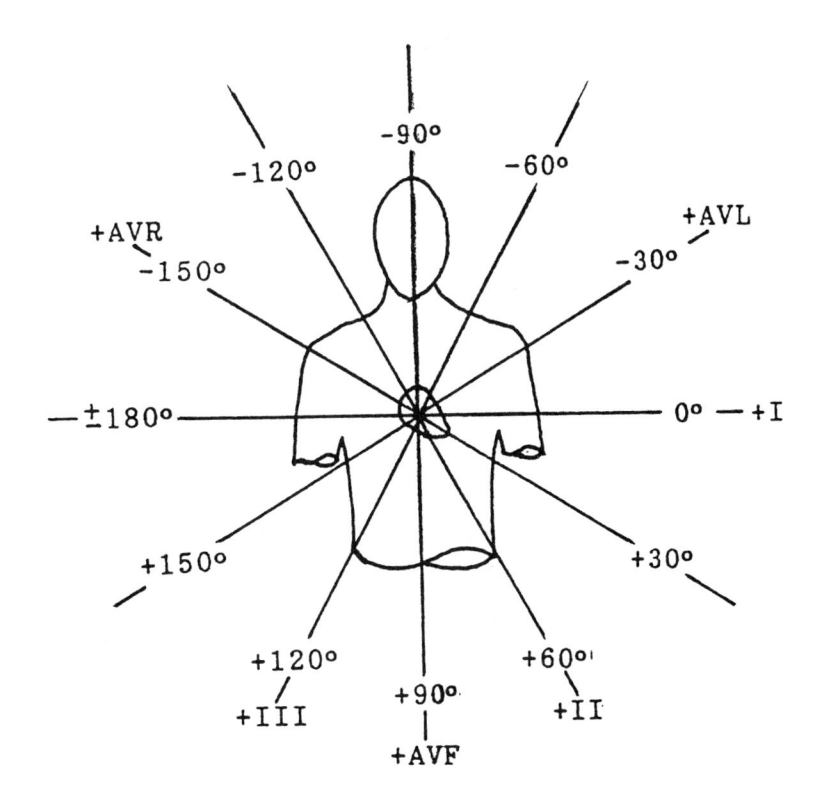

Chapter 3 — Location of the Frontal Plane Axis

HEXAXIAL REFERENCE SYSTEM

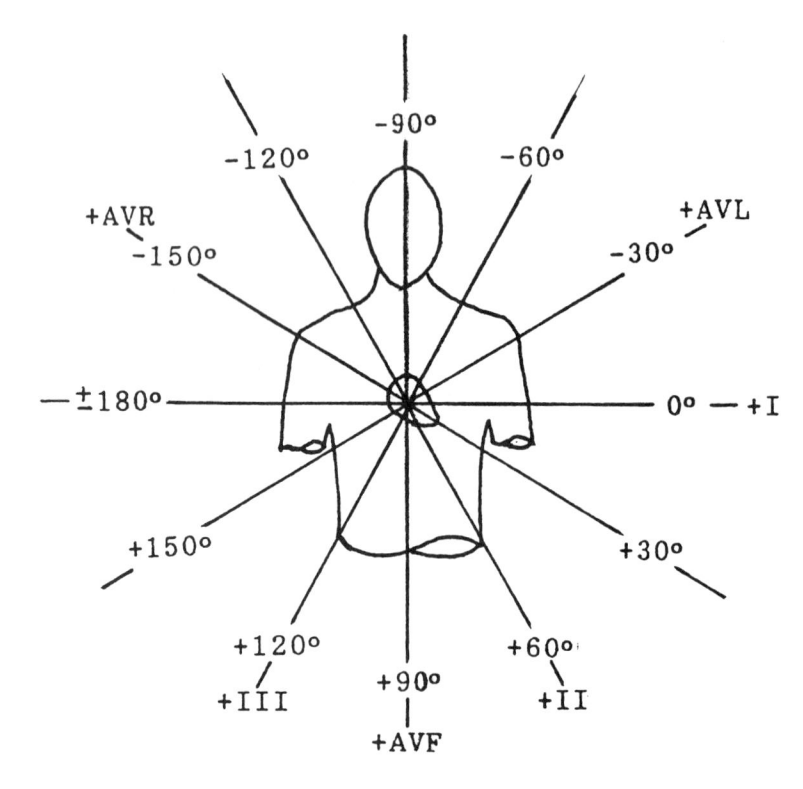

HEXAXIAL REFERENCE SYSTEM: The six frontal plane leads placed across the heart form the hexaxial reference system. This system is the means by which we communicate the location of the frontal plane axis. Please note:

Lead I is located at 0° and ±180°
Lead II is at +60° and -120°
Lead III +120° and -60°

QUESTION: Where is lead aVR located on the hexaxial figure?

ANSWER: Lead aVR is located at +30 and -150°.

Lead aVL is -30° and +150°.

Lead aVF is +90° and -90°.

NOTE: The positive (+) and negative (-) designation of the degrees of each lead are NOT related to the positive electrode. Notice that all the positive (+) degrees are on the inferior surface of the hexaxial figure and all the negative (-) degrees are on the superior surface of the hexaxial figure.

Chapter 3 -- Location of the Frontal Plane Axis

PERPENDICULAR LEADS

Take a few minutes to familiarize yourself with the hexaxial figure. Try to figure out which leads are perpendicular to each other.

QUESTIONS

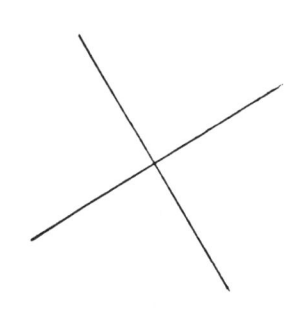

Which lead is perpendicular to lead I?

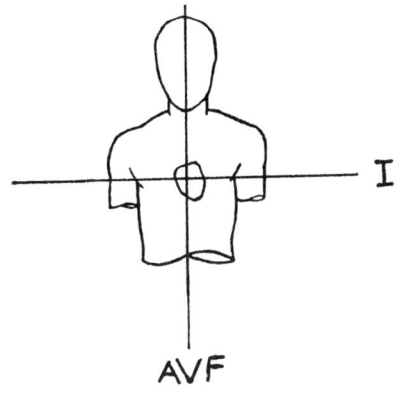

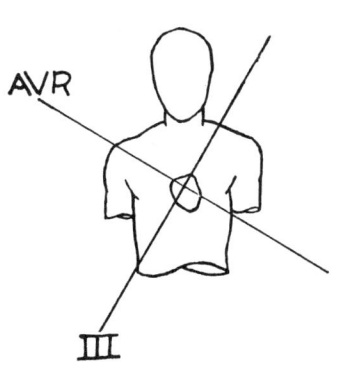

ANSWERS

Lead aVF is perpendicular to lead I.

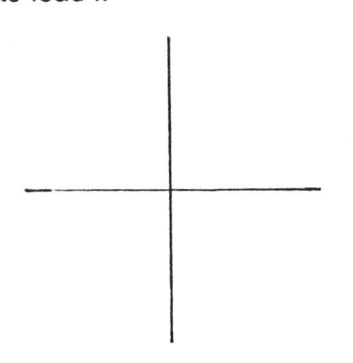

On the hexaxial figure, which lead is perpendicular to lead II?

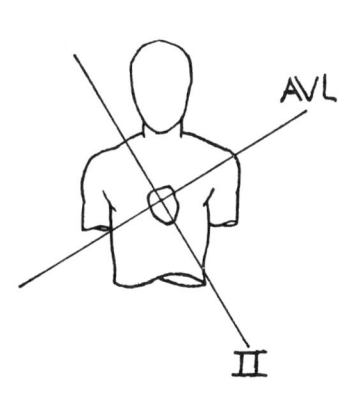

Lead aVL is perpendicular to lead II.

Which lead is perpendicular to lead III?

Lead aVR is perpendicular to lead III.

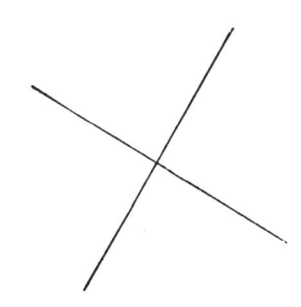

In review, the **PERPENDICULAR LEADS** are:

Lead I/aVF
Lead II/aVL
Lead III/aVR

Memorize which leads are perpendicular to each other. This will come in handy as you locate the frontal plane axis on your 12 lead ECGs.

Chapter 3 — Location of the Frontal Plane Axis

QUADRANTS

There are four quadrants in the hexaxial figure:

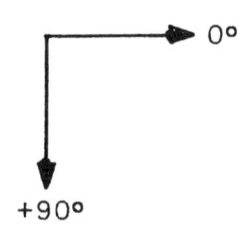

Normal quadrant is between 0° and +90°

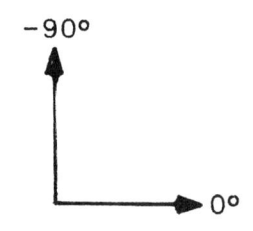

Left axis deviation quadrant is between 0° and -90°

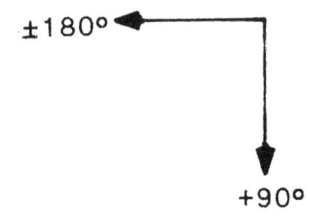

Right axis deviation quadrant is between +90° and ±180°

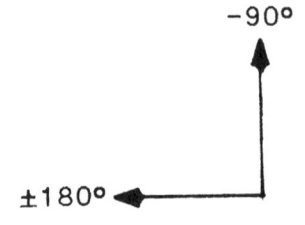

The quadrant located between ± 180° and -90° is "no man's land."

Chapter 3 -- Location of the Frontal Plane Axis

THREE PRINCIPLES OF ELECTROCARDIOGRAPHY: REVIEW

QUESTION: When the wave of depolarization travels towards the positive electrode of any lead the ECG stylus will inscribe a:

A. positive deflection
B. negative deflection

ANSWER: A. When the wave of depolarization travels towards the positive electrode, the ECG will inscribe a positive (upward) deflection:

QUESTION: When the wave of depolarization travels away from the positive electrode, the ECG will inscribe a:

A. positive deflection
B. negative deflection

ANSWER: B. When the wave of depolarization travels away from the positive electrode, the ECG will inscribe a negative (downward) deflection.

The above picture depicts the electrical wave of depolarization moving neither towards nor away from the positive electrode. It is moving perpendicular (at a right angle) to the positive electrode.

QUESTION: What kind of a complex would be inscribed in this case?

A. Positive
B. Negative
C. Biphasic

ANSWER: C.

A biphasic complex is inscribed when the electrical forces are moving perpendicular to the positive electrode. The waves of a biphasic complex are above and below the isoelectric line. When depolarization occurs exactly perpendicular to the positive electrode, an equiphasic complex or a straight line will be inscribed on the ECG.

Chapter 3 -- Location of the Frontal Plane Axis

QUESTION: Identify the biphasic complexes in the following:

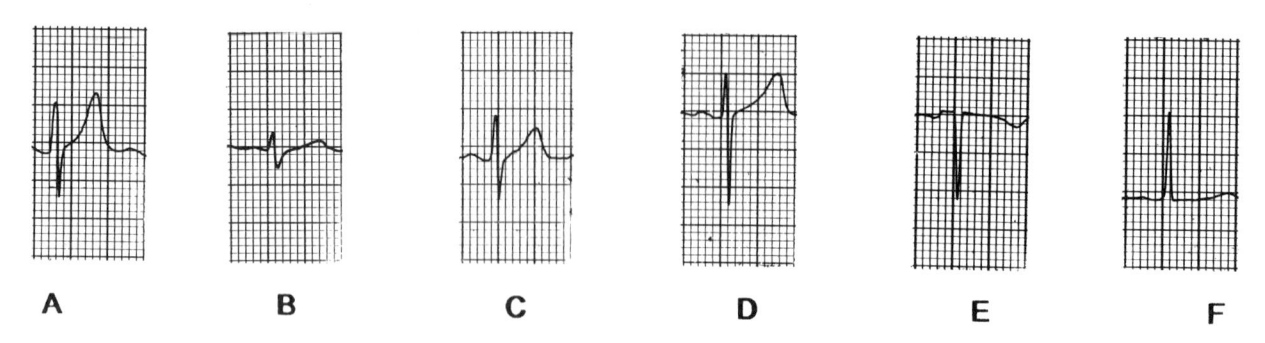

A	B	C	D	E	F

ANSWER: A,B,C, and D are **biphasic complexes.**

When the waves of the complex are equally phasic, that is, equally above and below the isoelectric line, the complex is *equiphasic*.

QUESTION: In the above examples, which leads have equiphasic complexes?

ANSWER: A,B, and C are **equiphasic complexes.**

In electrocardiography, the term vector is used to describe the direction of electrical current. Recall the definition of the frontal plane axis is the orientation of the heart's electrical activity in the frontal plane. Axis and vector are synonymous terms for all practical purposes.

All parts of the ECG have vectors or an axis. The P, T, U waves have an axis as well as the ST segment. We will be concerned only with the frontal plane axis of ventricular depolarization.

STEPS TO LOCATE THE FRONTAL PLANE AXIS

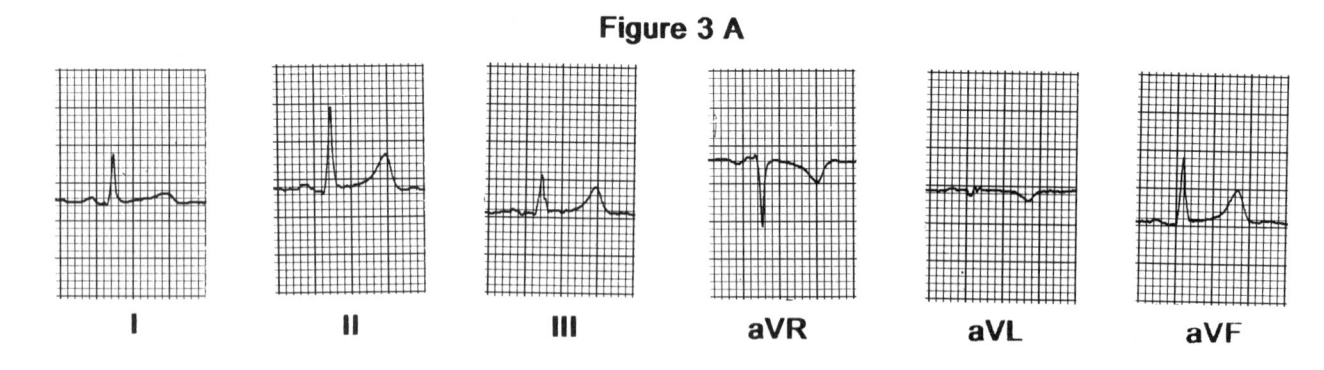

Figure 3 A

I	II	III	aVR	aVL	aVF

Figure 3 A. Use the above six frontal plane leads as you work through the four steps to locate the frontal plane axis.

Chapter 3 -- Location of the Frontal Plane Axis

STEP 1 The first step in location of axis is to ascertain if ventricular depolarization is moving from right to left or abnormally from left to right. **Step 1** asks the question, *Is ventricular depolarization moving from right to left or from left to right?*

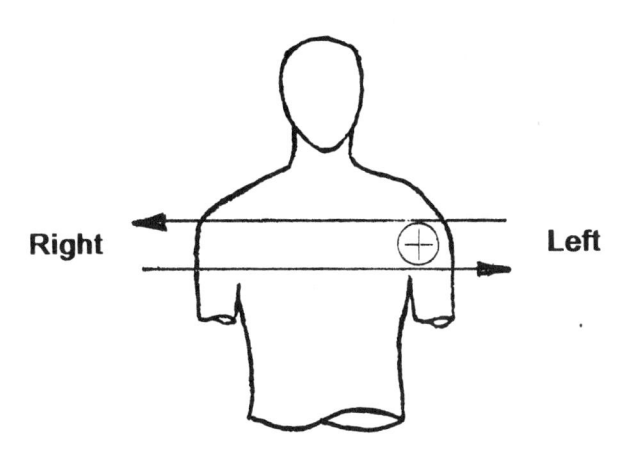

QUESTION: Which lead is in the best position to answer the right to left, left to right question?

ANSWER: lead I is in the best position to assess right to left, left to right forces. The positive electrode of lead I is situated to see forces moving towards it (right to left) or away from it (left to right).

Look at lead I in Figure 3 A. If the complex in lead I is mainly positive, depolarization is moving towards lead I; if the complex in lead I is mainly a negative deflection, depolarization is moving away from lead I.

Figure 3 A is repeated here for your convenience.

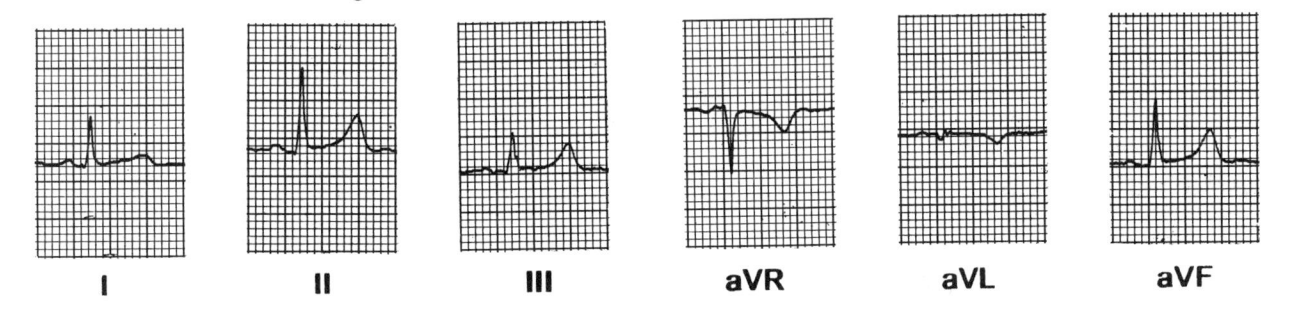

| I | II | III | aVR | aVL | aVF |

QUESTION: In Figure 3 A, the complex in lead I is a

A. positive deflection
B. negative deflection

ANSWER: A. The complex in lead I is a positive deflection, therefore the wave of ventricular depolarization is moving towards the positive electrode of lead I.

Chapter 3 — Location of the Frontal Plane Axis

RECALL: lead I lies at ± 180° ——— 0° + on the hexaxial figure.

⟶ + = ⋀

Draw an arrow from right to left to depict ventricular depolarization moving from right to left in Figure 3 A.

⟶

STEP 2 The second step is to ascertain if the wave of ventricular depolarization is moving from the heart towards the umbilicus or abnormally from the heart towards the head. Step 2 asks the question, *is the wave of ventricular depolarization moving from superior to inferior or from inferior to superior?*

QUESTION: Which lead is in the best position to answer the superior to inferior, inferior to superior question?

Superior

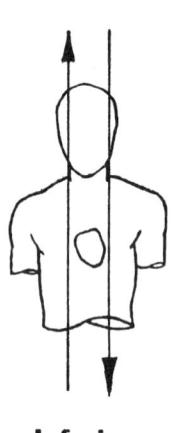

Inferior
aVF +

ANSWER: Lead aVF is in the best position to assess superior to inferior, inferior to superior forces (up to down or down to up).

Look at lead aVF in Figure 3 A on the following page. If the complex in lead aVF is a positive deflection, depolarization is moving towards the positive electrode of lead aVF. If the complex in lead aVF is a negative deflection, depolarization is moving away from the positive electrode of lead aVF.

Chapter 3 — Location of the Frontal Plane Axis

Figure 3 A is repeated here for your convenience.

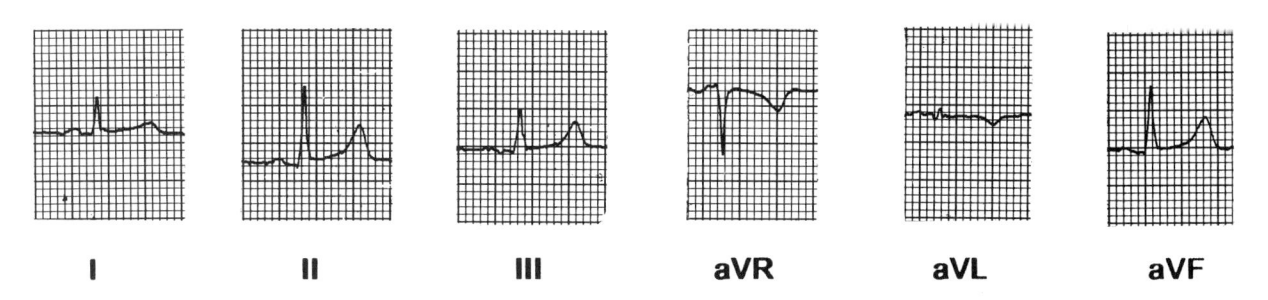

| I | II | III | aVR | aVL | aVF |

In Figure 3 A, the complex in lead aVF is positive, therefore, the wave of depolarization is moving towards the positive electrode of lead aVF.

Ventricular depolarization is moving from superior to inferior, so draw an arrow from superior to inferior. Connect this arrow to the right-to-left arrow that you previously drew as a result of Step 1:

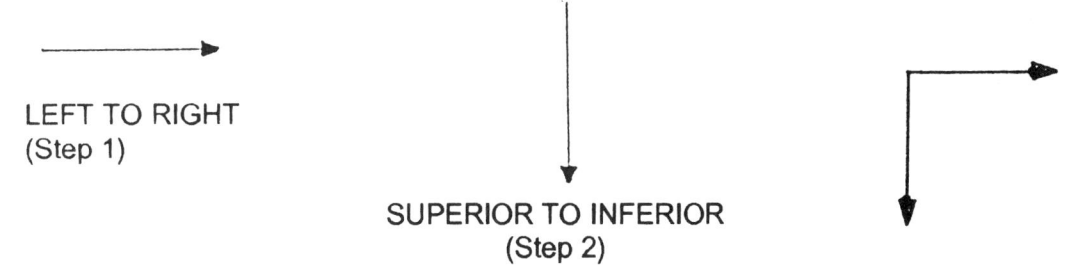

LEFT TO RIGHT
(Step 1)

SUPERIOR TO INFERIOR
(Step 2)

Now you know that the axis is located between 0° and +90° on the hexaxial figure. Recall this is the normal quadrant.

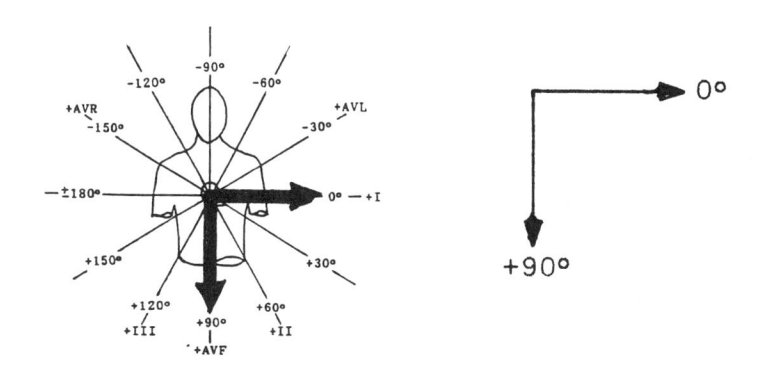

STEP 3 Step 3 uses the principle that a biphasic complex is inscribed when the wave of ventricular depolarization travels at a right angle (perpendicular) to the positive electrode.

RECALL THE PRINCIPLE:

$+ = \wedge$ or $-$

33

Chapter 3 -- Location of the Frontal Plane Axis

An equiphasic complex is inscribed when depolarization travels exactly perpendicular to the positive electrode. In Step 3, we work backwards with this principle. **Step 3** asks the question, *Which lead has the most equiphasic complex?*

QUESTION: Which lead in Figure 3 A has the most equiphasic complex?

Figure 3 A is repeated here for your convenience.

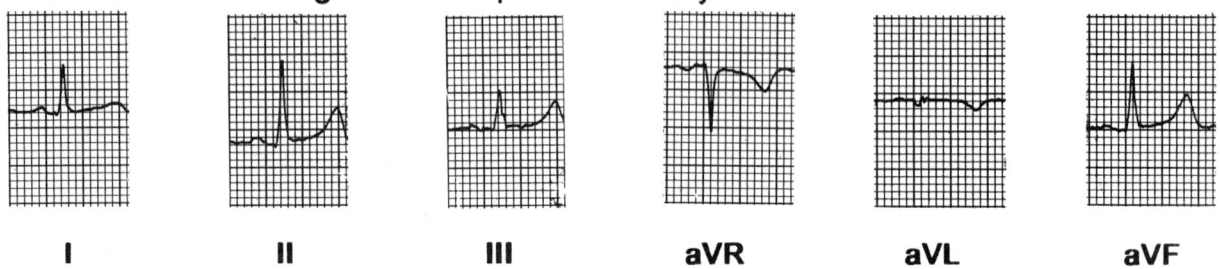

| I | II | III | aVR | aVL | aVF |

ANSWER: Lead aVL is the lead with the most equiphasic complex.

<u>**STEP 4**</u> Having identified the lead with the most equiphasic complex (aVL in Figure 3 A) and the quadrant (0° to +90°), identify which lead is perpendicular to lead aVL. **Step 4** asks the question, *which lead is perpendicular to the lead with the most equiphasic complex?*

QUESTION: Which lead in the hexaxial figure is perpendicular to lead aVL?

ANSWER: LEAD II.

Lead II in the normal quadrant is located at +60°: the frontal plane axis of Figure 3 A is +60°.

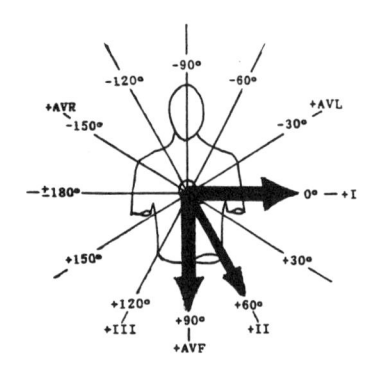

In review, the normal quadrant was identified by Steps 1 and 2.

aVL is the lead with the most equiphasic complex in Figure 3 A.

Lead II is perpendicular to lead aVL.

Lead II in the normal quadrant lies at +60°.

The frontal plane axis in Figure 3 A is +60°.

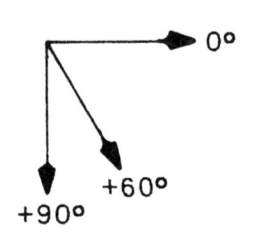

Chapter 3 -- Location of the Frontal Plane Axis

Remember, when locating the frontal plane axis, only the six frontal plane leads on the 12 lead ECG are considered.

Let's review the location of the frontal plane axis with the 12 lead ECG on the following page, Figure 3 B.

STEP 1 Determine right to left, left to right depolarization by looking at <u>lead I</u>. The complex in lead I in Figure 3 B is a positive deflection (R wave); draw the first arrow from right to left according to Principle #1.

⟶

STEP 2 Ascertain superior to inferior, inferior to superior depolarization by looking at <u>lead aVF</u>. The complex in lead aVF in Figure 3 B is a positive deflection; draw the second arrow superior to inferior, connecting it to the right to left arrow.

Once again, you have identified the frontal plane axis is between 0° and +90° on the hexaxial figure. This is the normal quadrant.

STEP 3 Decide which lead has the most equiphasic complex.

QUESTION: In Figure 3 B, which lead has the most equiphasic complex?

ANSWER: Lead III.

STEP 4 Identify the lead perpendicular to lead III on the hexaxial figure. Lead aVR is perpendicular to lead III.

The normal quadrant has already been identified. The axis in Figure 3 B is +30°.

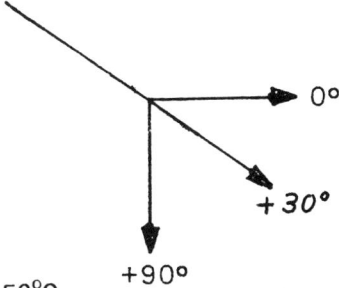

Lead aVR lies at +30° and -150° on the hexaxial figure.

QUESTION: How do you know the axis is +30° and not -150°?

ANSWER: The axis must be located within the normal quadrant identified by steps 1 and 2, and -150° is not in that quadrant; +30° is in the normal quadrant.

Figure 3 B

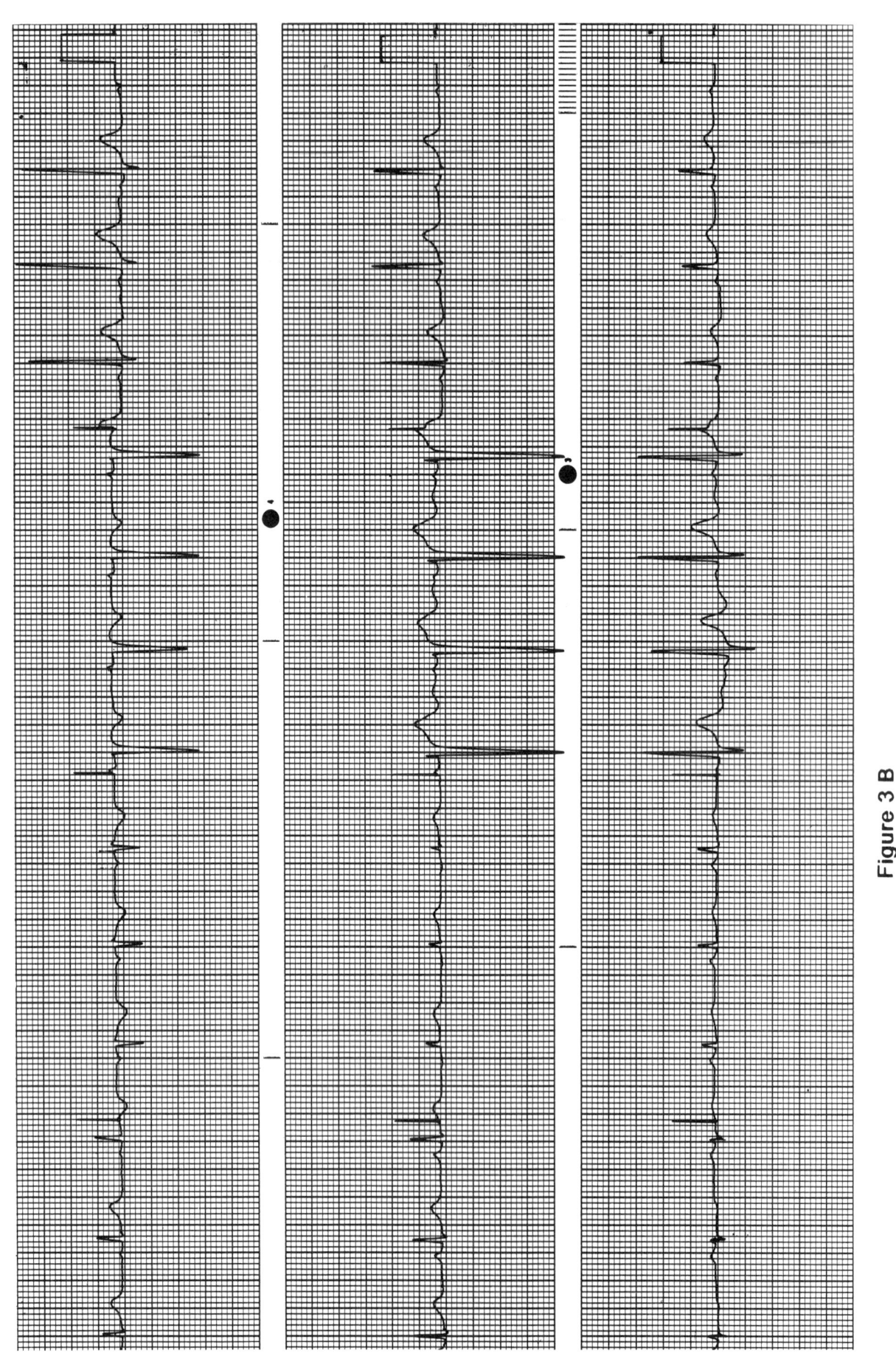

Chapter 3 — Location of the Frontal Plane Axis

Once more, review the steps in the location of the frontal plane axis with Figure 3 C.

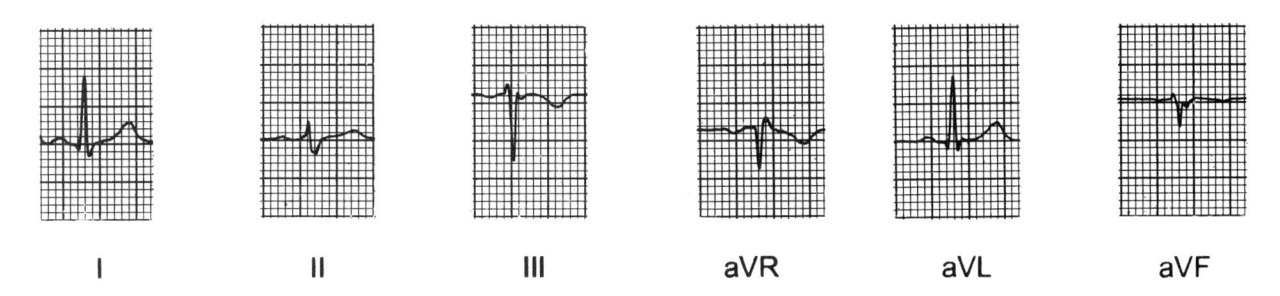

| I | II | III | aVR | aVL | aVF |

Figure 3 C

REFER TO FIGURE 3 C ABOVE FOR THE FOLLOWING DISCUSSION.

STEP 1 Decide right to left, left to right depolarization by looking at lead I. The complex in lead I is a positive deflection, so draw the first arrow from right to left.

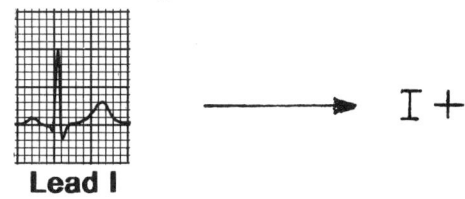

Lead I ⟶ I +

STEP 2 Ascertain superior to inferior, inferior to superior depolarization by looking at lead aVF. The complex in lead aVF is primarily a negative deflection.

QUESTION: Since aVF is a negative deflection, which way will the second arrow be drawn?

A. Up to down ↓

B. Down to up ↑

ANSWER: B. The forces are moving away from the positive electrode of aVF. Recall the location of the positive electrode of aVF is at the umbilicus. Ventricular depolarization is moving towards the head, away from the positive electrode of aVF.

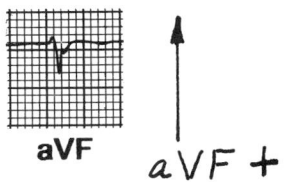

aVF   aVF +

37

Chapter 3 -- Location of the Frontal Plane Axis

The axis in Figure 3 C is located between 0° and -90°. This is the left axis deviation (LAD) quadrant.

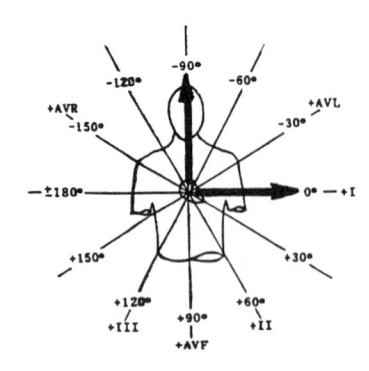

STEP 3 Identify the lead with the most equiphasic complex.

QUESTION: Which lead in Figure 3 C has the most equiphasic complex?

ANSWER: In Figure 3 C, lead II has the most equiphasic complex.

STEP 4 Identify the lead perpendicular to lead II on the hexaxial figure. Lead aVL is perpendicular to lead II.

The left axis deviation quadrant is already identified. The axis in Figure 3 C is -30°.

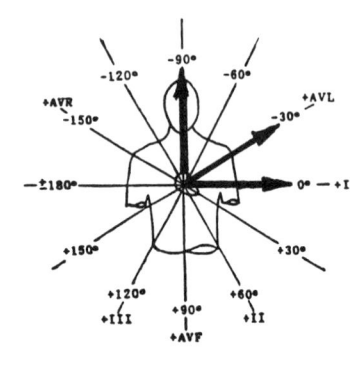

Chapter 3 -- Location of the Frontal Plane Axis

One more time, review the steps in the location of the frontal plane axis using Figure 3 D:

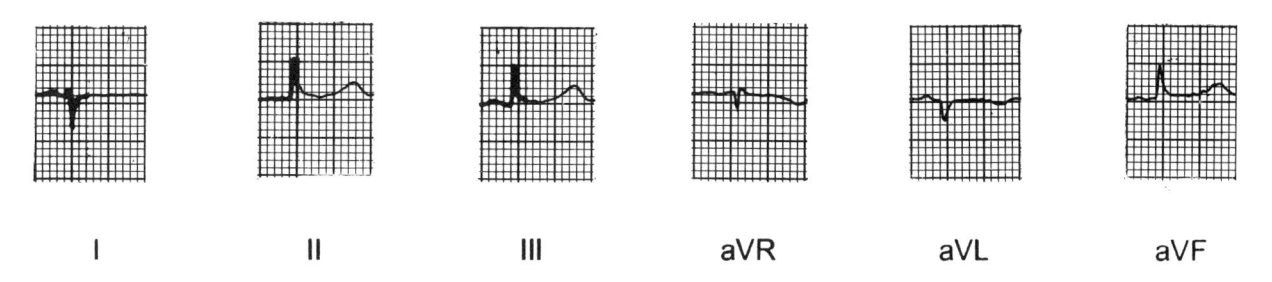

| I | II | III | aVR | aVL | aVF |

Figure 3 D

REFER TO FIGURE 3 D ABOVE FOR THE FOLLOWING DISCUSSION.

STEP 1 Decide right to left, left to right depolarization by looking at lead I. The complex in lead I is a negative deflection, so draw the first arrow from left to right.

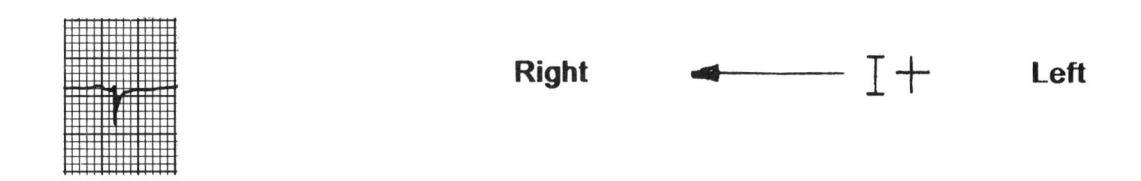

Right ←———— I+ ———— Left

Lead I Figure 3 D

STEP 2 Determine superior to inferior, inferior to superior depolarization by looking at lead aVF. The complex in lead aVF is a positive deflection, so draw the second arrow superior to inferior, connecting it to the left-to-right arrow.

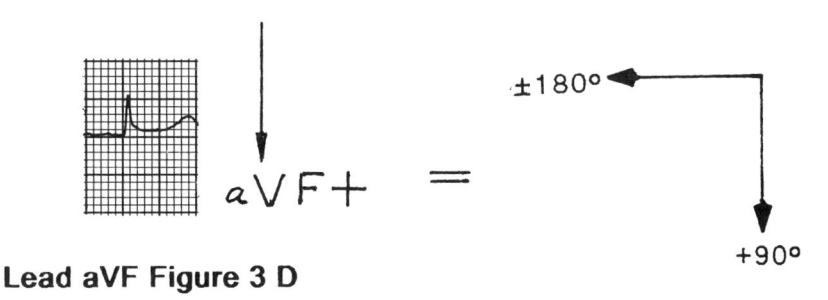

$aVF+$ = $\pm 180°$ ← ... ↓ $+90°$

Lead aVF Figure 3 D

The quadrant is located between $\pm 180°$ and $+90°$.
This is the right axis deviation (RAD) quadrant.

Chapter 3 — Location of the Frontal Plane Axis

STEP 3 Determine which lead has the most equiphasic complex. In Figure 3 D, lead aVR has the most equiphasic complex.

STEP 4 Identify the lead perpendicular to lead aVR on the hexaxial figure. Lead III is perpendicular to lead aVR. The quadrant is already identified. Lead III in the RAD quadrant is located at +120°. The axis in Figure 3 D is +120°.

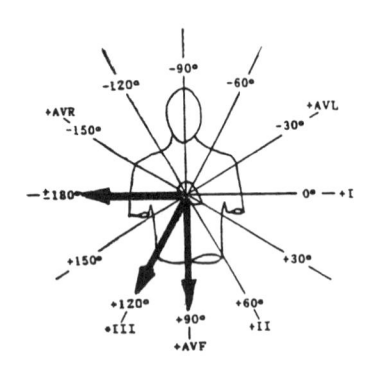

If you have trouble with the perpendicular leads, review them on page 27.

Students frequently ask, "When locating the frontal plane axis, do I always start with lead I?" The answer is, "Yes, if you are locating the frontal plane axis by this method, you always start with lead I" (Step 1). Next you assess lead aVF (Step 2). Next (Step 3) you determine which of the frontal plane leads has the most equiphasic complex. Steps 1 and 2 locate the quadrant. The lead perpendicular to the lead with the most equiphasic complex points to the location of the frontal plane axis in that quadrant (Step 4).

In step 3, if more than one lead has an equiphasic complex, choose the lead whose complex has the least amplitude.

In step 3, if there are no equiphasic complexes in any of the six frontal plane leads, choose the lead whose complex has the least amplitude.

Chapter 3 -- Location of the Frontal Plane Axis

Location of axis in the next example is a little different.

Figure 3 E

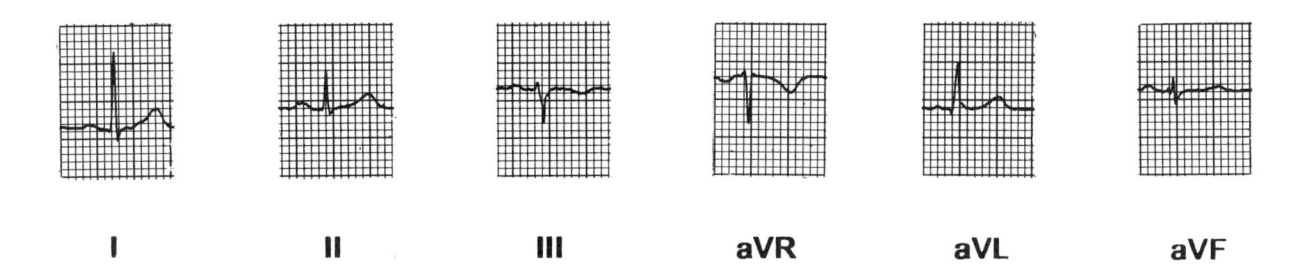

| I | II | III | aVR | aVL | aVF |

Lead I is a positive deflection, so the first arrow is drawn right to left:

⟶

Lead aVF has the most equiphasic complex. Lead I is perpendicular to lead aVF. The arrow is already drawn right to left. The axis is 0°.

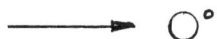

⟶ 0°

To review the above, consider the following examples:

Figure 3 F

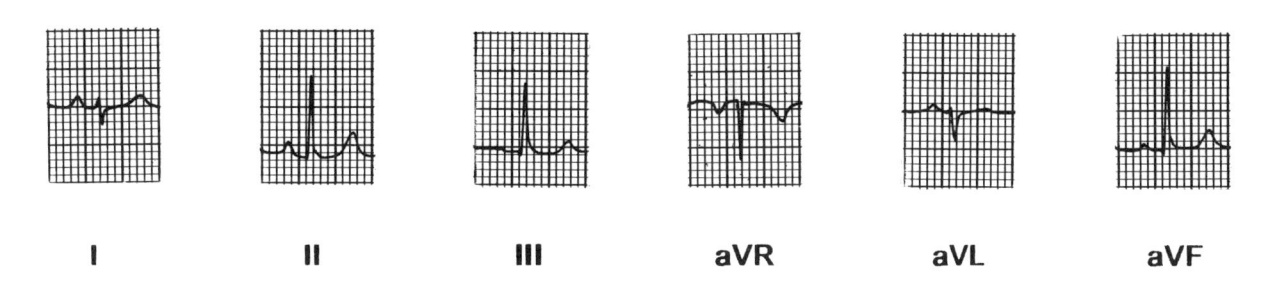

| I | II | III | aVR | aVL | aVF |

Lead I is the lead with the most equiphasic complex. aVF is perpendicular to lead I. The complex in aVF is positive so the arrow is drawn:

↓

The axis in Figure 3 F is +90°.

In review, when either lead I or aVF has the most equiphasic complex, you skip a step in the location of the frontal plane axis. You do not locate a quadrant, you locate the vector. Recall vector and axis are synonymous terms.

Chapter 3 -- Location of the Frontal Plane Axis

THE HEXAXIAL QUADRANTS

1. If lead I is ⋀

   and

   lead aVF is ⋀

   the quadrant is normal,
   0° to +90°

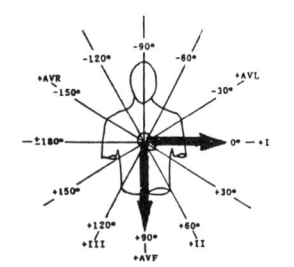

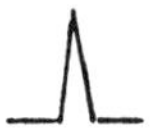

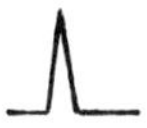

All cardiologists agree that between 0° and +90° is normal axis. There is some disagreement about how many degrees to extend this quadrant and still consider it normal. Most authorities agree that between -30° and +105° is within normal limits.

2. If lead I is ⋀

   and

   lead aVF is ⋁

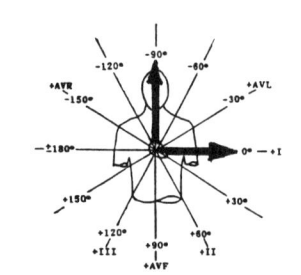

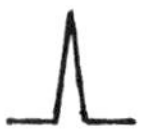

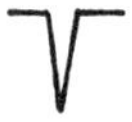

   This is left axis deviation (LAD) quadrant
   0° to -90°

3. If lead I is ⋁

   and

   lead aVF is ⋀

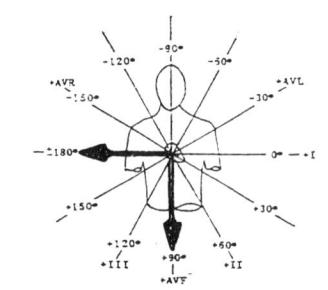

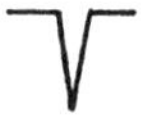

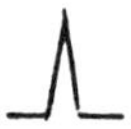

   This is right axis deviation (RAD) quadrant
   +90° to ±180°

4. If lead I is ⋁

   and

   lead aVF is ⋁

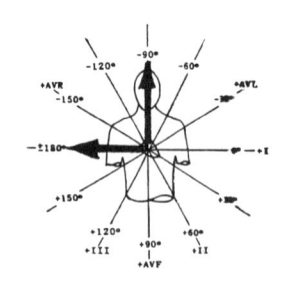

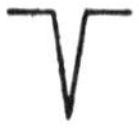

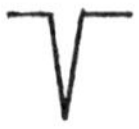

   This quadrant is often referred to as
   "no man's land"
   ±180° to -90°

This abnormal quadrant has many names: indeterminate axis, intermediate axis, northwest quadrant. We will use *no man's land* which aptly describes the abnormality of this quadrant.

Chapter 3 — Location of the Frontal Plane Axis

FRONTAL PLANE AXIS SUMMARY

Normal axis is present when either:

1. Both lead I and aVF have positive complexes.
2. Lead I has a positive complex and aVF has the most equiphasic complex.
3. aVF has a positive complex and lead I has the most equiphasic complex.

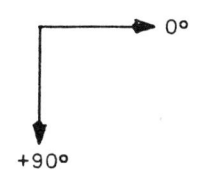

Clinically, it is not necessary to look for the exact degrees of a normal axis. Once you have ascertained that the axis is normal, that's all you need to do. Degrees will be included herein just for the sake of practice.

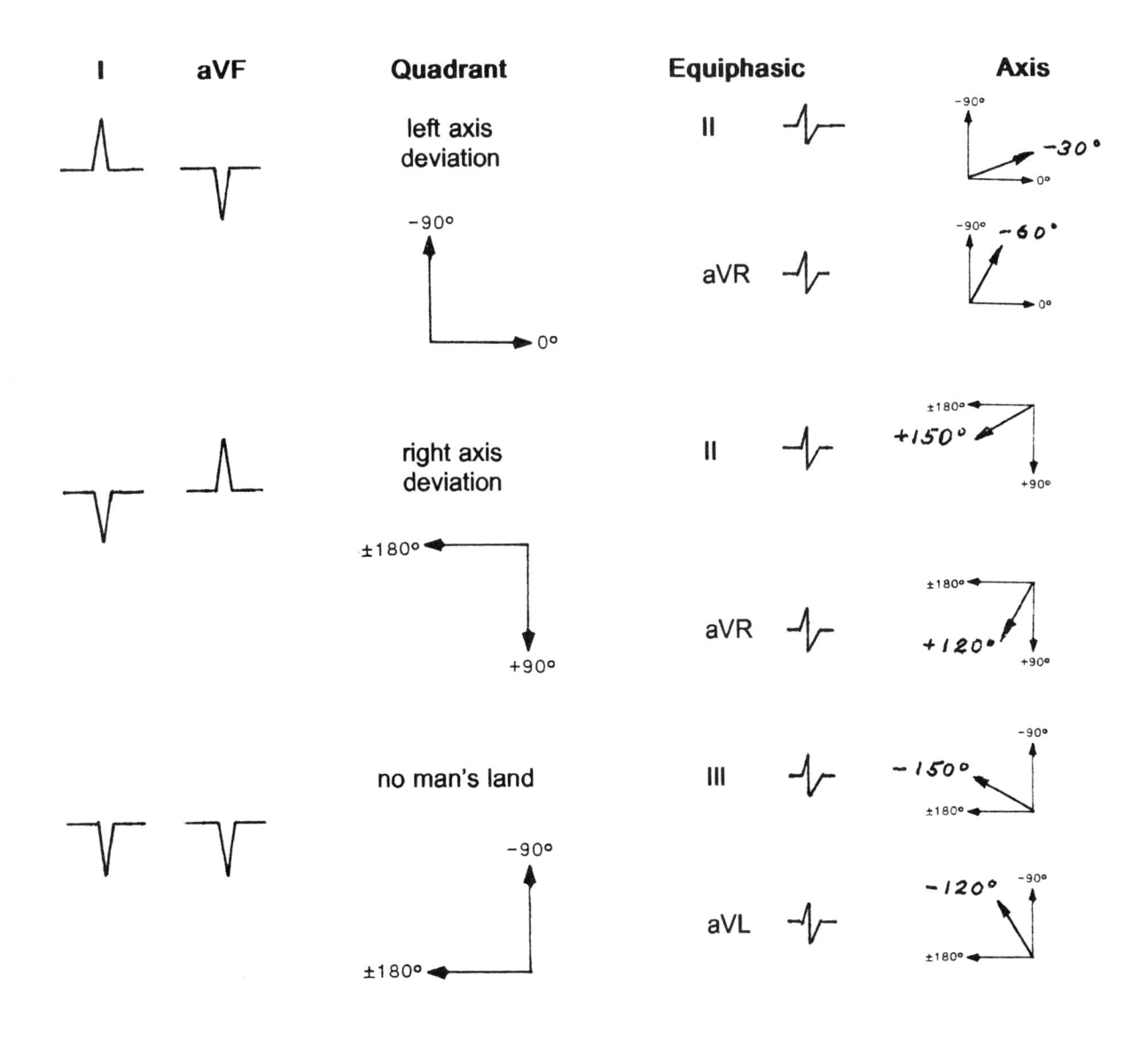

I	aVF	Quadrant	Equiphasic	Axis
positive	negative	left axis deviation	II	−30°
			aVR	−60°
negative	positive	right axis deviation	II	+150°
			aVR	+120°
negative	negative	no man's land	III	−150°
			aVL	−120°

43

Chapter 3 -- Location of the Frontal Plane Axis

CAUSES OF FRONTAL PLANE AXIS DEVIATION

Consider the heart, how it lies in the mediastinum, attached to the great vessels, supported by the surrounding structures: the lungs, the diaphragm, the abdominal cavity.

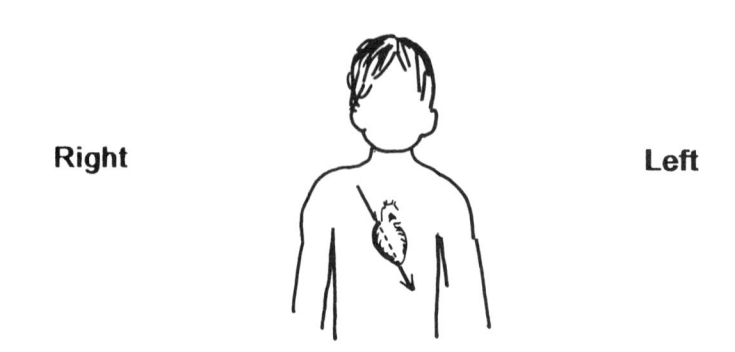

Right   **Left**

In the "normal" person, the wave of ventricular depolarization spreads from right to left and from superior to inferior, resulting in a frontal plane axis between $0°$ and $+90°$.

Consider another "normal" person, one who is shorter and stouter:

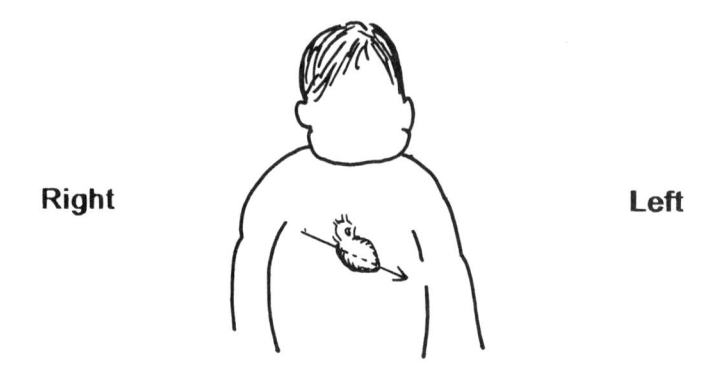

Right   **Left**

QUESTION: A short, stout person would tend to have an axis shifted towards the left.

A. True
B. False

ANSWER: A. True. The frontal plane axis of a short, stout person would be shifted towards the left as a normal variant.

Any condition which causes the abdominal contents to push up on the diaphragm, and thus the heart, would cause a frontal plane axis deviation to the left: pregnancy, ascites, abdominal tumors.

Chapter 3 — Location of the Frontal Plane Axis

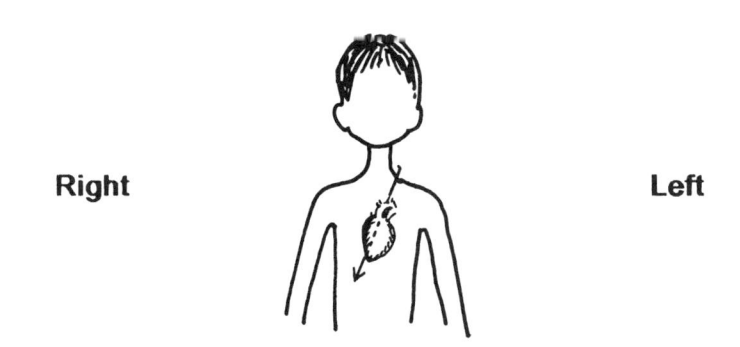

Right　　　　　　　　　　　　　　　　　　　　**Left**

QUESTION: A tall, thin person would tend to have the frontal plane axis shifted towards the right.

A. True
B. False

ANSWER: A. True. The frontal plane axis of a tall, thin person would shift towards the right as a normal variant.

CAUSES OF FRONTAL PLANE AXIS DEVIATION

RIGHT AXIS DEVIATION	**LEFT AXIS DEVIATION**
Normal variant	Normal variant
Right ventricular hypertrophy	Left ventricular hypertrophy
Right bundle branch block	Left bundle branch block
Left posterior hemiblock (LPH)	Left anterior descending hemiblock (LADH)
Left ventricular ectopy	Right ventricular ectopy
Dextrocardia	

Depending on the site and severity, myocardial infarction may also cause frontal plane axis deviation. Causes of frontal plane axis deviation will be discussed further in subsequent chapters.

In review, to interpret the 12 lead ECG you need to first assess the basic rhythm, then the frontal plane axis as listed on page 3. The next assessment is the progression of the R wave which we now turn to in Chapter 4.

CHAPTER 4
PROGRESSION OF THE R WAVE

The unipolar or V technique introduced by Frank Wilson is used in the horizontal plane with the chest or the precordial leads. The precordial leads consist of a positive electrode strategically placed on the chest. The position of the positive electrode for the six precordial leads are:

V_1 fourth intercostal space, right sternal border

V_2 fourth intercostal space, left sternal border

V_3 one-half way between V_2 and V_4 in a straight line with them

V_4 fifth intercostal space, left mid-clavicular line

V_5 fifth intercostal space, left anterior axillary line

V_6 fifth intercostal space, left midaxillary line

Leads V_1 through V_6 are Wilson's original V leads; they are not augmented.

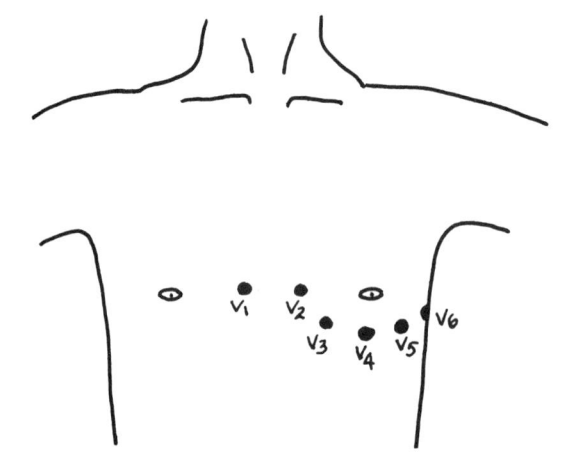

The normal ECG morphology of the complex in the V leads:

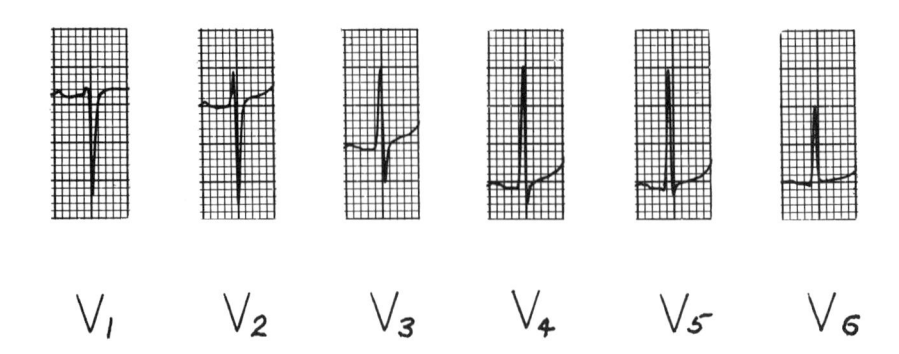

V_1 V_2 V_3 V_4 V_5 V_6

Chapter 4 — Progression of the R Wave

> V_1 is the septal lead.

QUESTION: Which wall of the ventricle depolarizes first?

ANSWER: The septum. If you missed this question please refer to page 17.

Recall that depolarization of the ventricular septum normally occurs from left-to-right. V_1 sees depolarization of the septum moving towards its positive electrode:

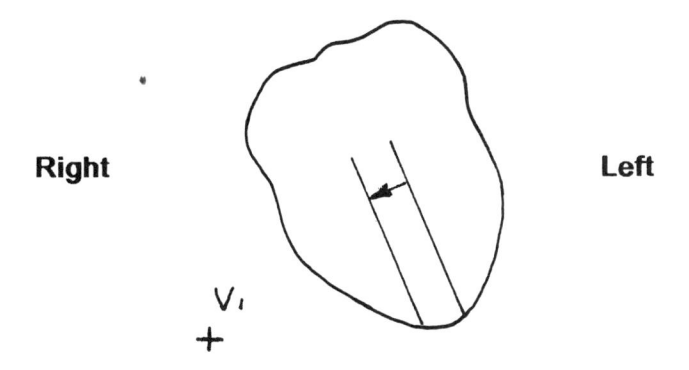

QUESTION: What kind of a wave will ventricular septum depolarization inscribe in V_1?

A. q
B. r
C. s

ANSWER: B. The septum is depolarizing towards the positive electrode of V_1 which will result in a positive deflection, an r wave. If you missed this question please refer to page 5.

The left and right ventricles depolarize almost simultaneously. The wall of the left ventricle is three times thicker than the right. The left ventricle actually is posterior in the chest.

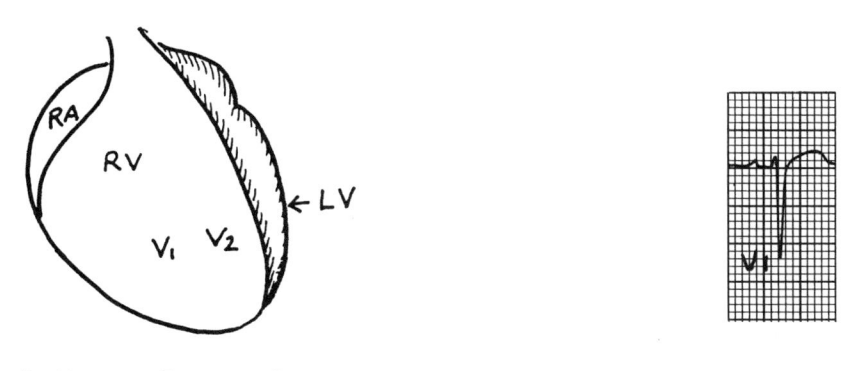

ANTERIOR VIEW

V_1, situated on the anterior wall of the chest, sees the posterior (left) ventricle depolarize away from it. An S wave is inscribed in V_1 because left ventricular depolarization is moving away from the positive electrode of V_1.

Chapter 4 — Progression of the R Wave

In summary, **the complex in V_1 normally has a small r wave followed by an S wave.**

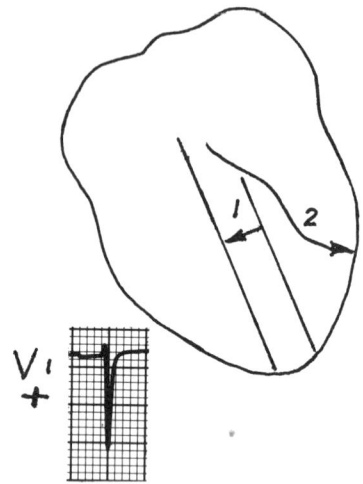

Recall that when the amplitude of the wave of the complex is less than 5 millimeters, it is denoted with a small letter, and an amplitude of 5 or more millimeters is denoted with a capital letter.

| V_2, V_3, and V_4 are the anterior leads. |

As depolarization spreads to the anterior wall of the left ventricle, the amplitude of the r waves in V_2, V_3, and V_4 increase.

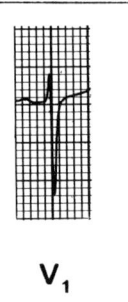

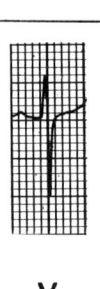

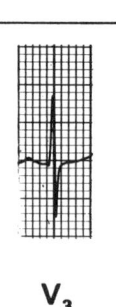

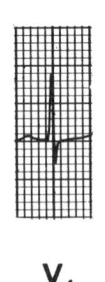

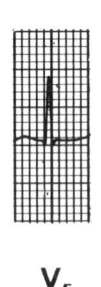

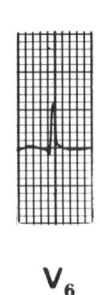

V_1 V_2 V_3 V_4 V_5 V_6

Transition occurs when the amplitude of the R wave becomes as big as, or bigger than the S wave. Transition normally occurs in V_3. Transition can also occur in V_2 or V_4 as a normal variant. Failure of the amplitude of the r wave to increase in V_2, V_3 is referred to as *loss of anterior forces*. Loss of anterior forces is an abnormal progression of the R wave.

QUESTION:

| V_5 and V_6 are left lateral leads. |

A. True
B. False

ANSWER: A. True

Recall that when the ventricular septum depolarizes, the wave of depolarization is moving away from the positive electrode of the left lateral leads (I, aVL, V_5, V_6). So ventricular septum depolarization inscribes a q wave in these left lateral leads. Then as the left ventricle depolarizes, an R wave follows the septal q wave in the left lateral leads.

Chapter 4 — Progression of the R Wave

In summary, the normal R wave progression in the precordial leads begins with a small r wave in V_1. The amplitude of the R wave increases in V_2 and V_3. Transition, the lead in which the amplitude of the R wave becomes as large as or larger than the S wave, normally occurs in V_3. As a normal variant, transition may occur in V_2 or V_4. The R waves persist left of the transition lead.

    V_1 is the septal lead
    V_2, V_3, V_4 are the anterior leads
    V_5, V_6 are left lateral leads

Assessment of the progression of the R wave is very helpful.

Normal progression of the R wave rules out many abnormalities:

- right ventricular hypertrophy
- right and left bundle branch blocks
- Wolff-Parkinson-White syndrome (WPW)
- myocardial infarction of the septum, anterior, and posterior walls of the left ventricle.

QUESTION: Describe the progression of the R wave as normal or abnormal in:

    Figure 1 A, page 2
    Figure 1 B, page 4
    Figure 3 B, page 36

ANSWER: The progression of the R wave is normal in all of the above examples.

PRACTICE 12 LEAD ECGs #1-12

Assess the following practice 12 lead ECGs using the following criteria:

Basic rhythm:
Frontal plane axis:
R wave progression:
Configuration and duration of the complex:
P wave:
ST segment (normal, elevated, depressed):
T wave:
Presence and size of U wave:
12 Lead ECG Interpretation:

If the basic rhythm, frontal plane axis, or the progression of the R wave is abnormal, interpretation of the 12 lead is abnormal. Interpret the following 12 lead ECGs as either normal or abnormal. We will return to the abnormal ones in subsequent chapters to make a more definitive interpretation.

Answers begin on page 59.

Chapter 4 — Progression of the R Wave

Practice 12 Lead ECG #1

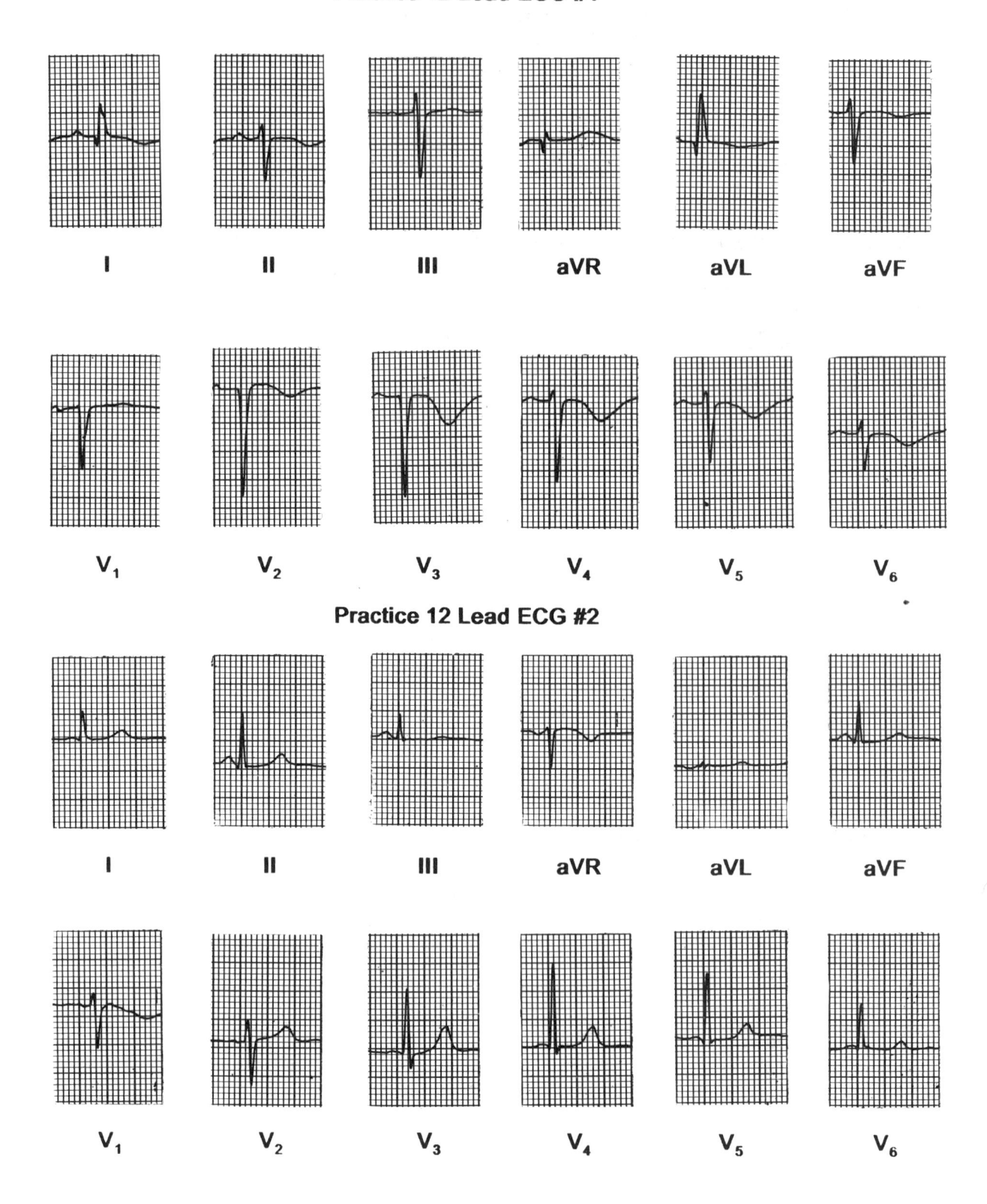

I II III aVR aVL aVF

V₁ V₂ V₃ V₄ V₅ V₆

Practice 12 Lead ECG #2

I II III aVR aVL aVF

V₁ V₂ V₃ V₄ V₅ V₆

Chapter 4 — Progression of the R Wave

Practice 12 Lead ECG #3

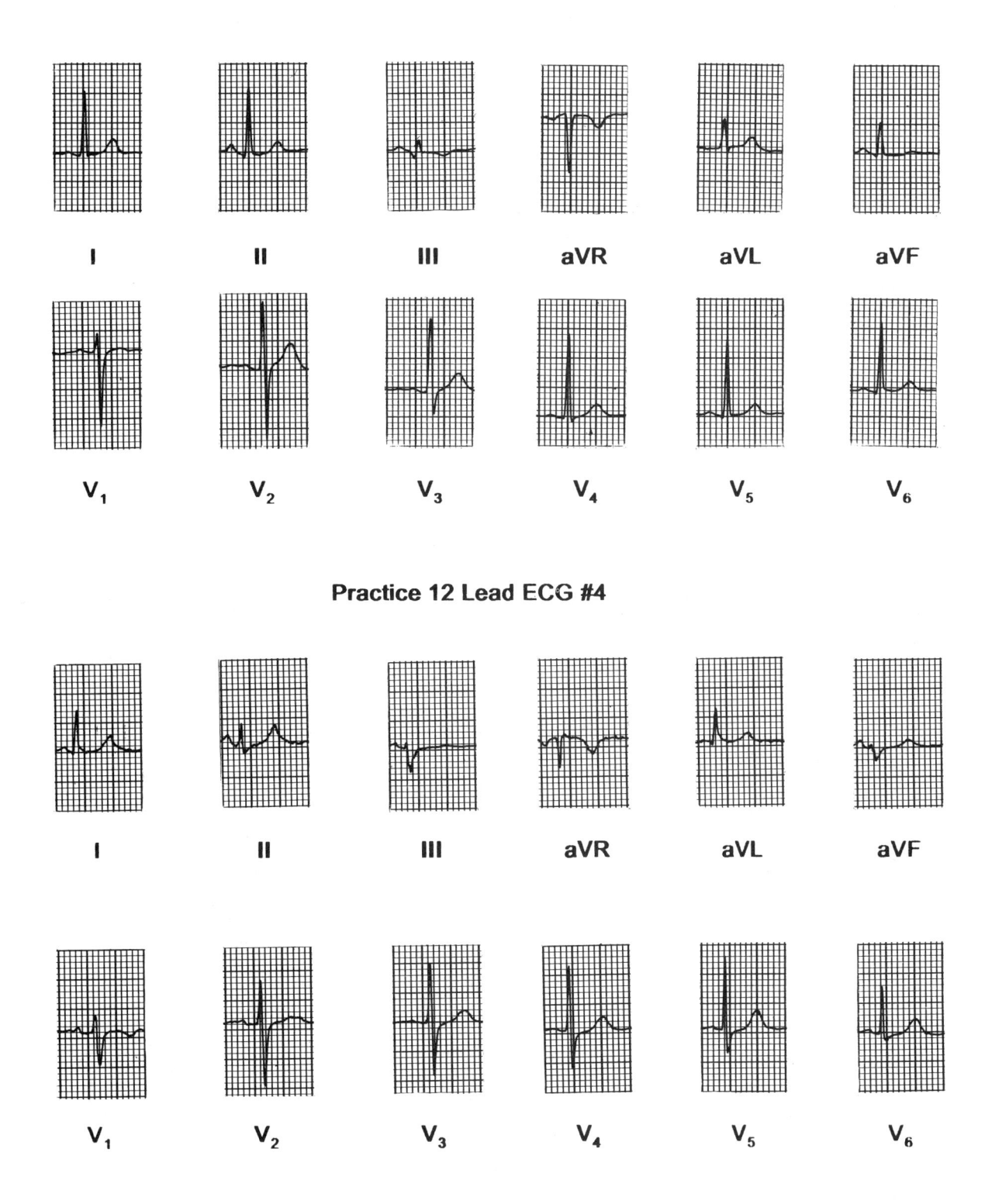

| I | II | III | aVR | aVL | aVF |

| V₁ | V₂ | V₃ | V₄ | V₅ | V₆ |

Practice 12 Lead ECG #4

| I | II | III | aVR | aVL | aVF |

| V₁ | V₂ | V₃ | V₄ | V₅ | V₆ |

Practice 12 Lead ECG #5

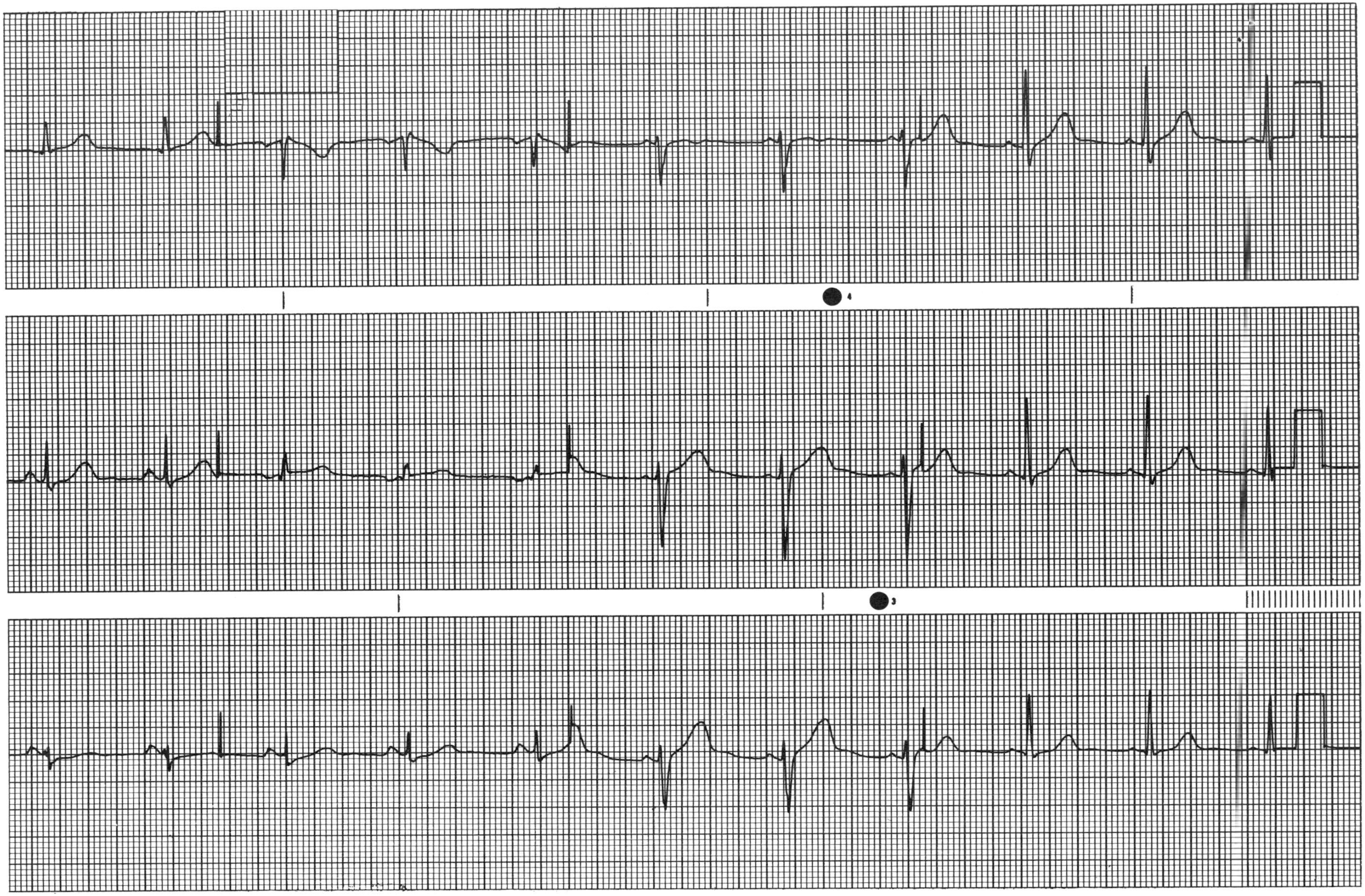

Practice 12 Lead ECG #6

Practice 12 Lead ECG #7

Chapter 4 — Progression of the R Wave

Practice 12 Lead ECG #8

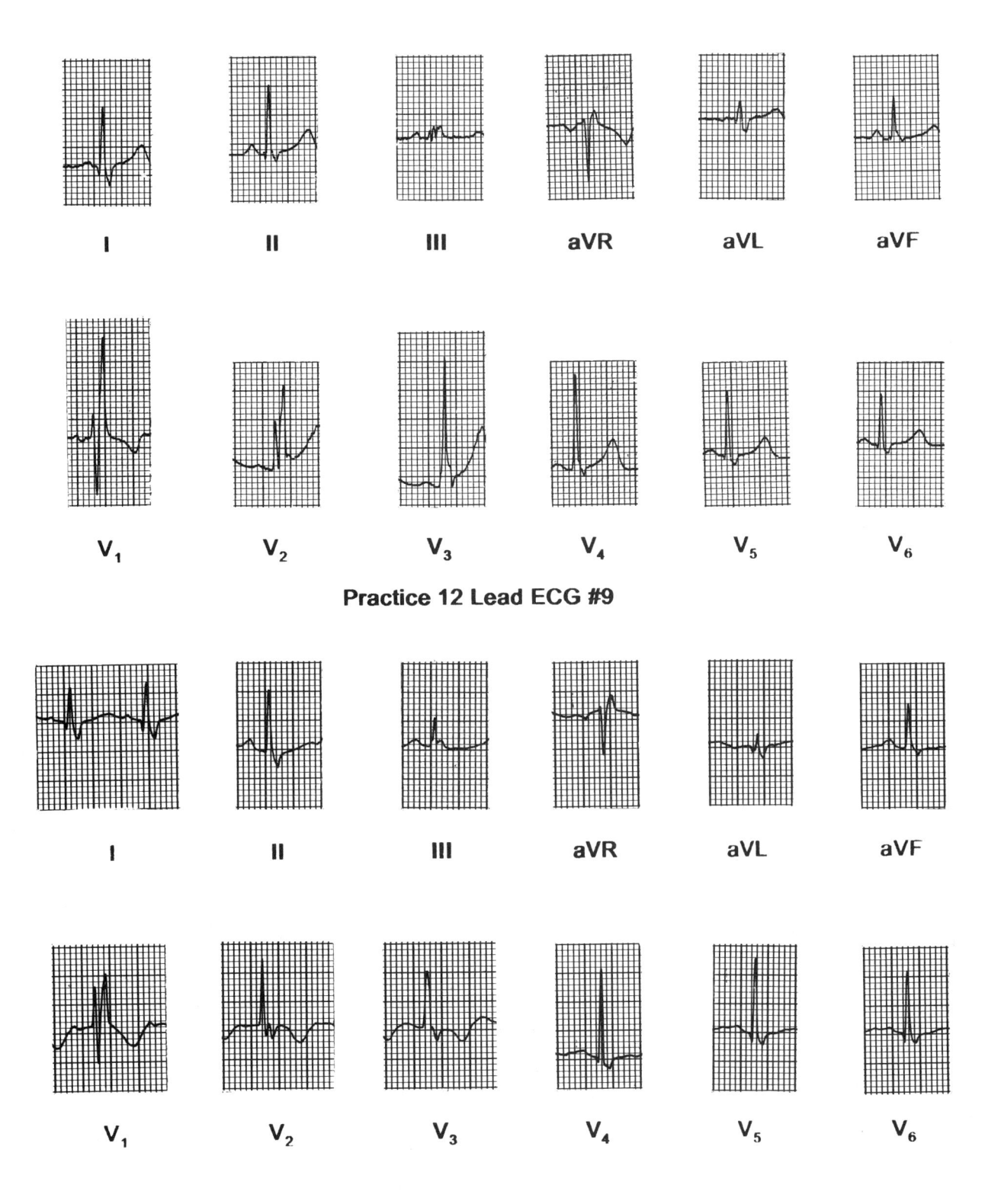

| I | II | III | aVR | aVL | aVF |

| V_1 | V_2 | V_3 | V_4 | V_5 | V_6 |

Practice 12 Lead ECG #9

| I | II | III | aVR | aVL | aVF |

| V_1 | V_2 | V_3 | V_4 | V_5 | V_6 |

Practice 12 Lead ECG #10

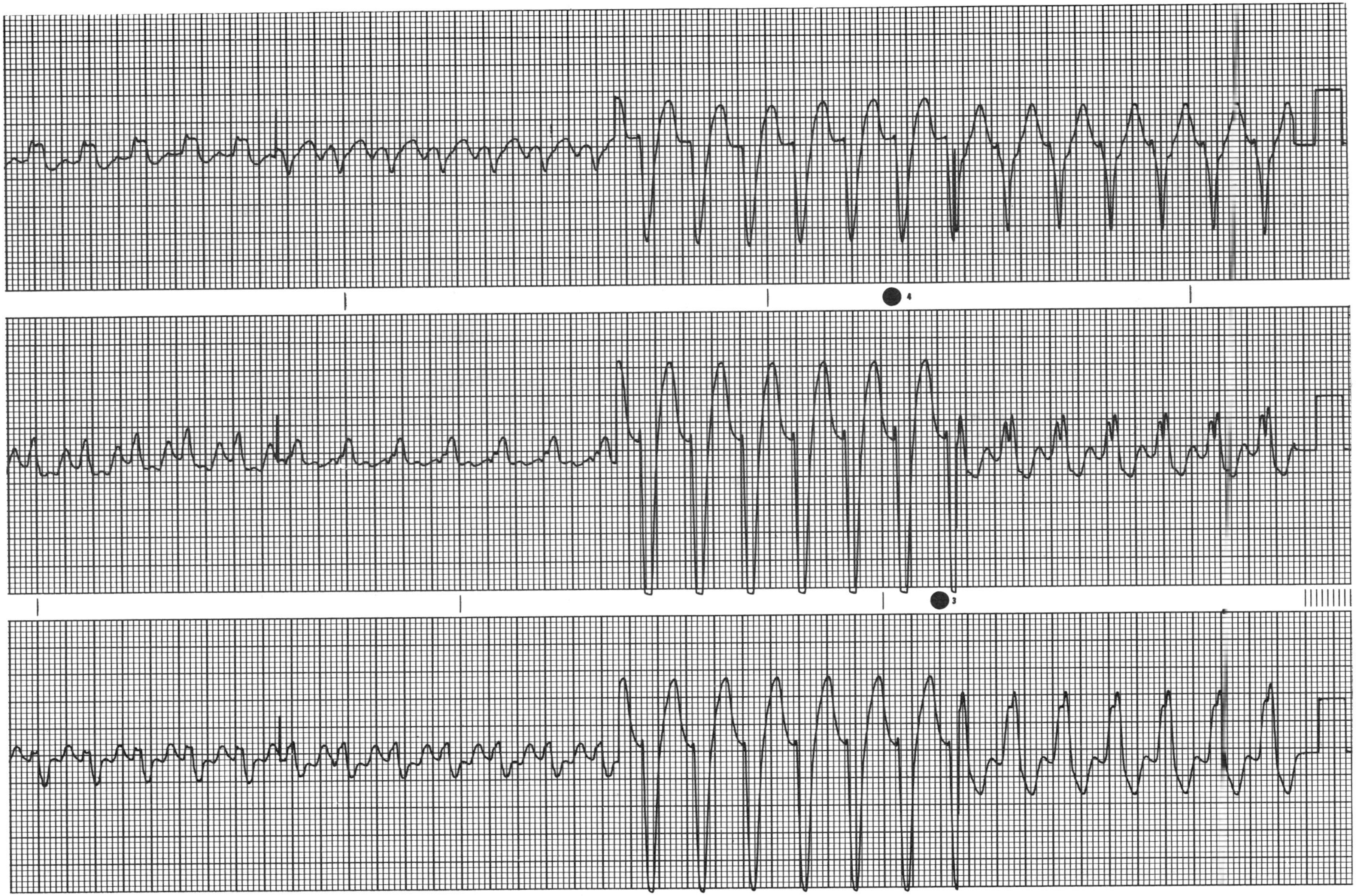

Practice 12 Lead ECG #11

Practice 12 Lead ECG #12

Chapter 4 — Progression of the R Wave

ANSWERS TO PRACTICE 12 LEAD ECGs #1-12

1. **Basic rhythm:** Sinus rhythm
   Frontal plane axis: LAD quadrant -60°
   R wave progression: Abnormal: there is a hint of an r wave in V_1 but it disappears in V_2. There is no r wave in V_3. A small r wave appears in V_4 but it is a very small r wave for this lead. The same is true for V_5 and V_6. Transition never occurs.
   Complex configuration: Abnormal as noted above
   Complex duration: Normal: 0.10 seconds
   P wave: Normal
   ST segment: Normal
   T wave: Abnormal: Inverted T waves in lead I, II, aVL, aVF, and V_2 through V_6
   U wave: None noted
   12 Lead ECG Interpretation: Abnormal

2. **Basic rhythm:** Sinus rhythm
   Frontal plane axis: Normal +60°
   R wave progression: Normal
   Complex configuration and duration: Normal
   P wave: Normal
   ST segment: Normal
   T wave: Normal. Inverted T waves in V_1 are a normal finding for this lead (Chapter 9).
   U wave: Normal U wave in V_2, V_3, V_4
   12 Lead ECG Interpretation: Normal

3. **Basic rhythm:** Sinus rhythm
   Frontal plane axis: Normal +30°
   R wave progression: Normal
   Complex configuration and duration: Normal
   P wave: Normal
   ST segment: Normal
   T wave: Normal
   U wave: Normal: U wave in V_2, V_3
   12 Lead ECG Interpretation: Normal

4. **Basic rhythm:** Sinus rhythm
   Frontal plane axis: Normal 0°
   R wave progression: Normal
   Complex configuration and duration: Normal
   P wave: Normal
   ST segment: Normal
   T wave: Normal
   U wave: ⊖
   12 Lead ECG Interpretation: Normal

Chapter 4 — Progression of the R Wave

5. **Basic rhythm:** Normal sinus rhythm
   Frontal plane axis: Normal +90°
   R wave progression: Normal: Transition occurs in V_4 which is a normal variant.
   Complex configuration and duration: Normal
   P wave: Normal
   ST segment: Normal
   T wave: Normal
   U wave: Normal: U wave in V_2, V_3, V_4
   12 Lead ECG Interpretation: Normal

6. **Basic rhythm:** Normal sinus rhythm
   Frontal plane axis: Normal +30°
   R wave progression: Normal: r wave in V_1; amplitude of r wave increases in V_2; r is sluggish in V_3 with transition in V_4 and normal R waves in V_5 and V_6. Remember that V_3 is placed one-half way between V_2 and V_4. Placement of V_3 is a judgment call by the technician doing the ECG and is therefore subject to technician error.
   Complex configuration and duration: Normal
   P wave: Normal
   ST segment: Normal
   T wave: Normal. Biphasic T waves in V_1 is a normal finding for this lead (Chapter 9).
   U wave: Normal: U waves in V_2, V_3, V_4
   12 Lead ECG Interpretation: Normal

7. **Basic rhythm:** Normal sinus rhythm
   Frontal plane axis: Normal +30°
   R wave progression: Abnormal: loss of anterior forces in V_2, V_3, V_4. Recall that failure of the amplitude of the r wave to increase in V_2 and V_3 is referred to as loss of anterior forces. Transition occurs in V_5 which is not a normal transition lead.
   Complex configuration: Abnormal as noted above and R^I in I, II, III, aVL, aVF, V_5, V_6
   Complex duration: Abnormal: 0.12 seconds
   P wave: Abnormal: tall and peaked in II, aVF
   ST segment: Elevated in V_1, V_2, V_3; slightly depressed in V_5, V_6
   T wave: Abnormal: Inverted in II, III, aVF, V_5, V_6
   U wave: ⊖
   12 Lead ECG Interpretation: Abnormal

8. **Basic rhythm:** Normal sinus rhythm
   Frontal plane axis: Normal +60°
   R wave progression: Abnormal: rSR^I in V_1; tall R in V_1 is abnormal progression of R wave; RR^I in V_2; Rr^I in V_3
   Complex configuration: Abnormal as noted above and wide s wave in V_5, V_6, I, aVL
   Complex duration: Abnormal: 0.12 seconds
   P wave: Normal
   ST segment: Slightly elevated in V_2
   T wave: Inverted in V_1. Recall that normal T waves may be as tall as 10 mm in the precordial leads.
   U wave: Normal: U wave in V_2, V_3
   12 Lead ECG Interpretation: Abnormal

Chapter 4 — Progression of the R Wave

9. **Basic rhythm:** Sinus tachycardia
   Frontal plane axis: Normal +60°
   R wave progression: Abnormal beginning in V_1 with RSR'. You don't have to spend too much time with this one. The tall R in V_1 tells you the progression of the R wave is abnormal.
   Complex configuration: Abnormal as noted above and wide s wave in V_5, V_6, I, aVL
   Complex duration: Abnormal: 0.12 seconds
   P wave: Normal
   ST segment: Depressed in V_1
   T wave: Abnormal in II, III, aVF, V_1, V_2, V_3, V_4, V_5, V_6. Recall that positive complexes should be accompanied by upright T waves.
   U wave: ⊖. U waves are not usually seen when the ventricular rate exceeds 90 BPM.
   12 Lead ECG Interpretation: Abnormal

10. **Basic rhythm:** Normal sinus rhythm
    Frontal plane axis: LAD quadrant -30°
    R wave progression: Abnormal: QS in V_1; r wave does not progress in V_2, V_3, V_4 (loss of anterior forces). Transition occurs in V_6 - too late!
    Configuration of the complex: As noted above and R' in leads I, aVL, V_6
    Duration of the complex: Abnormal: 0.14 seconds
    P wave: Normal
    ST segment: Elevated in V_1, V_2, V_3, V_4; depressed in I, aVL
    T wave: Normal
    U wave: Normal U wave in V_2 and V_3
    12 Lead ECG Interpretation: Abnormal

11. **Basic rhythm:** Sinus tachycardia
    Frontal plane axis: Normal 0°
    R wave progression: Abnormal: QS in V_1, r does not progress in V_2, V_3, V_4 = loss of anterior forces
    Complex: Configuration abnormal as noted above and r'/R' in I, II, aVL, V_5, V_6
    P wave: Abnormal: Tall and peaked in II, aVF
    ST segment: Abnormal: Depressed in I, II, V_4, V_5, V_6
    T wave: T wave assessment is difficult due to rapid ventricular rate and abnormal ST segments and T waves. The abnormal ST segments and T waves are secondary ST-T changes (Chapter 5).
    U wave: ⊖
    12 Lead ECG Interpretation: Abnormal

12. **Basic rhythm:** Normal sinus rhythm
    Frontal plane axis: Normal +60° (lead aVL is almost isoelectric)
    R wave progression: Normal
    Complex configuration and duration: Normal
    P wave: Normal
    ST segment: Slightly elevated in V_2
    T wave: Normal
    U wave: Normal U wave in V_2
    12 Lead ECG Interpretation: Normal

Chapter 4 — Progression of the R Wave

REVIEW OF THE 12 LEADS OF THE ECG

12 leads are advantageously placed around the heart to see the heart's electrical activity from twelve different points of view.

FRONTAL PLANE:

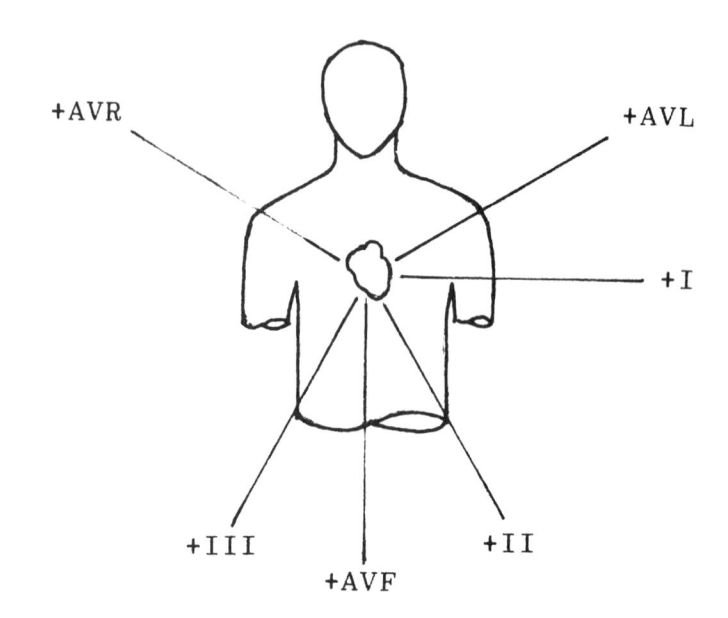

In the frontal plane, leads I and aVL are left lateral leads with their positive electrodes facing the lateral wall of the left ventricle.

QUESTION: Which two precordial leads are also left lateral leads?

ANSWER: V_5 and V_6 are the left lateral leads in the precordial plane. If you missed this question, please review page 18.

QUESTION: Leads II, III, and aVF are the inferior leads.

A. True
B. False

ANSWER: True. Notice the location of the positive electrode of leads II, III, aVF on the hexaxial figure. They are below the heart and looking up at the inferior surface.

On the hexaxial figure above, notice that the positive electrode of lead aVR looks at the base of the heart.

In summary, the frontal plane leads I and aVL are left lateral leads; leads II, III, and aVF are inferior leads; lead aVR looks at the base of the heart, i.e., the atria.

Chapter 4 — Progression of the R Wave

PRECORDIAL PLANE:

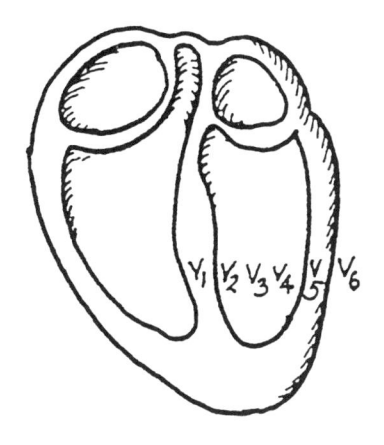

V_1 and (V_2) are septal leads.

(V_2), V_3, and V_4 are anterior leads.

(V_2 overlaps the septum and the anterior wall)

QUESTION: Leads V_5 and V_6 look at which part of the left ventricle?

ANSWER: V_5 and V_6 are left lateral leads.

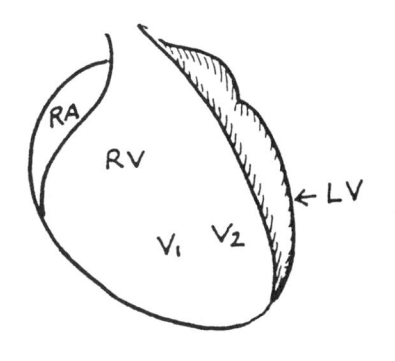

The left ventricle on the anterior/posterior plane is really the **posterior ventricle.**

ANTERIOR VIEW

Notice the location of V_1 and V_2. These two precordial leads sit right on top of the right ventricle. When there is trouble in the right ventricle it will be seen on the ECG in these two right ventricular leads - V_1 and V_2.

QUESTION: With right ventricular hypertrophy, you will see ECG changes in V_1 and V_2.

A. True
B. False

ANSWER: A. True. V_1 and V_2 are the right ventricular leads and record right ventricular activity whenever there is an abnormality affecting the right ventricle.

CHAPTER 5
CHAMBER ENLARGEMENTS

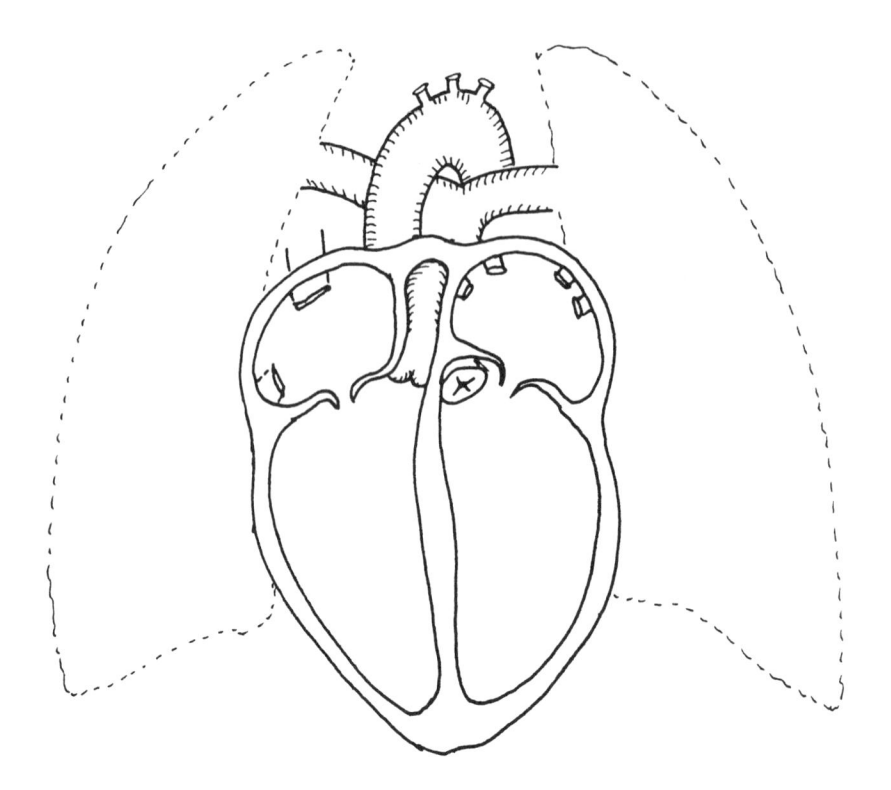

REVIEW OF CHAMBERS AND VALVES

Deoxygenated blood is returned to the right atrium by the superior and inferior vena cavae. The blood flows through the AV valve between the right atria and right ventricle. The tricuspid is the AV valve on the right side of the heart. The blood leaves the right ventricle via its outflow vessel, the pulmonary artery.

Between the right ventricle and the pulmonary artery there is a semilunar valve, the pulmonic valve. The deoxygenated blood leaves the right side of the heart on its journey to the lungs where, hopefully, it will be oxygenated.

Oxygenated blood is returned to the left atrium via the four pulmonary veins. The oxygenated blood passes through the AV valve between the left atria and left ventricle. The AV valve on the left side of the heart is the bicuspid (mitral) valve. The bicuspid valve is called the mitral valve because the two cusps resemble a miter, the headdress worn by bishops.

The blood leaves the left ventricle via its outflow vessel, the aorta. Between the left ventricle and the aorta there is a semilunar valve, the aortic valve. The oxygenated blood leaves the left side of the heart on its way to the systemic circulation to oxygenate the cells of the body.

The four valves of the heart are easy to remember: starting on the right side, as the blood begins its journey through the heart, you always want to "try" (tricuspid) before you "buy" (bicuspid).

The semilunars are named for the outflow vessels they serve. On the right side, the outflow vessel is the pulmonary artery served by the pulmonic valve. On the left side, the outflow vessel is the aorta, served by the aortic valve.

Chapter 5 — Chamber Enlargements

CAUSES OF CHAMBER ENLARGEMENTS

Chamber enlargements occur because the forward flow of blood is impeded. Blood is then forced to back up, resulting in chamber enlargement. To ascertain the causes of chamber enlargement, look forward of that chamber for possible causes of impediment to blood flow.

LEFT VENTRICULAR HYPERTROPHY

QUESTION: What valve is forward of the left ventricle?

ANSWER: The aortic valve is forward of the left ventricle.

Aortic stenosis or insufficiency can cause left ventricular hypertrophy.

The systemic circulation is forward of the left ventricle. Systemic hypertension and congestive heart failure can cause left ventricular hypertrophy. Coarctation of the aorta also causes an impediment to blood flow that can cause left ventricular hypertrophy.

In summary, left ventricular hypertrophy can be caused by:

- systemic hypertension
- congestive heart failure
- coarctation of the aorta
- aortic valve disease
- cardiomyopathies

LEFT ATRIAL ENLARGEMENT

QUESTION: As the blood courses through the heart, what is forward of the left atrium?

ANSWER: Everything forward of the left ventricle is forward of the left atrium. Causes of left atrial enlargement are the same as left ventricular hypertrophy, with one additional cause: mitral valve disease.

QUESTION: What valve is between the left atrium and the left ventricle?

ANSWER: The bicuspid valve. Mitral insufficiency or stenosis can cause left atrial enlargement.

In summary, left atrial enlargement can be caused by:

- systemic hypertension
- congestive heart failure
- coarctation of the aorta
- aortic valve disease
- cardiomyopathies
- mitral valve disease

Chapter 5 — Chamber Enlargements

RIGHT VENTRICULAR HYPERTROPHY

QUESTION: As blood flows through the heart, what is forward of the right ventricle?

ANSWER: Everything forward of the left ventricle and left atrium is forward of the right ventricle. Right ventricular hypertrophy may be caused by all of the above plus pathology of the structures that are forward of the right ventricle. The lungs and the pulmonary artery with its semilunar valve are forward of the right ventricle.

QUESTION: What is the most common cause of right ventricular failure?

ANSWER: The most common cause of right ventricular failure is left ventricular failure.

QUESTION: What is the second most common cause of right ventricular failure?

ANSWER: The second most common cause of right ventricular failure is pulmonary pathology.

In summary, right ventricular hypertrophy may be caused by:

- systemic hypertension
- congestive heart failure
- coarctation of the aorta
- aortic valve disease
- cardiomyopathies
- mitral valve disease
- pulmonary pathology such as pulmonary hypertension or lung disease
- pulmonic valve disease

RIGHT ATRIAL ENLARGEMENT

QUESTION: As the blood flows through the heart, what is forward of the right atrium?

ANSWER: Everything forward of the left ventricle, the left atrium, and the right ventricle is forward of the right atrium with the addition of the tricuspid valve. **Right atrial enlargement may be caused by all of the above plus pathology of the tricuspid valve.**

NOTE: Chamber enlargements may be identified on the ECG. However, they are more accurately diagnosed with an echocardiogram.

Chapter 5 -- Chamber Enlargements

ATRIAL ENLARGEMENT

Atrial depolarization inscribes the P wave on the ECG.

QUESTION: When atrial enlargement occurs, what wave(s) on the ECG would you expect to be affected?

A. P
B. qRs
C. T
D. U

ANSWER: A. The P wave is the result of atrial depolarization. Therefore, the P wave will be affected when atrial enlargement is present. Recall that the normal P wave is round and small.

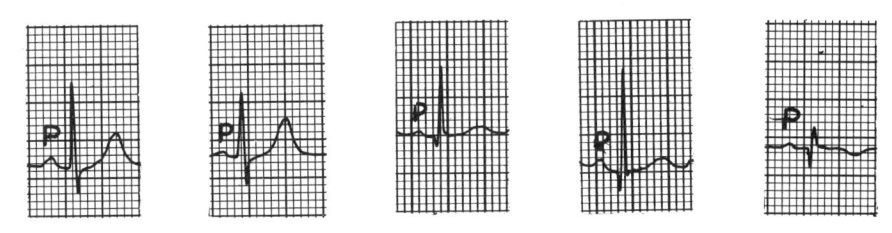

NORMAL P WAVES

QUESTION: The normal P wave is round and no more than $2^1/_2$ millimeters in either direction.

A. True
B. False

ANSWER: A. True. Since each millimeter on the horizontal plane is 0.04 seconds, $2^1/_2$ millimeters is equal to 0.10 seconds. Each millimeter on the vertical plane is 0.10 millivolt; $2^1/_2$ millimeters is equal to 0.25 millivolts. Recall that voltage is usually expressed in millimeters.

Chapter 5 — Chamber Enlargements

Normally, the sinus node initiates depolarization. Atrial depolarization spreads across the atria from superior to inferior, and from right to left in the frontal plane:

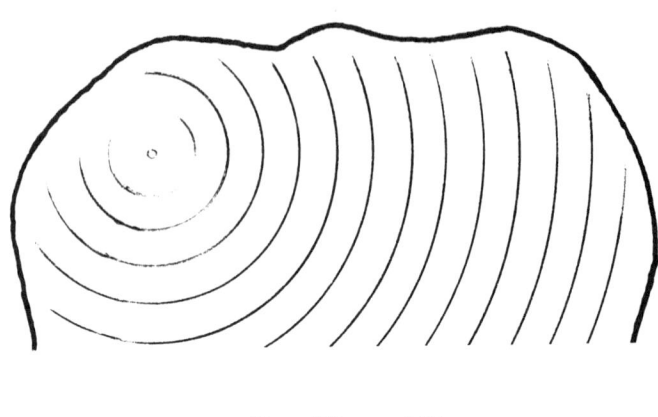

II   III   aVF

NOTE: In the frontal plane, the best leads to assess atrial depolarization are the inferior leads II, III, and aVF. These inferior leads are looking up and see the atrial wave of depolarization moving towards their positive electrodes.

NOTE: In the precordial plane, the best lead to assess atrial depolarization is lead V_1. V_1 sees the right atrium depolarization coming towards the positive electrode of V_1, and then the left (posterior) atrium depolarizes, moving away from the positive electrode of V_1.

QUESTION: The P wave in V_1 may be biphasic.

A. True
B. False

right atrium depolarizes + V_1 left atrium depolarizes = biphasic P wave

ANSWER: A. True. V_1 sees right atrial depolarization coming towards it and inscribes an upward deflection, then left atrial depolarization moving away from the positive electrode of V_1 and a downward deflection is inscribed resulting in a biphasic P wave in V_1. Recall biphasic T waves may also be seen in V_1.

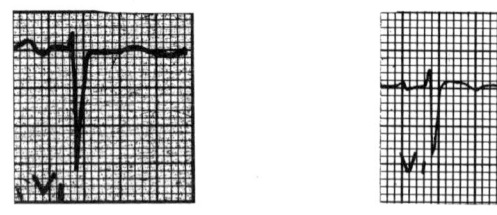

It is not abnormal to have a biphasic P wave in V_1 and V_2 with a positive/negative configuration. However, the terminal negative part of the P wave should not be greater than the initial positive part of the P wave. The negative part of the P wave is called *P terminal.*

P terminal should be no more than 0.04 seconds in duration or 1.0 millimeter in depth.

Chapter 5 — Chamber Enlargements

RIGHT ATRIAL ENLARGEMENT

Right atrial enlargement is *P pulmonale.* When the right atrium is enlarged the P wave loses its round configuration, becomes pointed, and the amplitude may increase. The pointed configuration and increased amplitude of P pulmonale are best seen in the inferior leads II, III, aVF, and V_1. To diagnose atrial enlargement, you do not need to see the changes in all four of the above mentioned leads. To be significant, however, the changes should be evident in at least two of the leads.

Practice 12 lead ECG # 7 and 11 on pages 54 and 56 are examples of right atrial enlargement with tall, peaked P waves in the inferior leads II, III, and aVF.

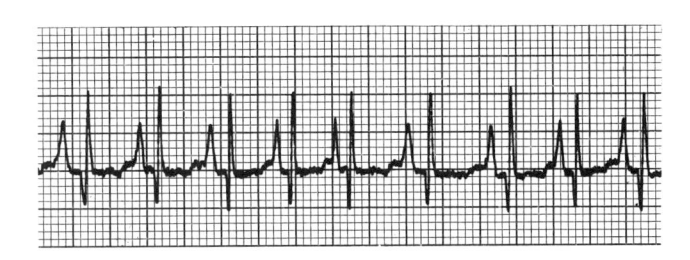

NOTE the tall, pointed P wave in the above strip — ECG characteristics of P pulmonale.

LEFT ATRIAL ENLARGEMENT

Left atrial enlargement is *P mitrale*. When the left atrium enlarges, the P wave increases in width and often becomes notched. This wide, notched P wave can best be seen in the inferior leads II, III, and aVF. **Helpful hint:** An easy way to remember P Mitrale is that the P wave resembles an **M** in the inferior leads due to the notched appearance: **M = M**.

P mitrale causes the P terminal to increase in lead V_1. Recall that the P terminal in V_1 is the result of depolarization of the left atria. No wonder this part of the P wave increases when the left atrium is enlarged! A P terminal that is larger than the initial positive part of the P wave or more than one millimeter deep or wide is abnormal and characteristic of P mitrale.

To diagnose P mitrale, you do not need to see the changes in all four of the above mentioned leads. To be significant, however, the changes should be evident in at least two of the leads.

| II | III | aVF | V_1 |

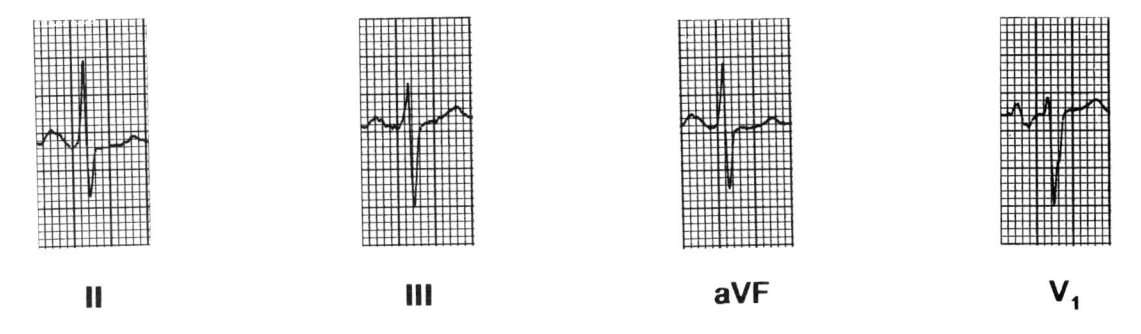

NOTE the wide, notched P wave in the inferior leads and the deep, wide P terminal in V_1 in the above leads. These are the ECG characteristics of P mitrale.

Chapter 5 — Chamber Enlargements

BIATRIAL ENLARGEMENT

When both atria are enlarged, the P wave becomes peaked, tall, wide, and it may be notched in the inferior leads. In V_1, an abnormally large P terminal may be evident.

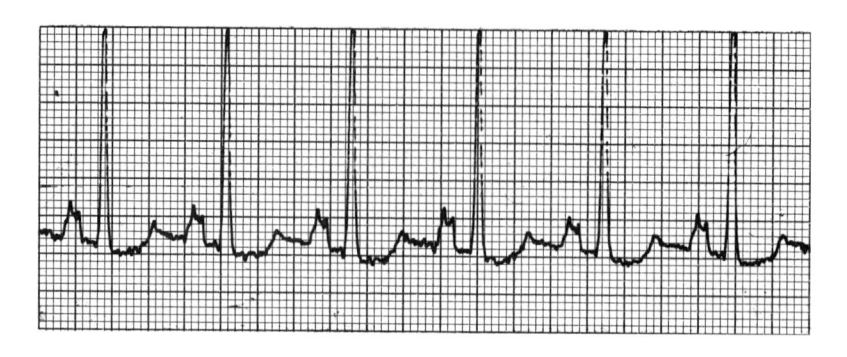

NOTE: the tall, peaked, wide, and notched P wave. These are the ECG characteristics of biatrial enlargements.

Biatrial enlargement is evident in Figure 5 A on the following page. Note the tall, wide P wave in lead II, the wide Ps in II, III, aVF, and the huge P terminal in V_1. The P wave in lead I is also wide and notched.

QUESTION: What is the frontal plane axis in Figure 5 A on page 71?

ANSWER: RAD quadrant +120°.

QUESTION: Describe the progression of the R wave in Figure 5 A.

ANSWER: The R wave progression is abnormal with large R waves in V_1.

QUESTION: Figure 5 A is an abnormal 12 lead ECG.

A. True
B. False

ANSWER: A. True.

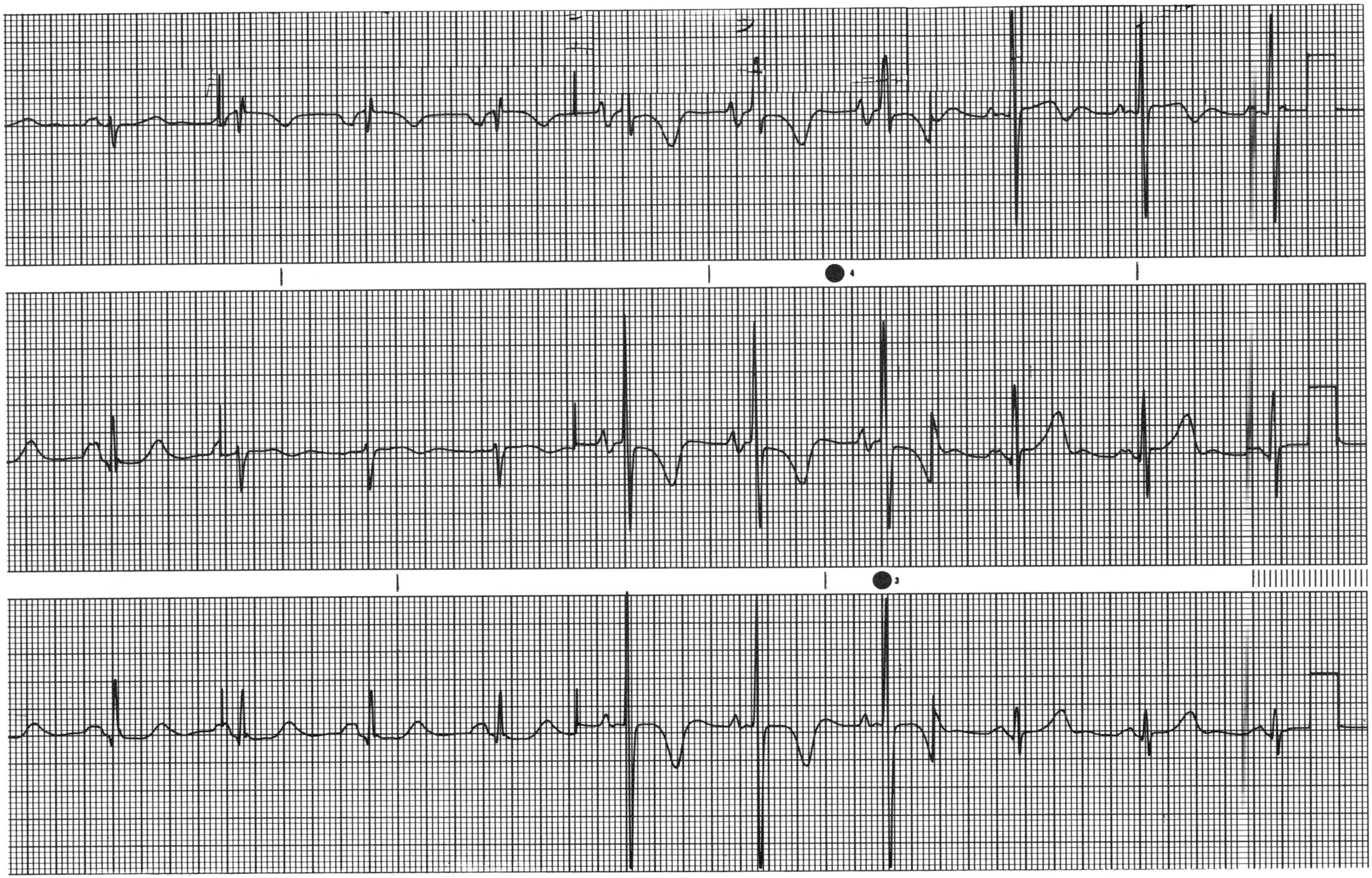

Figure 5 A

Chapter 5 — Chamber Enlargements

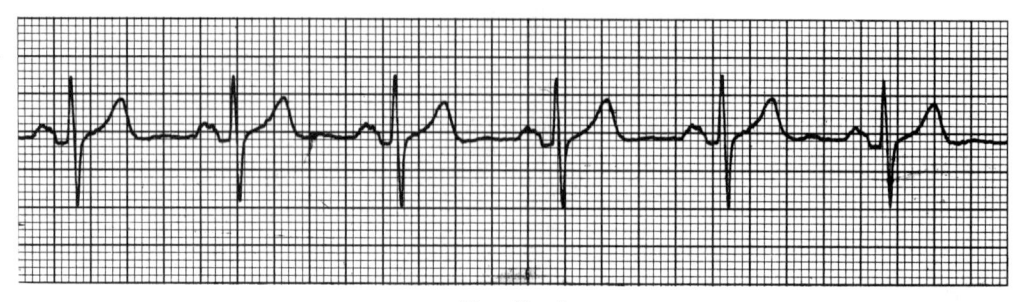

P mitrale

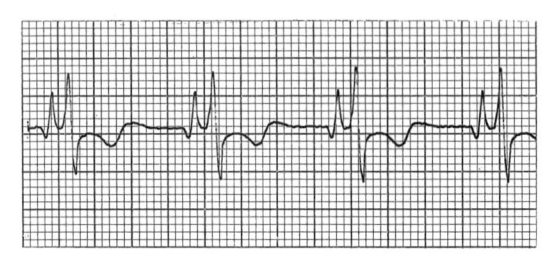

P pulmonale

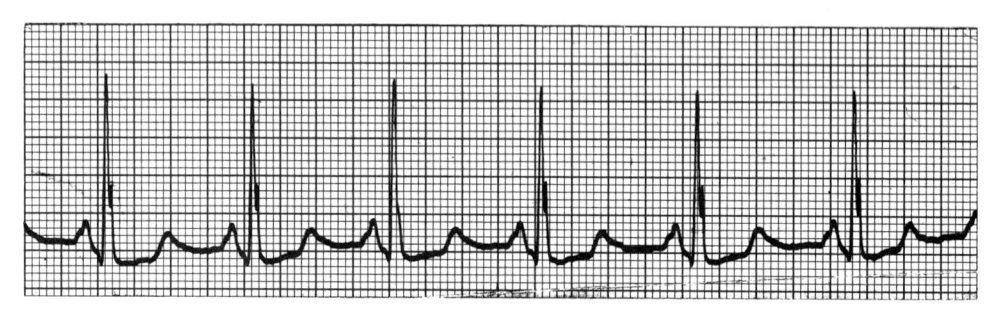

Biatrial enlargement

The chart on the following page summarizes the ECG criteria of right, left, and biatrial enlargement. The solid line depicts right atrial activity and the dotted line is the left atrial activity.

The top box shows how the normal P wave is inscribed in the inferior leads II, II, aVF, and V_1. The middle box displays right atrial enlargement. The enlarged right atrium overshadows the normal left atrial depolarization resulting in the tall pointed P wave characteristic of P pulmonale in the inferior leads and V_1.

The lower box shows left atrial enlargement. The large left atrium (dotted line) rises above the normal right atrial depolarization resulting in the wide notched P wave seen in the inferior leads; In V_1, the enlarged left atria depolarizes away from the positive of V_1 inscribing the large negative portion of the P wave (P terminal).

Chapter 5 -- Chamber Enlargements

ATRIAL ENLARGEMENT

KEY:
 Solid line: RA
 Dotted Line: LA

	II, III, aVF	V$_1$
Normal P wave		
Right atrial enlargement		
Left atrial enlargement		

ECG CRITERIA

Right atrial enlargement
P peaked in II, III, aVF, V$_1$
P > 2.5 mm tall in II, III, aVF

Left atrial enlargement
Notched P   II, III, aVF
P > 0.10 seconds

Prominent negative terminal
P wave deflection in V$_1$ > 1:1

Biatrial enlargement
Peaked P   II, III, aVF
P > 2.5 mm tall
Wide P > 0.10 seconds
Notched P

Large P terminal in V$_1$

Chapter 5 — Chamber Enlargements

PRACTICE STRIPS #13-20

In the following practice strips identify any atrial enlargements that are present. Answers begin on page 76.

13.

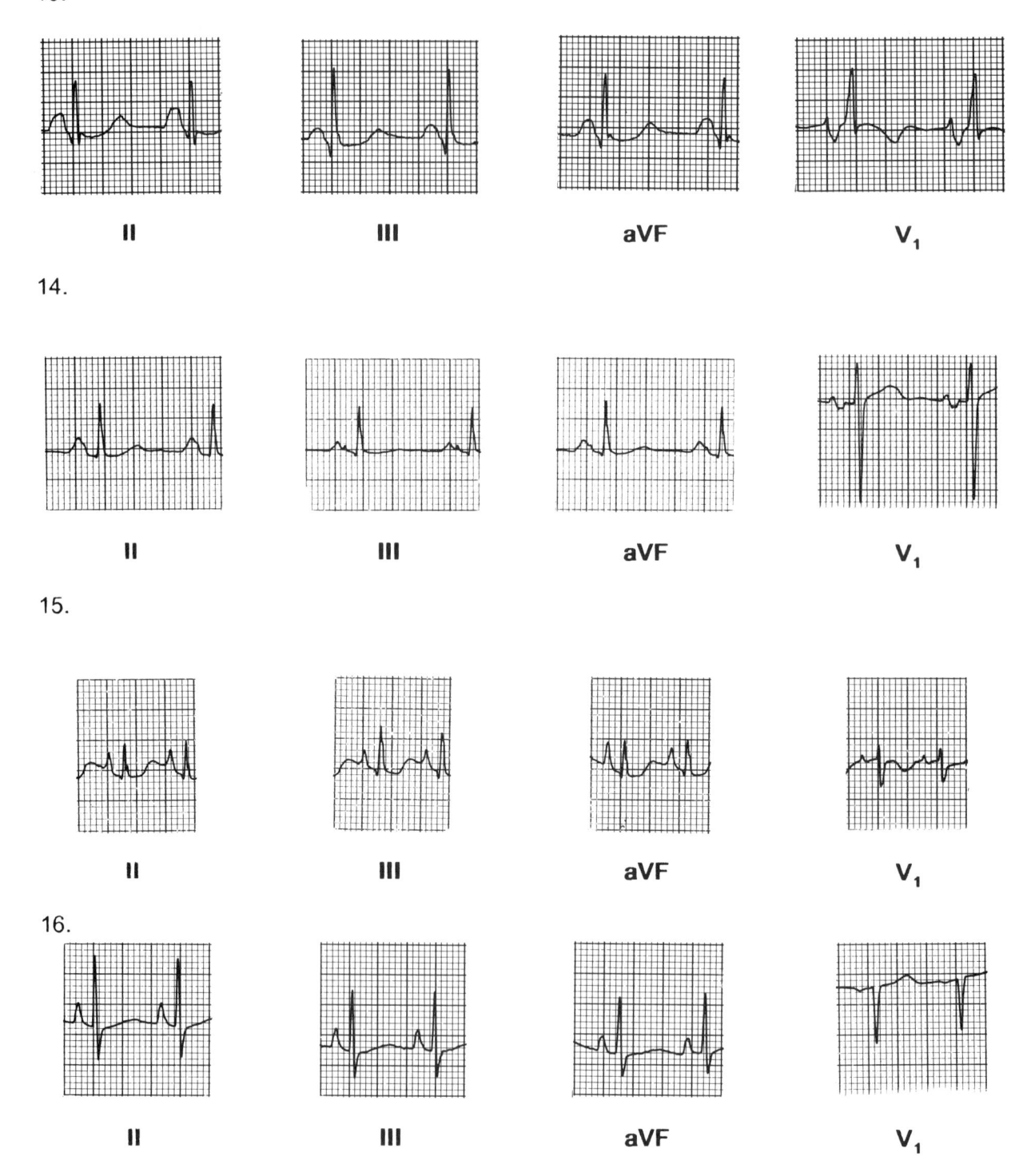

    II   **III**   **aVF**   **V$_1$**

14.

    II   **III**   **aVF**   **V$_1$**

15.

    II   **III**   **aVF**   **V$_1$**

16.

    II   **III**   **aVF**   **V$_1$**

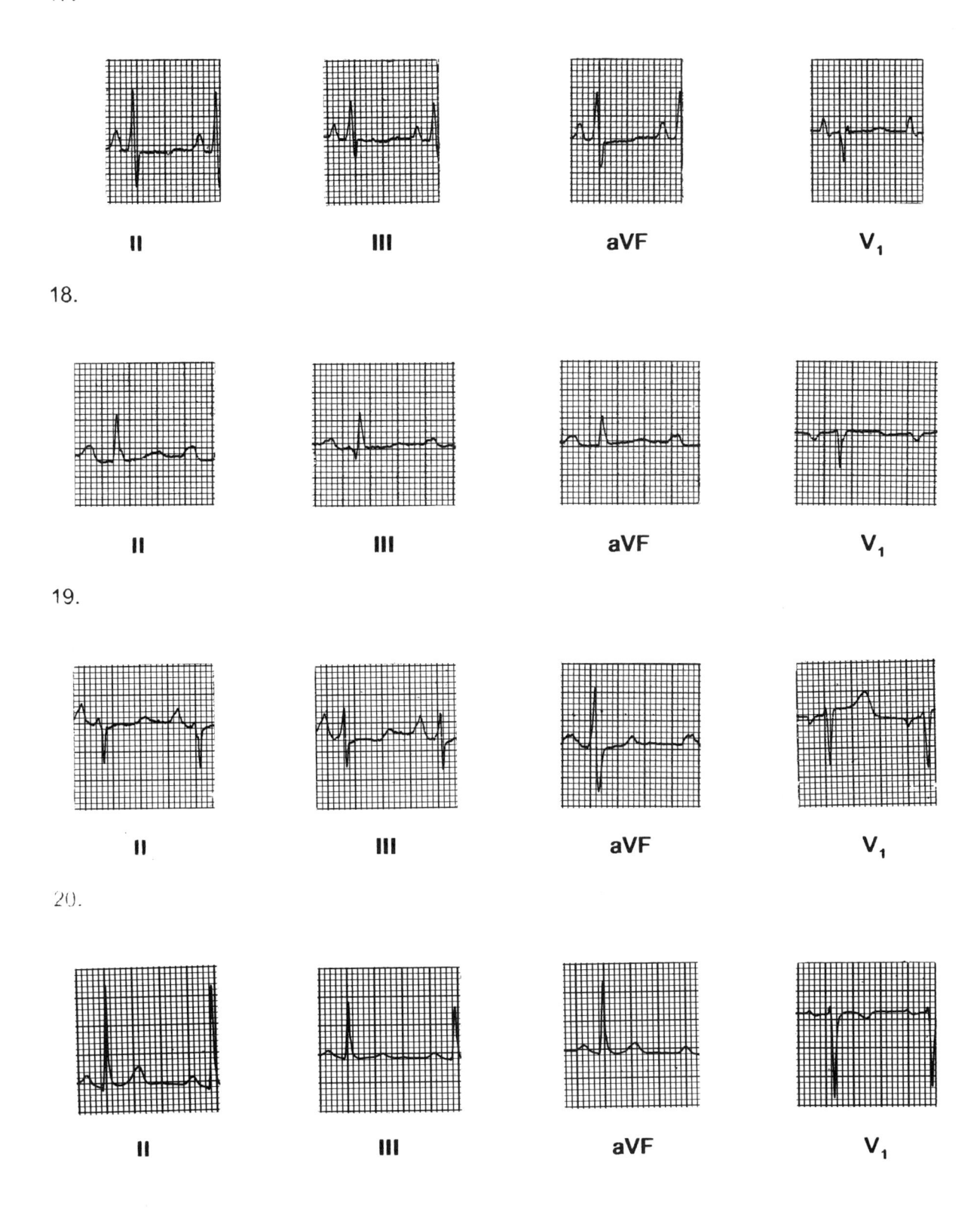

Chapter 5 -- Chamber Enlargements

17.

| II | III | aVF | V₁ |

18.

| II | III | aVF | V₁ |

19.

| II | III | aVF | V₁ |

20.

| II | III | aVF | V₁ |

Chapter 5 — Chamber Enlargements

ANSWERS TO PRACTICE STRIPS #13-20

13. **Size of the P wave:** Wide P waves in II, III, aVF; tall in II, aVF; large P terminal in V_1
    P wave interpretation: Abnormal
    - Biatrial enlargement

14. **Size of the P wave:** Wide and notched in II, III, aVF; large P terminal in V_1
    P wave interpretation: Abnormal
    - P mitrale

15. **Size of the P wave:** Tall in II and peaked in II, III, aVF; peaked in V_1
    P wave interpretation: Abnormal
    - P Pulmonale

16. **Size of the P wave:** Tall and peaked in II, III; peaked in aVF
    P wave interpretation: Abnormal
    - P Pulmonale

17. **Size of the P wave:** Tall and peaked in II; peaked in III, aVF, V_1
    P wave interpretation: Abnormal
    - P Pulmonale

18. **Size of the P wave:** Wide and notched II, III, aVF; abnormal P terminal in V_1
    P wave interpretation: Abnormal
    - P Mitrale
    - First degree AV heart block

19. **Size of the P wave:** Tall, peaked, wide, and notched in II, III, aVF; abnormal P terminal in V_1
    P wave interpretation: Abnormal
    - Biatrial enlargement

20. **Size of the P wave:** Normal
    P wave interpretation: Normal

Chapter 5 — Chamber Enlargements

VENTRICULAR HYPERTROPHY

Ventricular depolarization results in the waves of the complex (qRs) on the ECG. Therefore, it is no surprise that ventricular hypertrophy causes changes in the waves of the complex. ECG changes are also seen in the ST segment and the T wave because ventricular repolarization is altered by abnormal ventricular depolarization.

To assess ventricular hypertrophy, we primarily assess the precordial leads. However, the frontal plane leads are also used to aid in the interpretation of ventricular hypertrophy.

LEFT VENTRICULAR HYPERTROPHY ECG CHARACTERISTICS

1. **Increased voltage in the precordial leads.** Since the size of the left ventricle has increased, the waves on the ECG inscribed due to left ventricular depolarization will increase in amplitude.

Recall that in V_1 the initial wave (small r) is the result of ventricular septum depolarization moving towards the positive electrode of V_1. This small r is followed by an S wave. The S wave is the result of depolarization of the left (posterior) ventricle. Normally V_1 and V_2 have fairly large S waves. When the size of the left ventricle increases, these fairly large S waves increase and become *very large S waves*. These large S waves in V_1 and V_2 represent increased voltage moving away from the positive electrodes of these leads. An S wave of 25 millimeters or more in V_1 and/or V_2 is one ECG characteristic of left ventricular hypertrophy.

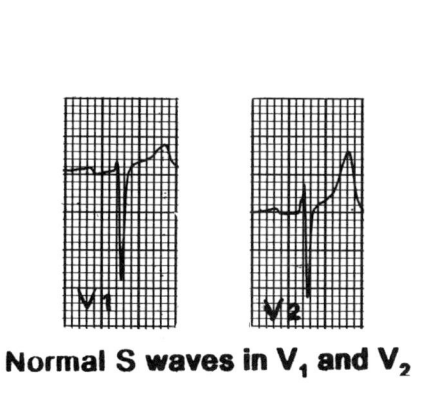

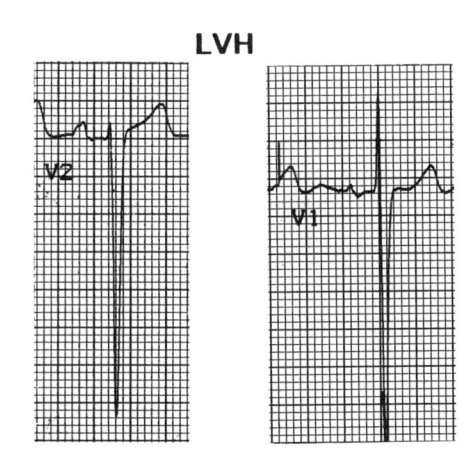

Normal S waves in V_1 and V_2

LVH

Increased amplitude of S waves in V_1 and V_2

Chapter 5 -- Chamber Enlargements

Normally the initial wave (small q wave) in V_5 and V_6 is the result of septal depolarization moving away from the positive electrodes of V_5 and V_6. The small q is followed by a tall R wave in the left lateral leads (V_5, V_6) due to depolarization of the left ventricle. When the size of the left ventricle increases, the voltage of these large R waves increase and they become *very large R waves*. These very large R waves represent increased voltage moving towards the positive electrodes of V_5 and V_6. An R wave of 25 millimeters or more in V_5 and/or V_6 is one ECG characteristic of left ventricular hypertrophy.

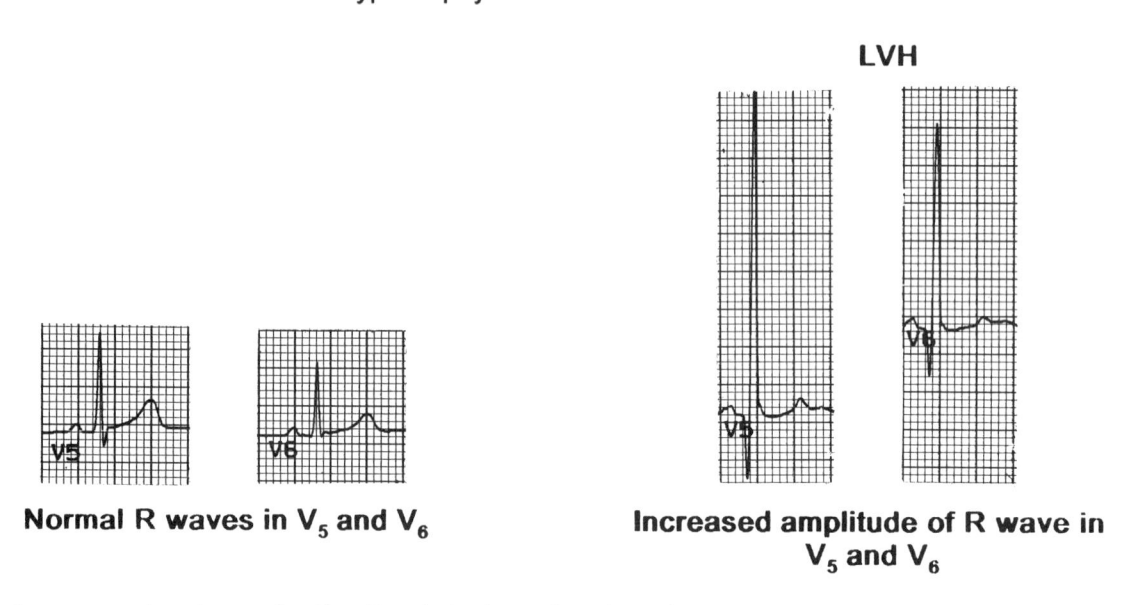

LVH

Normal R waves in V_5 and V_6

Increased amplitude of R wave in V_5 and V_6

2. **Increased voltage in the frontal plane leads.** Since the size of the left ventricle has increased, the amplitude of the complex in the frontal plane may increase. Any R wave or any S wave 20 millimeters or more in the frontal plane leads is one ECG characteristic of left ventricular hypertrophy. This particular voltage change is infrequently seen with hypertrophy.

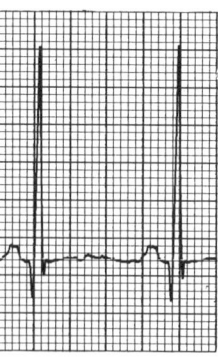

Lead II (for example)

NOTE: DO NOT expect to see all of these voltage changes in all the above mentioned leads in any one 12 lead ECG.

Chapter 5 — Chamber Enlargements

3. **Secondary ST-T wave changes.** Secondary ST-T wave changes occur in hypertrophy due to altered repolarization of the ventricle. Repolarization is abnormal because depolarization is abnormal. These changes are seen in the ST segment and/or the T wave. The ST segment is depressed and the T wave is inverted with an upright complex; the ST segment is elevated and the T wave is upright with essentially negative complexes. Recall that the normal ST segment is isoelectric and the normal T is in the same direction as its complex.

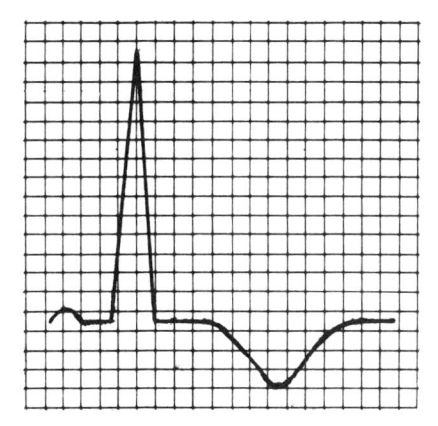

These ST-T wave changes are "secondary" because repolarization is abnormal secondarily to altered depolarization. They are <u>not</u> primary changes. "Strain" pattern is another term for these secondary ST-T wave changes. This strain pattern is also commonly seen with digitalized patients. In left ventricular hypertrophy these ST-T changes are seen in the precordial left lateral leads V_5 and V_6.

4. **Left axis deviation** may be present in left ventricular hypertrophy. Left axis deviation is one ECG characteristic of left ventricular hypertrophy; however, it is <u>not always</u> present.

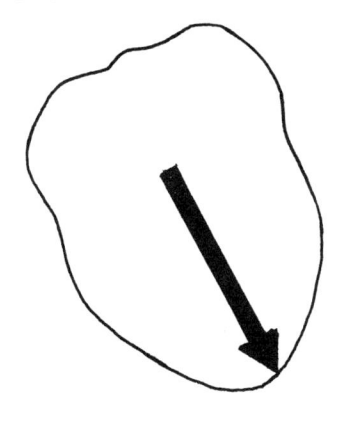

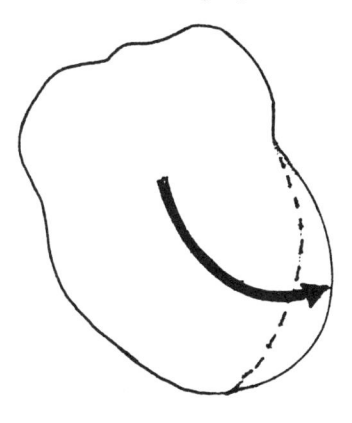

Normal Axis   **LVH Axis**

5. **Increase in the qRs interval.** Since the size of the left ventricle has increased, the duration of ventricular depolarization may increase. A qRs complex <u>of 0.09 seconds or greater</u> is one ECG characteristic of left ventricular hypertrophy.

Chapter 5 — Chamber Enlargements

6. **Increased ventricular activation time in the precordial left lateral leads.**

QUESTION: The precordial left lateral leads are V_5 and V_6.

A. True
B. False

ANSWER: A. True. V_5 and V_6 are the precordial left lateral leads. In the frontal plane, leads I and aVL are also left lateral leads.

The <u>V</u>entricular <u>A</u>ctivation <u>T</u>ime, or the VAT, is also known as the intrinsicoid deflection. It sounds complicated, but it really is not. The VAT is simply the time it takes from the beginning of ventricular depolarization to the crest of the wave of depolarization.

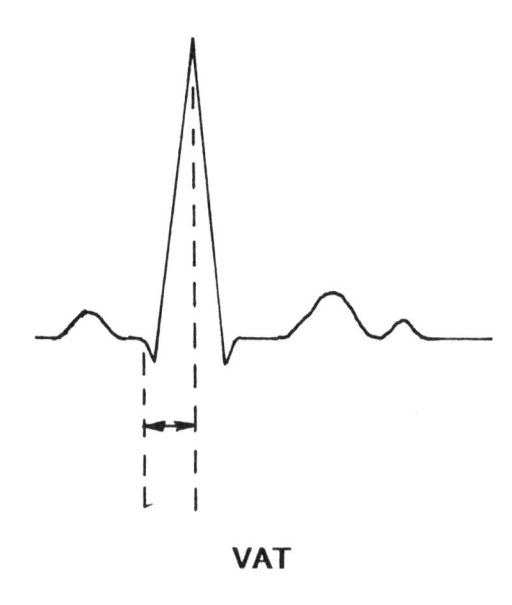

VAT

QUESTION: The VAT is a time measurement, therefore it is measured on the horizontal line.

A. True
B. False

ANSWER: A. True.

Normally the VAT in the precordial left lateral leads is 0.04 seconds. VAT in V_5 and/or V_6 greater than 0.04 seconds is one ECG characteristic of left ventricular hypertrophy.

7. **Evidence of left atrial enlargement.** Left atrial enlargement is one ECG characteristic of left ventricular hypertrophy, since they often occur together.

There are a considerable number of ECG characteristics for left ventricular hypertrophy. To simplify the interpretation, Doctor Estes developed a scoring system. This system assigns points for the presence of ECG characteristics as follows:

Chapter 5 — Chamber Enlargements

ESTES SCORING SYSTEM FOR LVH

ECG CHARACTERISTICS		POINTS

Voltage:

S in V_1 or V_2: 25 mm or more
R in V_5 or V_6: 25 mm or more   All or any one   3
R or S in any frontal plane lead: ≥ 20 mm

Secondary ST-T changes:

    Patient not on digitalis   3
    Patient on digitalis   2

Abnormal P Terminal in V_1   3

Left axis deviation: -30° or more leftwards   2

qRs interval: 0.09 seconds or more   1

VAT in V_5 and/or V_6: 0.05 seconds or more   1

4 POINTS IS PROBABLE LVH

5 POINTS OR MORE STRONGLY INDICATES LVH

Figure 5 B on the following page is an example of LVH. The patient is not on digitalis.

Please assess Figure 5 B on page 82.

QUESTION: How many points does Figure 5 B rate according to the Estes scoring system?

ANSWER: The answer is on page 83.

Figure 5 B

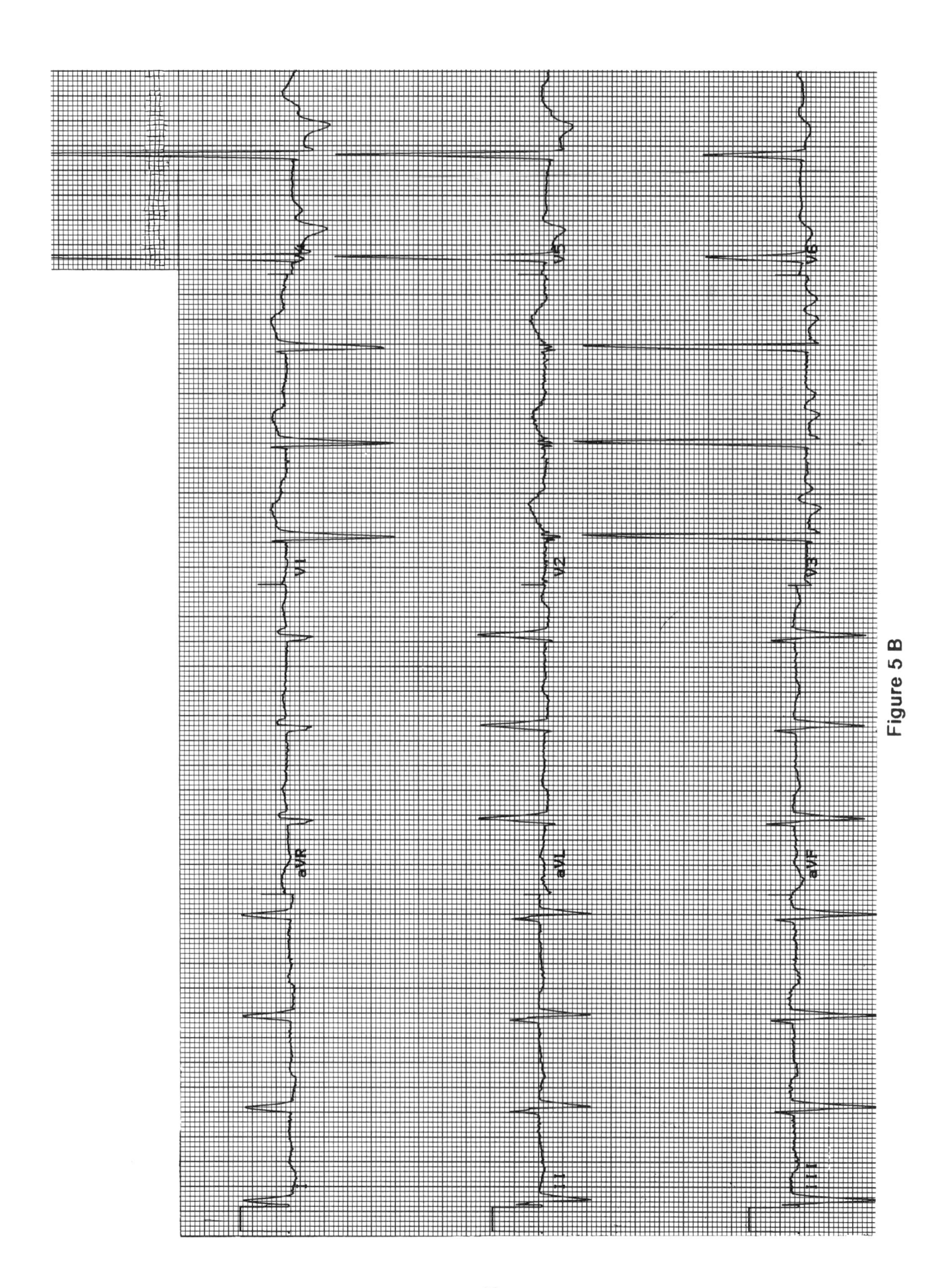

Chapter 5 – Chamber Enlargements

Figure 5 B assessment:

Basic rhythm: Atrial fibrillation with controlled ventricular rate (78 BPM)
Frontal plane axis: LAD quadrant -60°
R wave progression: Abnormal: V_2 is abnormal
Complex configuration: Abnormal as noted above and R voltage is greater than 25 mm in V_3, V_4, V_5
Complex duration: Abnormal: 0.12 seconds
P wave: θ
Secondary ST-T changes: Seen in leads I, II, V_3, V_4, V_5, V_6
12 Lead ECG Interpretation: Abnormal
  - Left ventricular hypertrophy (LVH)

ANSWER: Figure 5 B

Estes Score for LVH for this patient:	Points
Voltage criteria	3
Secondary ST-T changes	3
Left axis deviation greater than -30°	2
Complex interval 0.09 seconds or greater	1
VAT in V_5 greater than 0.05 seconds	1
TOTAL	10 points

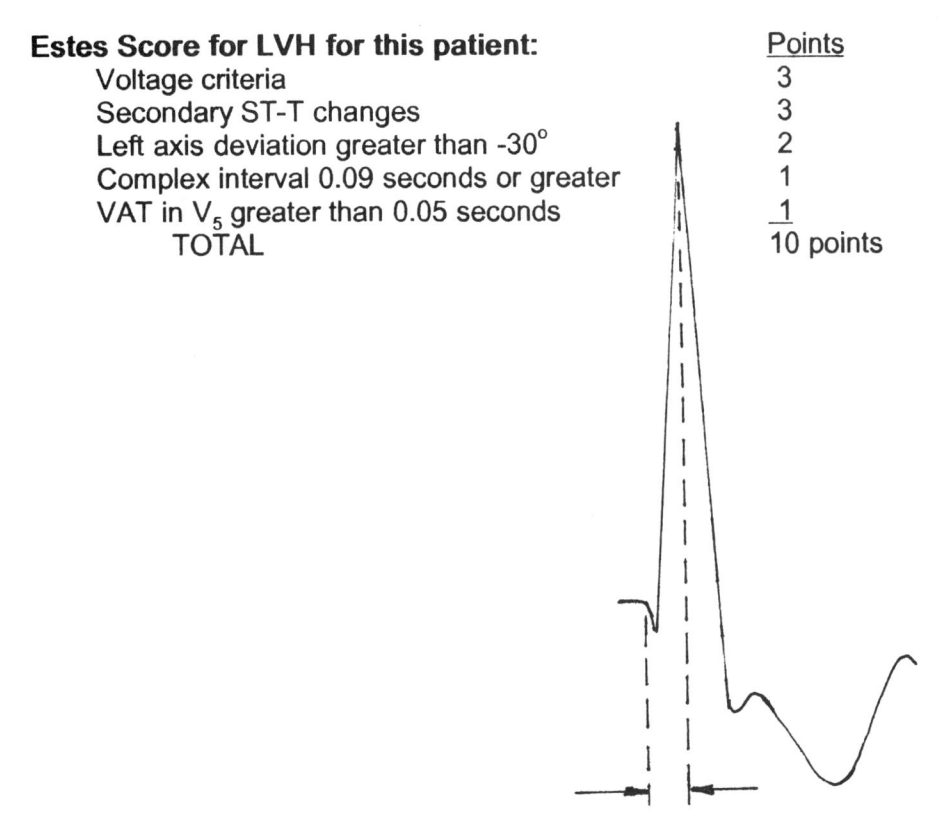

Figure 5 B VAT in V_5

NOTE that from the beginning of the complex to the crest of the R wave, the distance is greater than 1 small box (0.04 seconds) on the horizontal line.

Figure 5 C on the following page is another example of LVH. The patient is digitalized.

Figure 5 C

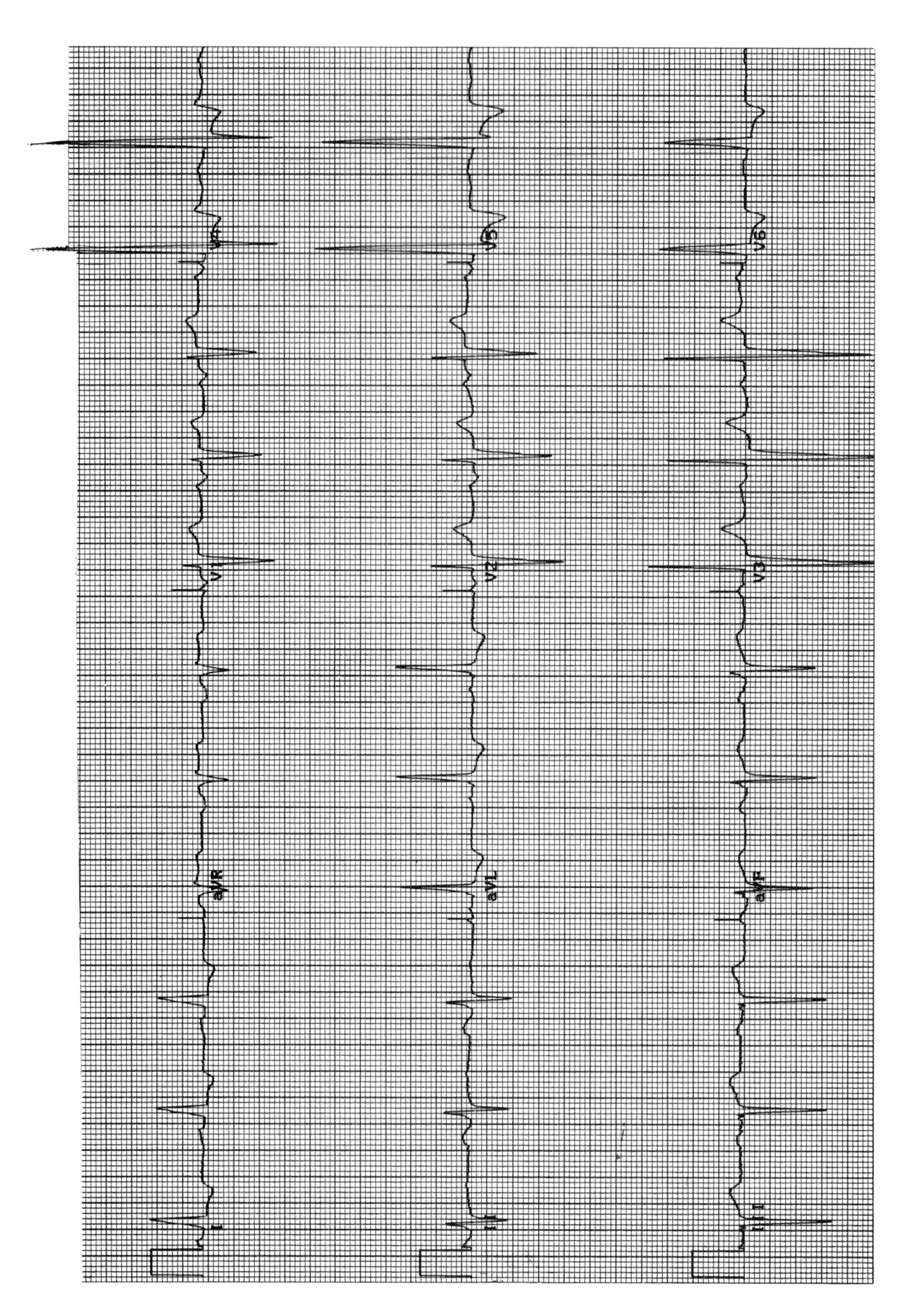

Chapter 5 — Chamber Enlargements

Figure 5 C assessment:

Basic rhythm: Normal sinus rhythm
Frontal plane axis: LAD quadrant -30°
R wave Progression: Normal with transition in V_4
Complex configuration: R voltage 25 mm in V_5
Complex duration: Normal: 0.11 second
P waves: Wide and notched II, III, aVF; abnormal P terminal in V_1
Secondary ST-T changes: I, aVL, V_5, V_6
12 Lead ECG Interpretation: Abnormal
 - Left ventricular hypertrophy
 - P mitrale

QUESTION: How many points does figure 5 C rate according to the Estes scoring system?

ANSWER: Estes score for LVH for this digitalized patient:

Voltage criteria	3
Secondary ST-T changes	2
Left axis deviation -30°	3
Complex interval 0.09 seconds or greater	1
Abnormal P terminal	3
TOTAL	12 points

Recall in the Estes Scoring System:

4 points = probable LVH
5 points or more = strongly indicates LVH

Chapter 5 -- Chamber Enlargements

RIGHT VENTRICULAR HYPERTROPHY ECG CHARACTERISTICS

1. **Increased r waves in the right precordial leads.** Since the right ventricle has increased, the amplitude of the waves inscribed due to right ventricular depolarization will increase. The amplitude of the r waves will increase in the right precordial leads.

QUESTION: The right precordial leads are V_1 and V_2.

A. True
B. False

ANSWER: A. True. V_1 and V_2 are the right precordial leads. Normally, we do not see right ventricular depolarization because the right ventricle is overshadowed by the larger left ventricle on the ECG. When there is trouble in the right ventricle it is seen in the right precordial leads V_1 and V_2.

Recall that V_1 normally has a small r followed by an S wave. The small r is due to depolarization of the septum moving towards V_1 and the S wave is due to depolarization of the left ventricle moving away from V_1. When the right ventricle hypertrophies this increased wave of depolarization is seen in V_1 and V_2 and large R waves are inscribed in these leads.

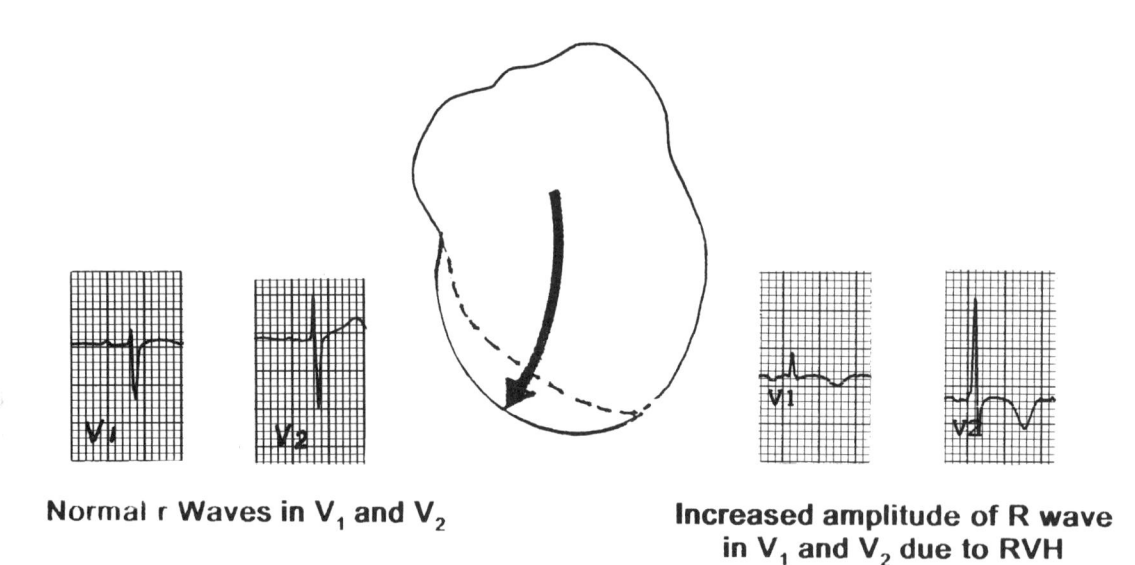

Normal r Waves in V_1 and V_2 Increased amplitude of R wave
                                              in V_1 and V_2 due to RVH

How large is a "large" R wave? The amplitude of the r wave in V_1 should be less than or equal to the S wave in V_1. If the r wave is one millimeter tall and the s wave is ½ millimeter deep:

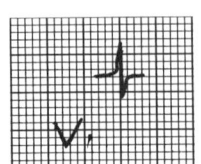

THIS IS A GIANT R WAVE FOR LEAD V_1.

The r wave in V_1 is relative to the S wave in V_1.

Chapter 5 — Chamber Enlargements

Examples of tall r waves in V_1:

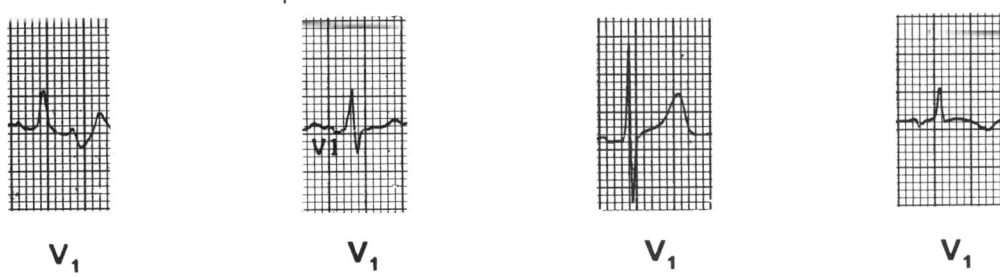

V_1 V_1 V_1 V_1

2. **Increased amplitude of the s wave in V_5 and V_6**

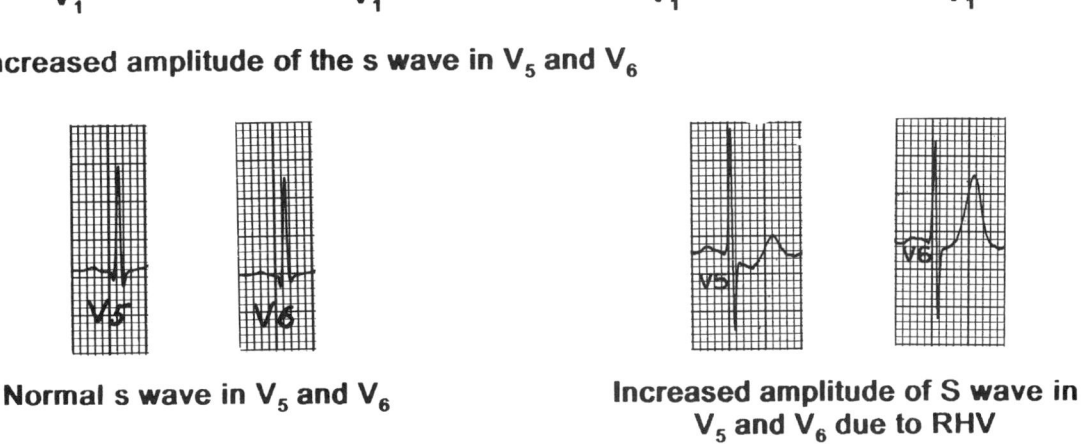

Normal s wave in V_5 and V_6   **Increased amplitude of S wave in V_5 and V_6 due to RHV**

The s waves in V_5 and V_6 normally result from right ventricular depolarization. The s waves in V_5 and V_6 normally are very small or non-existent because the right ventricle is overshadowed by the larger left ventricle. In right ventricular hypertrophy, that is no longer the case. As the large right ventricle depolarizes away from the positive electrodes of V_5 and V_6, large S waves are inscribed in these left lateral leads.

3. **Secondary ST-T wave changes**

Secondary ST-T changes occur in right ventricular hypertrophy due to abnormal repolarization of the right ventricle. These changes are seen in ST segment depression and/or T wave inversion.

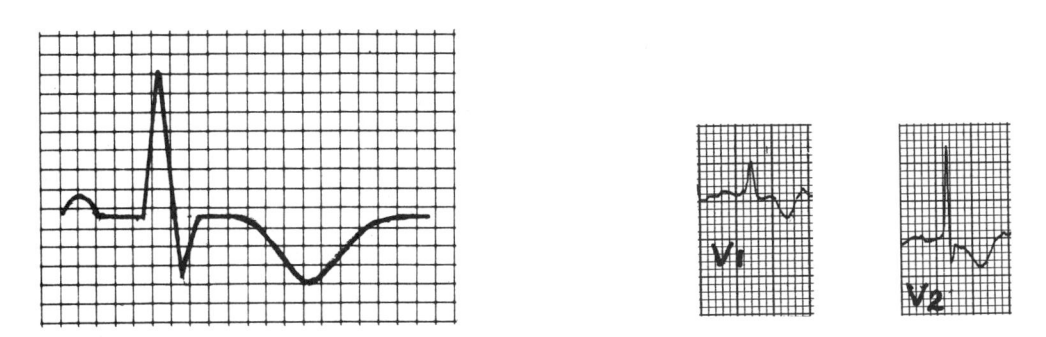

These ST-T wave changes are "secondary" because abnormal repolarization occurs secondarily to abnormal depolarization. Recall that these changes are also referred to as strain pattern.

Chapter 5 -- Chamber Enlargements

QUESTION: Where are the secondary ST-T changes seen in <u>left</u> ventricular hypertrophy?

ANSWER: The left lateral leads (I, aVL, V_5, V_6)

The secondary ST-T changes in <u>right</u> ventricular hypertrophy will be seen in the right ventricular leads, V_1 and V_2.

4. Right Axis Deviation

Axis deviation may or may not be present in right ventricular hypertrophy. If present it is usually around +100° or more rightward. Recall that +100° or more rightward is in the right axis deviation quadrant:

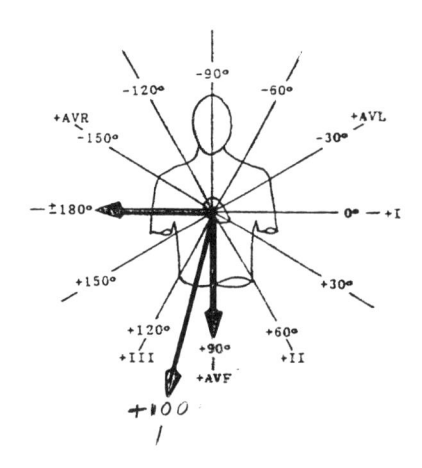

5. Increased ventricular activation time (VAT) in the right precordial leads

QUESTION: The right precordial leads are V_1 and V_2.

A. True
B. False

ANSWER: A. True. V_1 and V_2 are the right precordial leads. When there are abnormalities in the right ventricle, such as right ventricular hypertrophy, changes will be seen in these leads. One of the changes is an increase in the ventricular activation time (VAT).

Chapter 5 — Chamber Enlargements

Normally the VAT in the right ventricular leads is 0.02 seconds. It is measured from the beginning of the r wave to the crest of the r wave on the horizontal line. You can see that this is a very short period of time. VAT in V_1 or V_2 greater than 0.02 seconds is one ECG characteristic of right ventricular hypertrophy.

Normal V_1   **Increased VAT V_1**

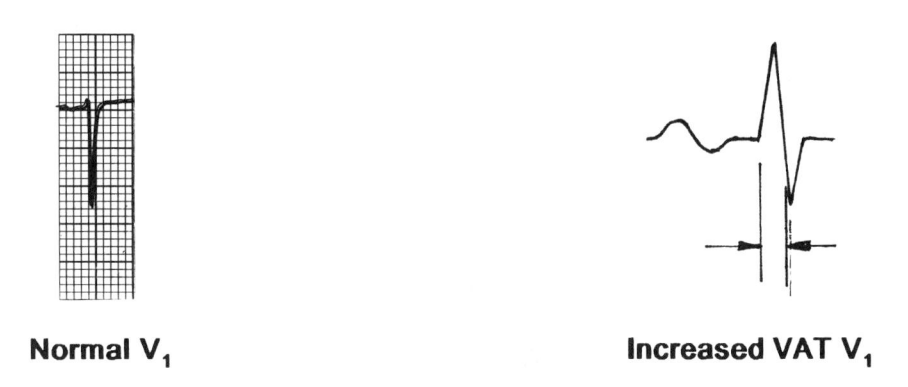

Figure 5 D on the following page is an example of right ventricular hypertrophy (RVH).

QUESTION: Which of the following five ECG characteristics for RVH can you identify in Figure 5 D?

1. Increased voltage of the r waves in the right precordial leads V_1 and/or V_2

2. Increased voltage of the s wave in V_5 and/or V_6

3. Secondary ST-T wave changes in the right precordial leads V_1 and/or V_2

4. Right axis deviation +100° or more rightward.

5. VAT greater than 0.02 seconds in V_1 and/or V_2

ANSWER: On page 91.

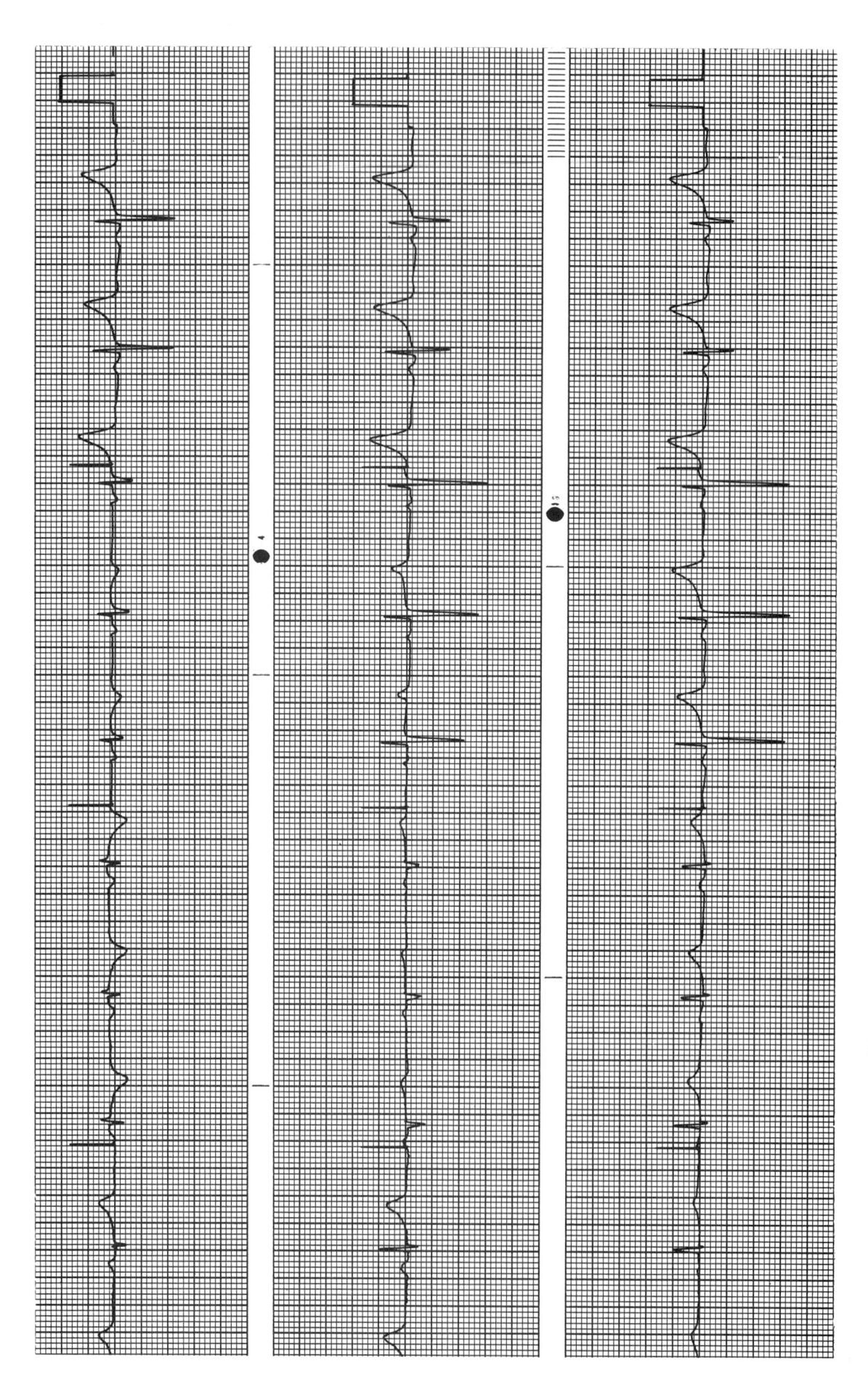

Figure 5 D. Right ventricular hypertrophy

Chapter 5 — Chamber Enlargements

Figure 5 D assessment:

Basic rhythm: Normal sinus rhythm
Frontal plane axis: RAD quadrant +120°
R wave progression: Abnormal: tall r in V_1 and loss of anterior forces. Recall that when the r wave in V_1 is greater than the s wave, it is a giant r.
Complex configuration: Abnormal as noted above and deep S/s waves in V_5, V_6, I, aVL
Complex duration: Normal
P wave: Normal
ST segment: Normal
T wave: Normal
Secondary ST-T changes: In V_1
12 Lead ECG Interpretation: Abnormal
 - Right ventricular hypertrophy

ANSWER:
1. Increased r wave voltage in V_1
2. Increased voltage of the S wave in V_5 and V_6
3. Secondary ST-T changes in V_1
4. Right axis deviation +120°

Please refer back to Figure 5 A on page 71. Previously, Figure 5 A was interpreted as biatrial enlargement plus right axis deviation and abnormal R wave progression with tall R waves in V_1 and V_2. Figure 5 A is also an example of right ventricular hypertrophy.

PRACTICE 12 LEAD ECGs #21-35

Assess the following practice 12 lead ECGs using these guidelines:

Basic rhythm:
Frontal plane axis:
R wave progression:
Complex configuration and duration:
P wave:
ST segment:
T wave:
Secondary ST changes:
Increased VAT:
12 lead ECG Interpretation:

Interpret the practice 12 lead ECGs as normal or abnormal and identify any chamber enlargements that are present. Answers begin on page 106.

Practice 12 Lead ECG #21

Practice 12 Lead ECG #22

Practice 12 Lead ECG #23

Practice 12 Lead ECG #24

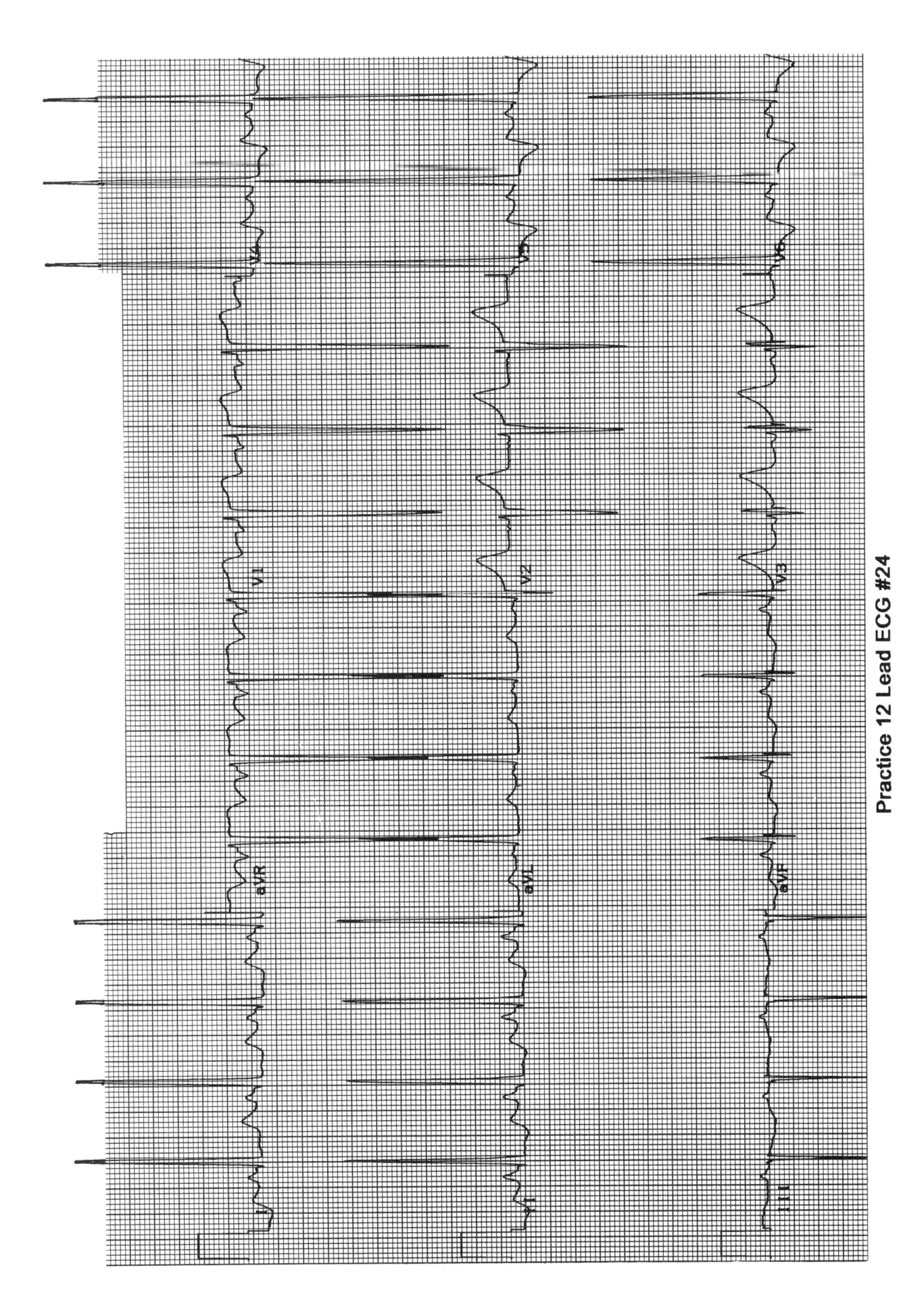

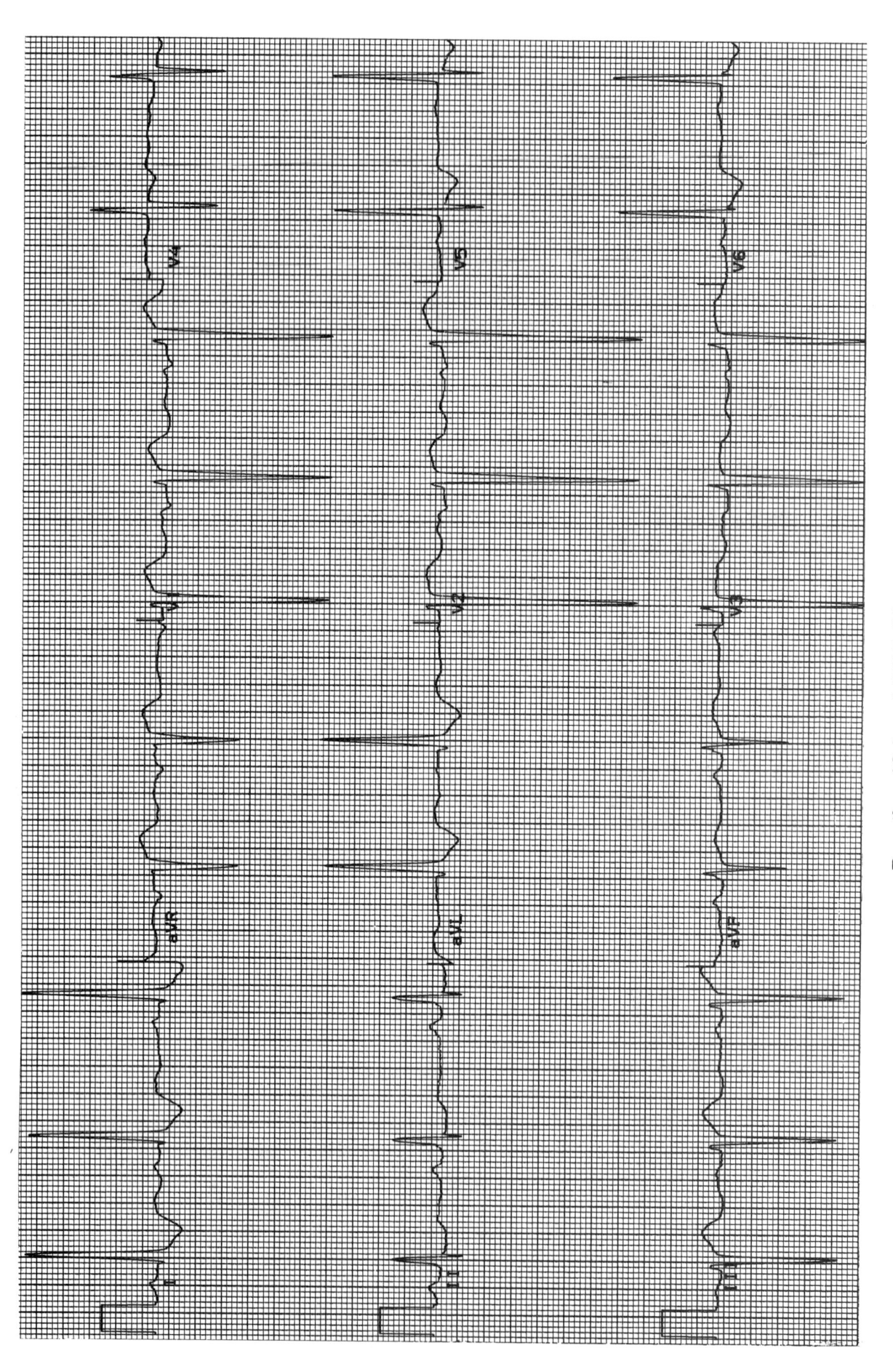

Practice 12 Lead ECG #25

Chapter 5 -- Chamber Enlargements

Practice 12 Lead ECG #26

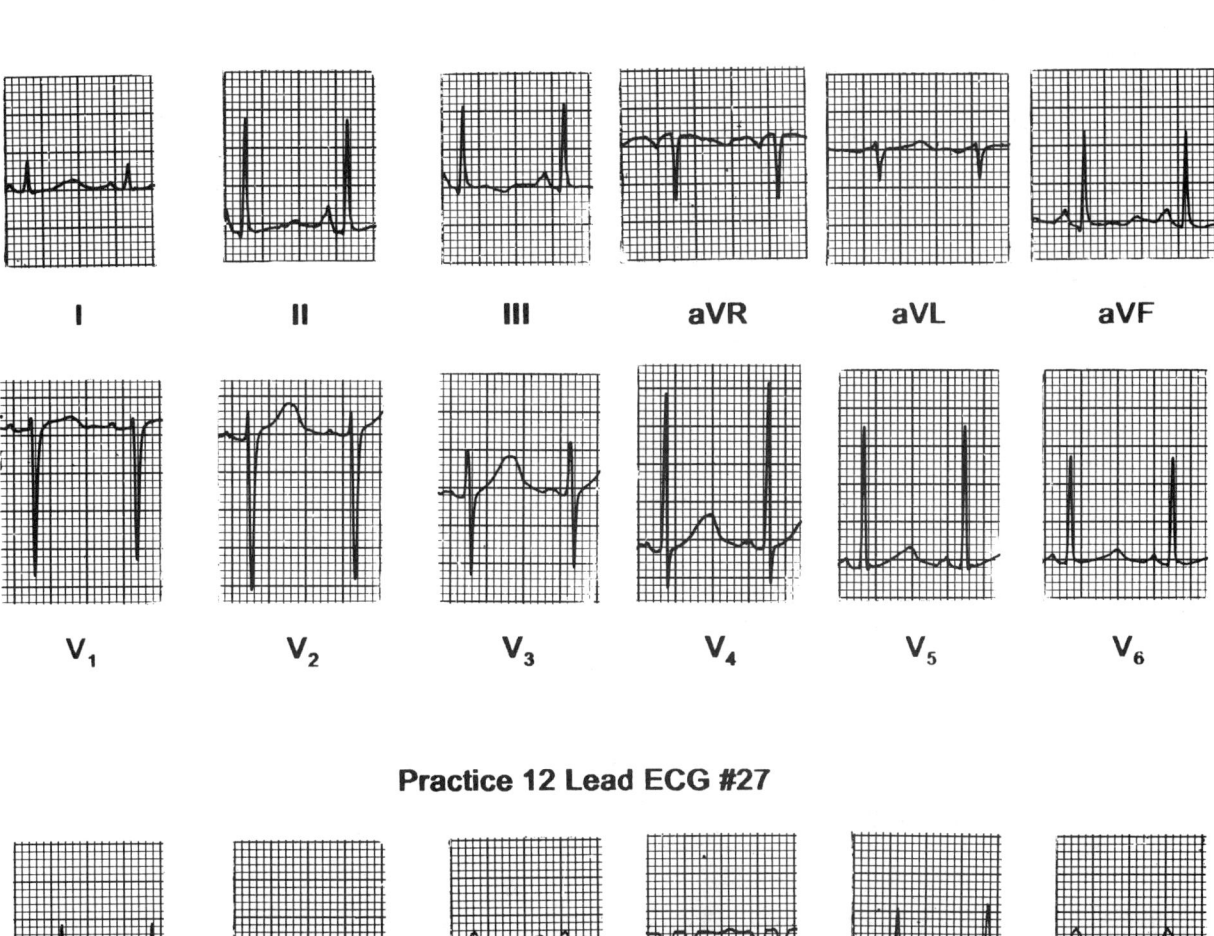

I II III aVR aVL aVF

V_1 V_2 V_3 V_4 V_5 V_6

Practice 12 Lead ECG #27

I II III aVR aVL aVF

V_1 V_2 V_3 V_4 V_5 V_6

Practice 12 Lead ECG #28

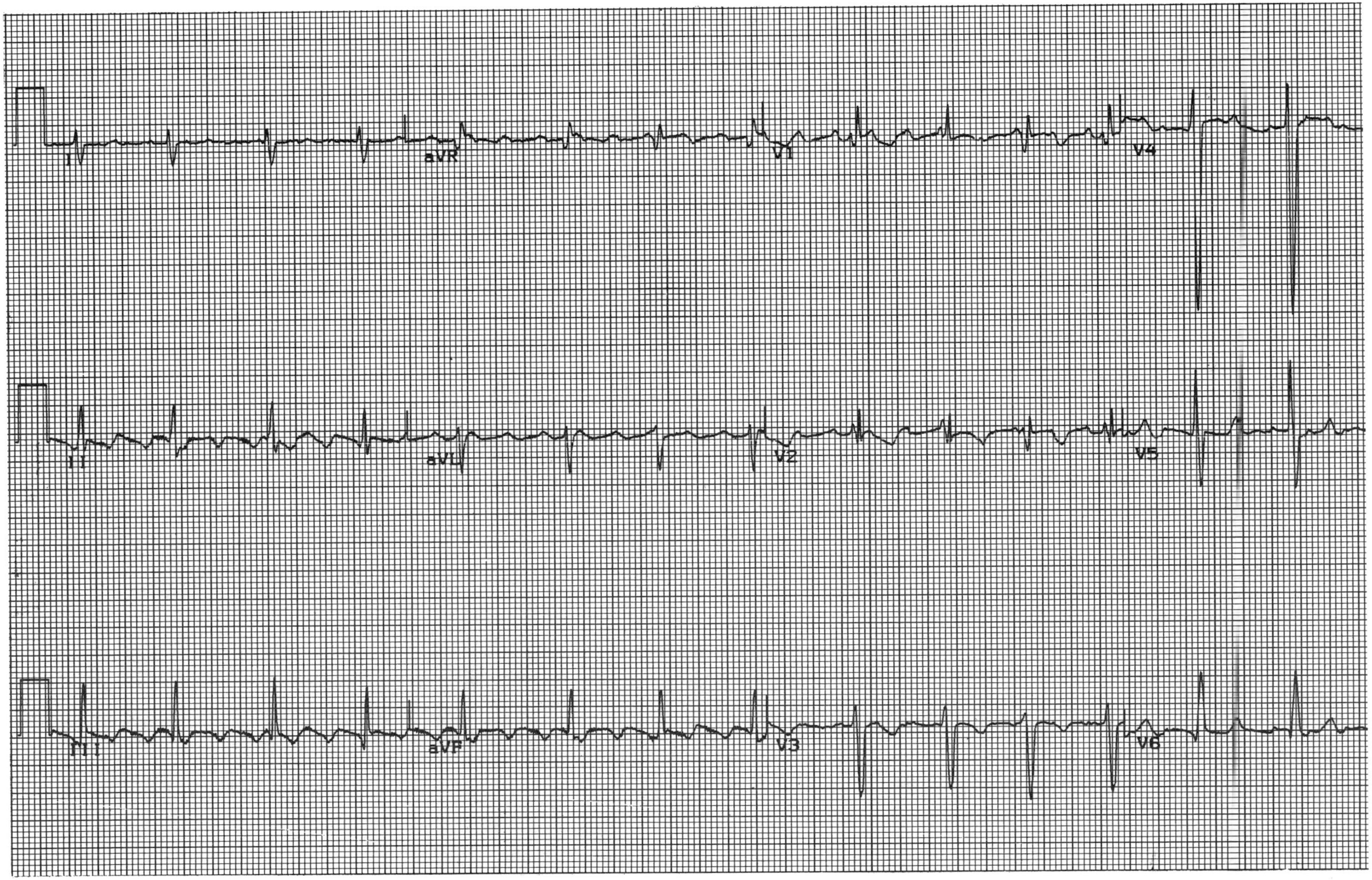

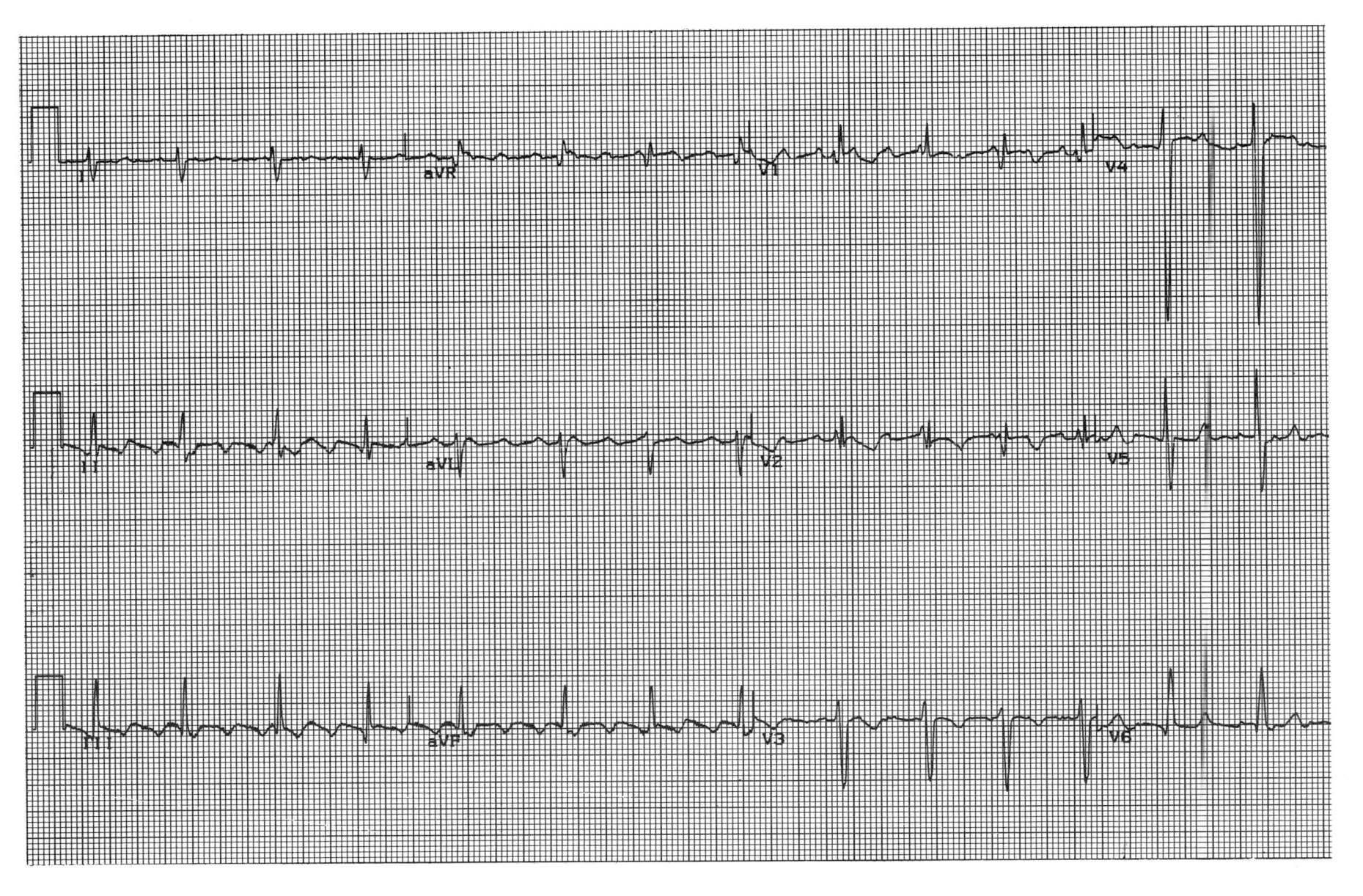

Practice 12 Lead ECG #29

Practice 12 Lead ECG #30: patient is on digitalis

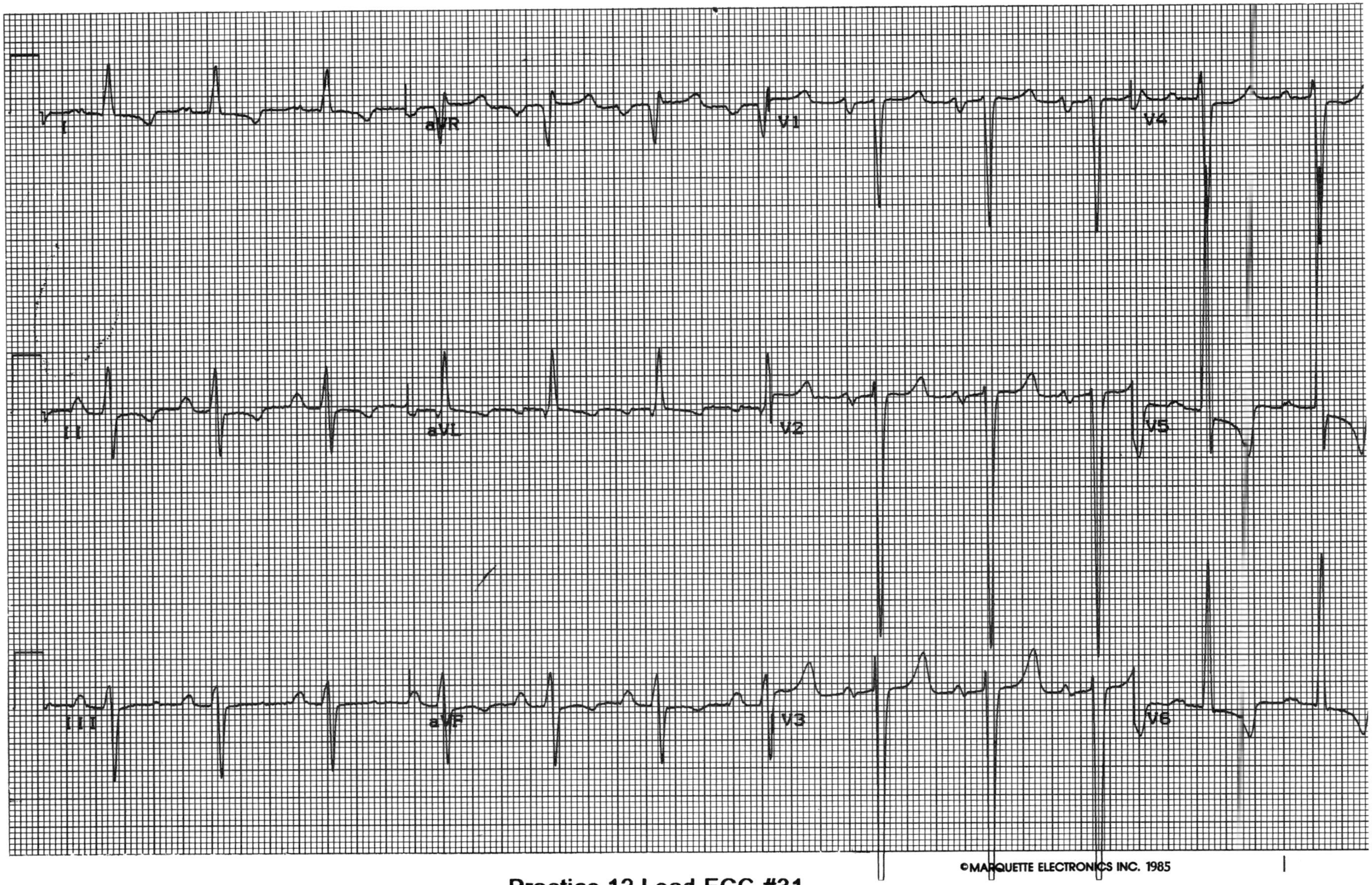

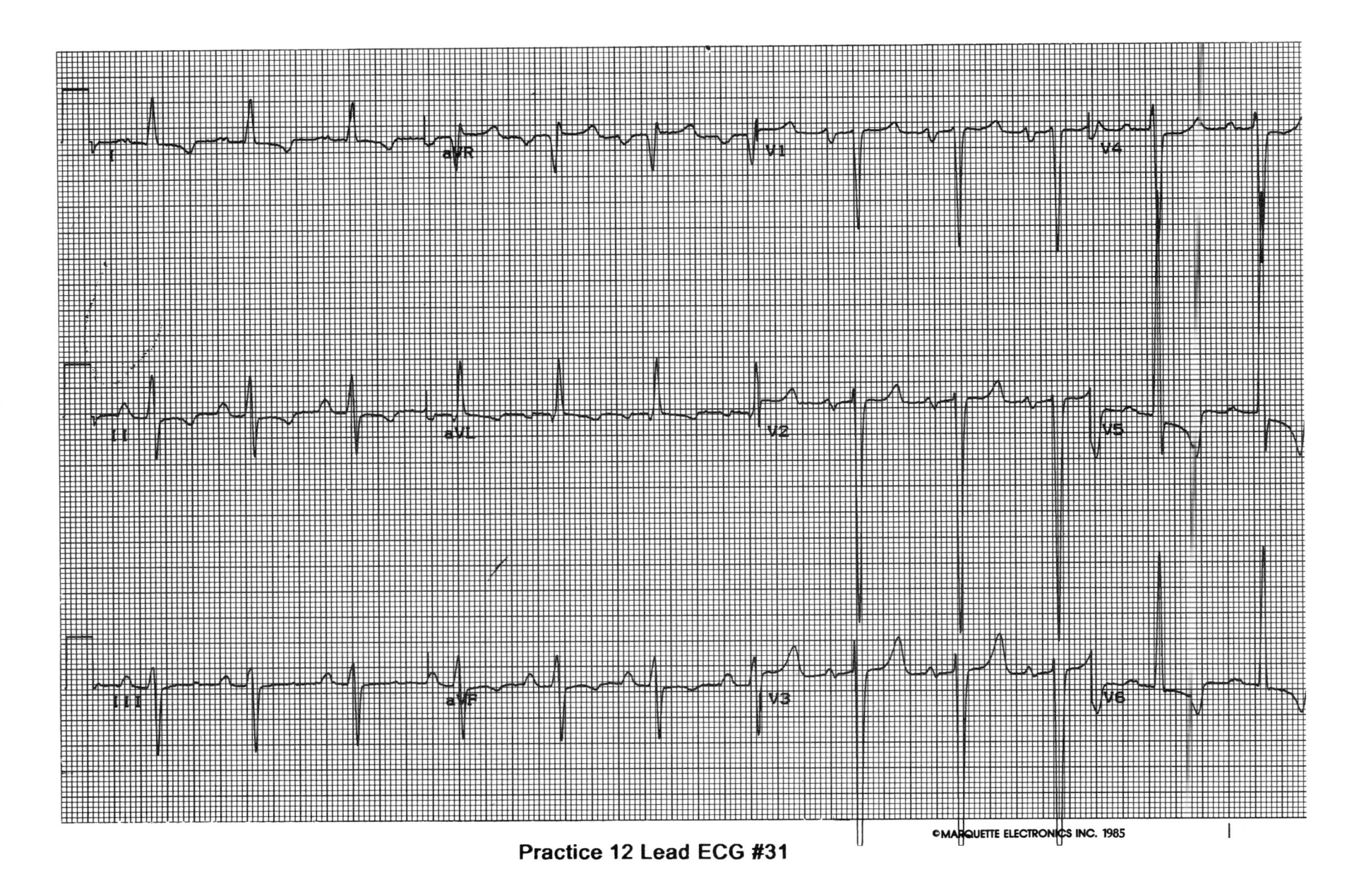

Practice 12 Lead ECG #31

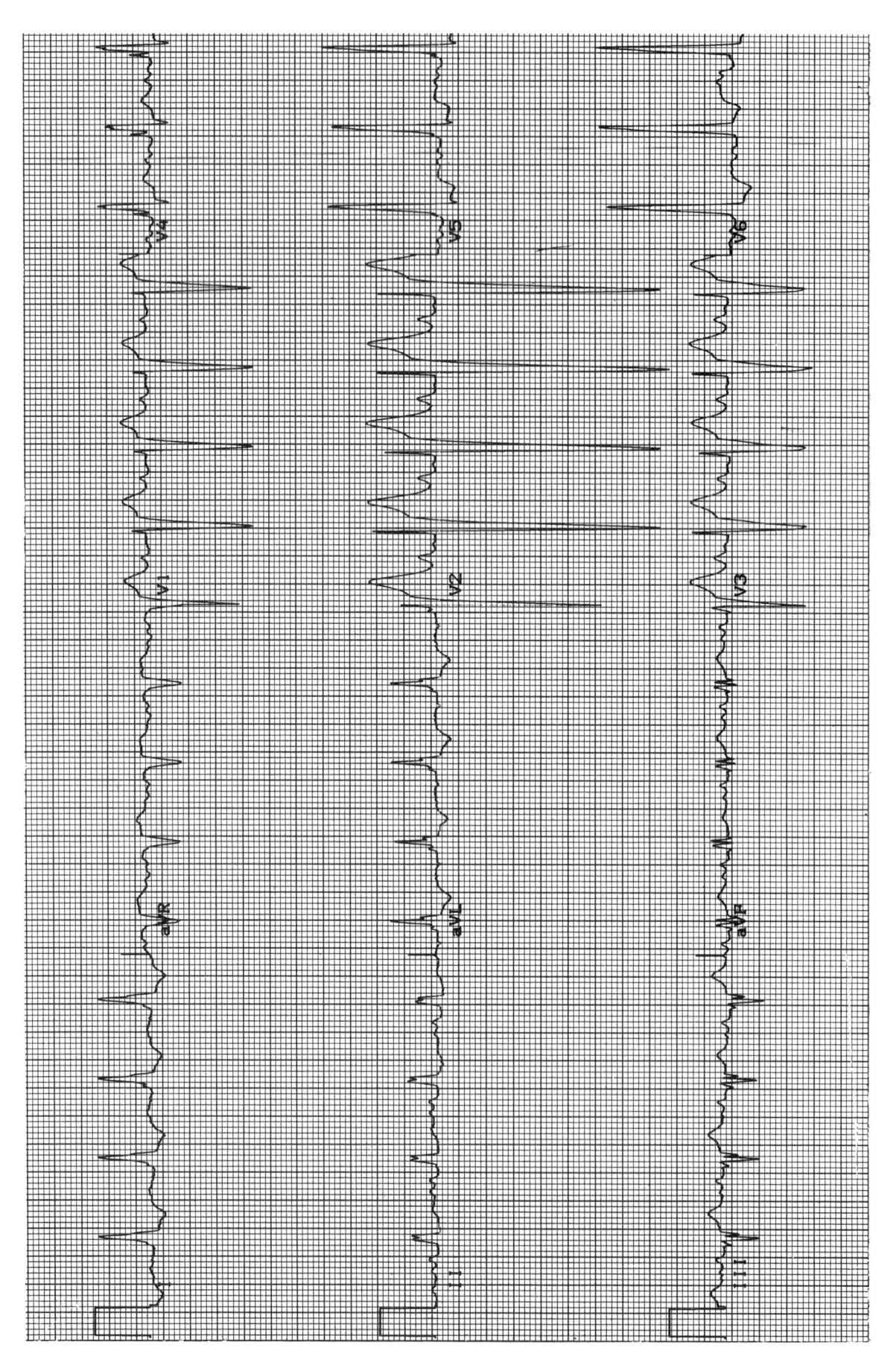

Practice 12 Lead ECG #32

Practice 12 Lead ECG #33

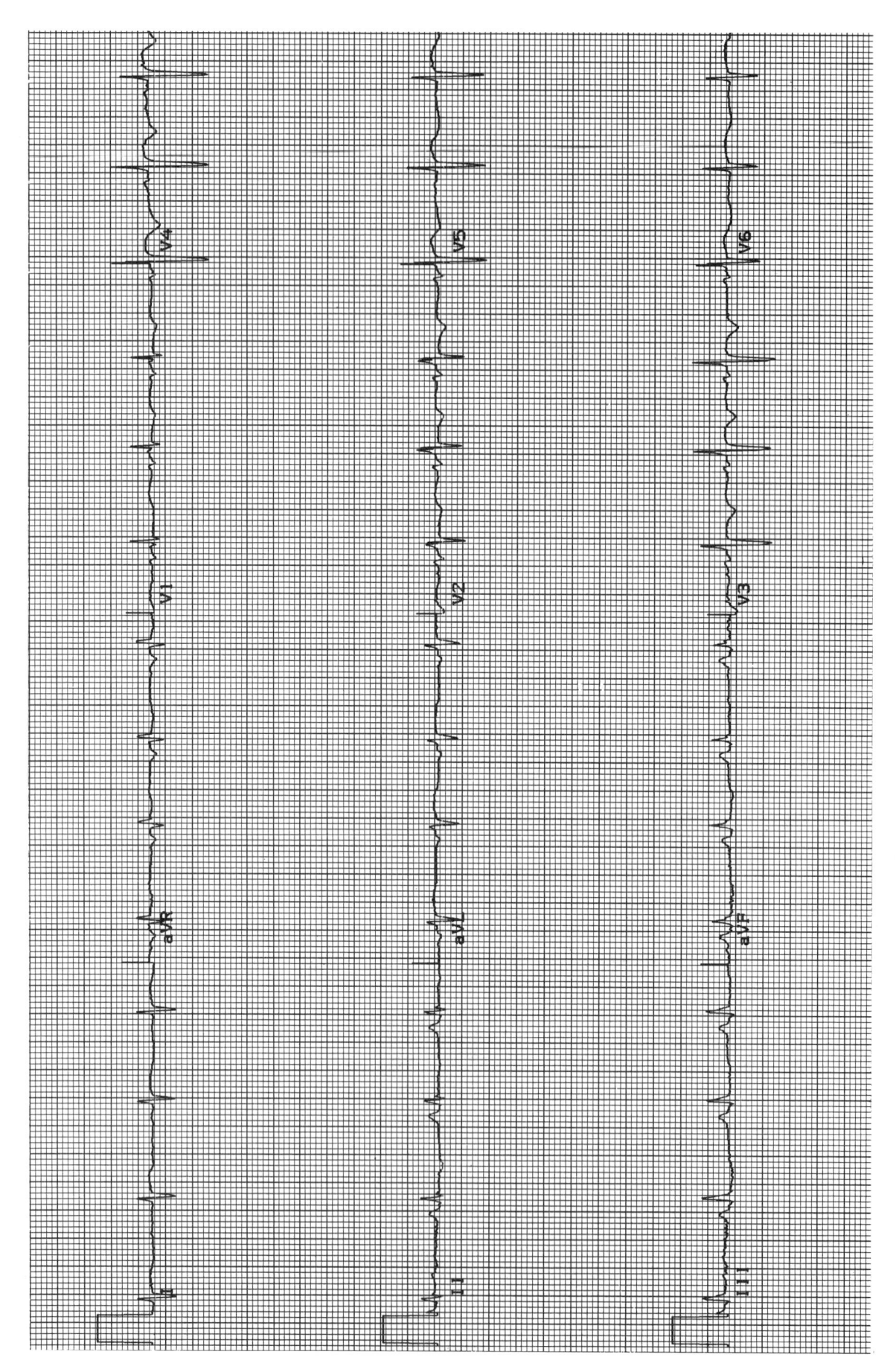

Practice 12 Lead ECG #34

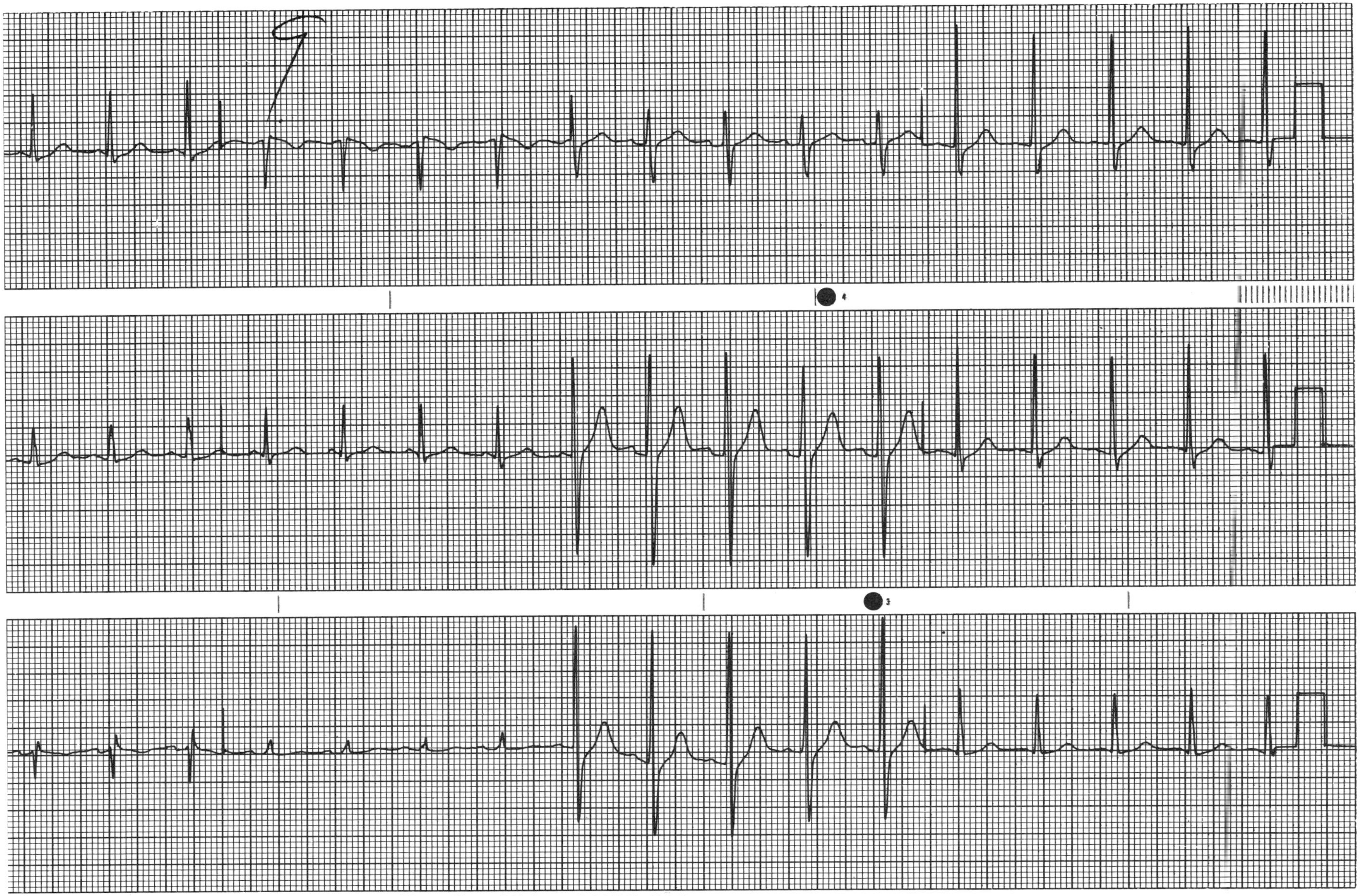

Practice 12 Lead ECG #35

Chapter 5 — Chamber Enlargements

ANSWERS TO PRACTICE 12 LEAD ECGs #21-35

21. **Basic rhythm:** Normal sinus rhythm
    Frontal plane axis: Normal 0°
    R wave progression: Normal
    Complex configuration and duration: Normal
    P wave: Normal
    ST segment: Normal
    T wave: Normal
    12 Lead ECG Interpretation: Normal

22. **Basic rhythm:** Sinus tachycardia
    Frontal plane axis: LAD quadrant -60°
    R wave progression: Normal except for loss of anterior forces in V_3 (possibly technician error)
    Complex configuration: Abnormal: $S \geq 25$ mm in V_1, V_2; $R \geq 25$ mm in V_5, V_6
    Complex duration: 0.11 seconds (normal, but greater than 0.09 seconds)
    P wave: Tall, wide, and notched in II, III, aVF; large P terminal in V_1
    Secondary ST-T changes: I, V_5, V_6
    Other: VAT greater than 0.04 seconds in V_5, V_6
    12 Lead ECG Interpretation: Abnormal
    - Sinus tachycardia
    - Biatrial enlargement
    - Left ventricular hypertrophy

    Estes score for LVH for this patient:
Voltage criteria	3
Secondary ST-T changes (patient on digitalis)	2
Left axis deviation -30° or more leftward	2
Complex interval 0.09 seconds or greater	1
Increased VAT V_5, V_6	1
Abnormal P terminal V_1	3
TOTAL	12

23. **Basic rhythm:** Sinus tachycardia (this is a normal rate for this patient: see interpretation)
    Frontal plane axis: RAD quadrant +150°
    R wave progression: Abnormal: large R in V_1, V_2; deep S in V_5, V_6
    Complex configuration: Abnormal as noted above
    Complex duration: Normal
    P wave: Normal
    ST segment: Depressed in V_1, V_2
    T wave: Normal
    Other: VAT greater than 0.02 seconds V_1, V_2
    12 Lead ECG Interpretation: This is the normal 12 lead ECG of a 7-day-old infant. The newborn has a pattern similar to right ventricular hypertrophy with tall R waves in the right precordial leads V_1 and V_2. Infants are born with right ventricular hypertrophy due to high pulmonary vascular resistance during fetal life. The left ventricle has not become dominant at this early age.

Chapter 5 — Chamber Enlargements

24. **Basic rhythm:** Normal sinus rhythm
    Frontal plane axis: Normal 0°
    R wave progression: Abnormal: loss of anterior forces. V_1 has an initial r wave which is smaller in V_2; V_3 shows an even smaller initial r followed by $SR'S'$, an abnormal finding for V_3.
    Complex configuration: As you look at the complex it is impossible not to notice the increased voltage in I, II, aVR, aVL, V_1, V_4, V_5, V_6. You should be thinking of left ventricular hypertrophy.
    Complex duration: Normal: 0.10 seconds.
    P wave: Peaked, tall, and notched in lead II; peaked in lead I, aVF; abnormal P terminal in V_1 — criteria for right and left atrial enlargement.
    Secondary ST-T changes: In the left precordial leads V_5 and V_6 due to LVH.
    ST-T changes: In II, III, aVF are probably due to digitalis effect (Chapter 9).
    U wave: There are biphasic T waves in V_4, V_5, V_6 that could be mistaken for U waves
    12 Lead ECG Interpretation: Abnormal
    - Biatrial enlargement
    - Left ventricular hypertrophy

    Estes score for LVH for this patient
Voltage criteria	3
Secondary ST-T changes (patient on digitalis)	2
Complex interval 0.10 seconds	1
Increased VAT V_5, V_6	1
Abnormal P terminal V_1	3
TOTAL	10

25. **Basic rhythm:** Normal sinus rhythm with first degree AV heart block (PRI is 0.22 seconds)
    Frontal plane axis: Normal 0°
    R wave progression: Abnormal: loss of anterior forces in V_2, V_3; transition in V_5 - too late!
    Complex configuration: Abnormal as noted above and $S \geq 25$ mm in V_1, V_2; R = 24 mm in lead I
    Complex duration: Normal: 0.11 seconds
    P wave: Wide and notched in II, III, aVF
    Secondary ST-T changes: I, aVL, V_5, V_6
    12 Lead ECG Interpretation: Abnormal
    - P mitrale
    - Left ventricular hypertrophy

    Estes score for LVH for this patient:
Voltage criteria	3
Secondary ST-T (not on digitalis)	3
Complex interval greater than 0.09 seconds	1
TOTAL	7

Chapter 5 — Chamber Enlargements

26. **Basic rhythm:** Sinus tachycardia (106 BPM)
    Frontal plane axis: Normal +60°
    R wave progression: Normal: transition in V_4 is a normal variant
    Complex configuration and duration: Normal
    P wave: Peaked in II, III, V_1
    ST segment: Normal
    T wave: Abnormal: Biphasic in II, III, aVF
    12 Lead ECG Interpretation: Abnormal
    - Sinus tachycardia
    - P pulmonale

27. **Basic rhythm:** Sinus tachycardia (120 BPM)
    Frontal plane axis: Normal 0°
    R wave progression: Normal with transition in V_4
    Complex configuration and duration: Normal except for r r^I in II
    P wave: Abnormal: wide and notched in II, aVF; abnormal P terminal in V_1
    ST segment: Normal
    T wave: Inverted in I, aVL, V_5, V_6
    12 Lead ECG Interpretation: Abnormal
    - Sinus tachycardia
    - P mitrale
    - Possible lateral ischemia (Chapter 7)

28. **Basic rhythm:** Sinus tachycardia
    Frontal plane axis: Normal 0°
    R wave progression: Normal
    Complex configuration and duration: Normal
    P wave: Normal
    ST segment: Normal
    T wave: Normal
    U wave: θ
    12 Lead ECG Interpretation: Normal except for sinus tachycardia

29. **Basic rhythm:** Atrial flutter 3:1
    Frontal plane axis: RAD quadrant +120°
    R wave progression: Abnormal with rsR^I in V_1, V_2; transition in V_5
    Complex configuration: Abnormal: As noted above and increased amplitude of S in V_5
    Complex duration: Normal
    P wave: Flutter waves
    Secondary ST-T changes: V_1, V_2, V_3
    T wave: Often obscured by the flutter waves
    12 Lead ECG Interpretation: Abnormal
    - Atrial flutter 3:1
    - Right ventricular hypertrophy

Chapter 5 — Chamber Enlargements

30. **Basic rhythm:** Normal sinus rhythm
    Frontal plane axis: Normal +30°
    R wave progression: Normal
    Complex configuration: S wave 25 mm+ in V_2
    P wave: Normal
    Secondary ST-T changes: I, aVL
    12 Lead ECG Interpretation: Abnormal
      - Left ventricular hypertrophy

    Estes score for LVH for this patient:
Voltage criteria	3
Secondary ST-T (not on digitalis)	3
TOTAL	6

    Recall that 5 or more points strongly indicates LVH according to the Estes scoring system.

31. **Basic rhythm:** Normal sinus rhythm
    Frontal plane axis: LAD quadrant -30°
    R wave progression: Abnormal: Loss of anterior forces and transition in V_5
    P wave: Wide and notched in II, III, aVF; abnormal P terminal in V_1
    Complex configuration: Abnormal: S waves greater than 25 mm in V_2; R ≥ 25 mm in V_5, V_6
    Complex duration: Normal: 0.10 seconds
    Secondary ST-T changes: I, aVL, V_5, V_6
    T wave: Inverted in II, aVF
    12 Lead ECG Interpretation: Abnormal
      - P mitrale
      - Left ventricular hypertrophy

    Estes score for LVH for this patient:
Voltage criteria	3
Secondary ST-T (patient on digitalis)	2
Left axis deviation -30°	2
Abnormal P terminal in V_1	3
TOTAL	10

Chapter 5 — Chamber Enlargements

32. **Basic rhythm:** Sinus tachycardia (106 BPM)
    Frontal plane axis: Normal: 0°
    R wave progression: Normal except for V_3 where R voltage decreases — this could be due to technician error.
    Complex configuration: S voltage greater than 25 mm in V_2; R voltage = 25 mm in V_6
    Complex duration: Normal: 0.11 seconds
    P wave: Wide and notched in II, III, aVF
    Secondary ST-T changes: I, aVL, V_5, V_6
    VAT: greater than 0.04 seconds in V_5, V_6
    12 Lead ECG Interpretation: Abnormal
    - Sinus tachycardia
    - P mitrale
    - Left ventricular hypertrophy

    Estes score for LVH for this patient:

Voltage criteria	3
Secondary ST-T (digitalized)	2
Complex duration $\geq$ 0.09	1
Increased VAT V_5, V_6	1
TOTAL	7

33. **Basic rhythm:** Sinus tachycardia
    Frontal plane axis: RAD quadrant +120°
    R wave progression: Abnormal: Large R wave in V_1
    Complex configuration: Abnormal as stated above and deep S wave in V_5, V_6
    Complex duration: Normal: 0.08 seconds
    P wave: Wide and notched in II, III, aVF
    Secondary ST-T changes: V_1, V_2
    T wave: Inverted in V_3, V_4; flat in II, III, aVF
    12 Lead ECG Interpretation: Abnormal
    - Sinus tachycardia
    - Right ventricular hypertrophy
    - Non-specific T wave abnormality (Chapter 9)

34. **Basic rhythm:** Normal sinus rhythm
    Frontal plane axis: RAD quadrant +120°
    R wave progression: Abnormal: Tall R in V_1; loss of anterior forces with transition in V_6
    Complex configuration: Abnormal as noted above and deep S waves in V_5 and V_6
    Complex duration: Normal
    P wave: Normal
    Secondary ST-T changes: V_1 and V_2
    ST segment: Normal
    T wave: Abnormal: Inverted in V_3, V_4
    12 Lead ECG Interpretation: Abnormal
    - Right ventricular hypertrophy
    - Consider anterior ischemia (Chapter 7)

Chapter 5 — Chamber Enlargements

35. **Basic rhythm:** Sinus tachycardia
    Frontal plane axis: Normal 0°
    R wave progression: Normal
    Complex configuration and duration: Normal
    P wave: Normal
    ST segment: Normal
    T wave: Normal
    U wave: θ
    12 Lead ECG Interpretation: Normal except for sinus tachycardia

CHAPTER 6
INTRAVENTRICULAR CONDUCTION DEFECTS (IVCD)

Recall the intraventricular conduction system of the heart.

    Bundle of His
    Right bundle branch (RBB)
    Left bundle branch (LBB)
        - Left anterior descending fascicle (LADF)
        - Left posterior fascicle (LPF)

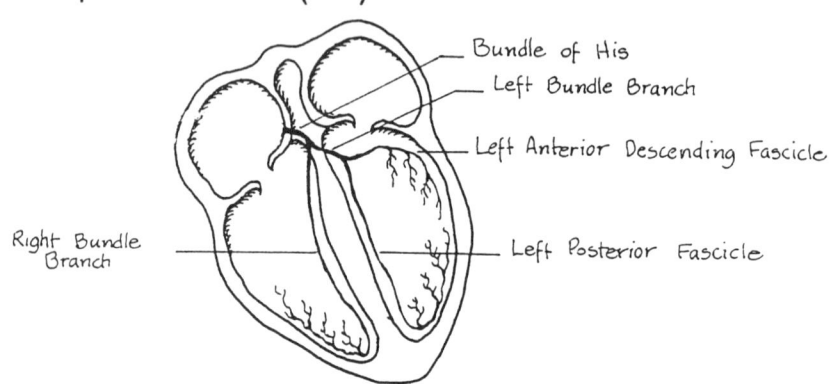

QUESTION: The left anterior descending fascicle is also called the left anterior superior fascicle.

A. True
B. False

ANSWER: A. True, and the posterior fascicle is also called the inferior fascicle.

An IVCD (**i**ntra**v**entricular **c**onduction **d**efect) occurs when part of the intraventricular conduction system is blocked.

Example:

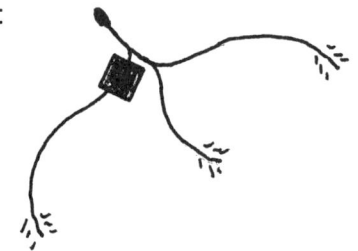

This is right bundle branch block.

Example:

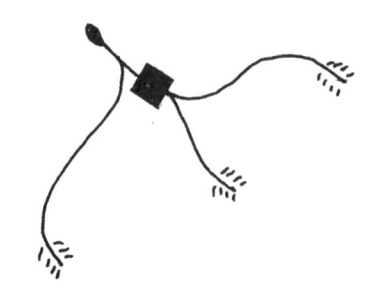

This is left bundle branch block.

Chapter 6 -- Intraventricular Conduction Defects (IVCD)

QUESTION: What is the term when both the right and left bundle branches are blocked?

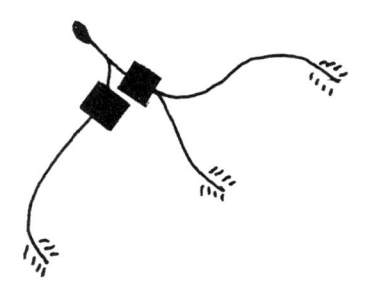

ANSWER: **Third degree (complete) AV heart block.**

In review, right bundle branch block (RBBB) means the right bundle is unable to conduct; left bundle branch block (LBBB) means the left bundle is unable to conduct. When neither the right nor the left bundle branch can conduct, third degree heart block exists.

QUESTION: What is the definitive treatment for third degree AV heart block?

ANSWER: Insertion of a pacemaker.

HEMIBLOCKS

Example:

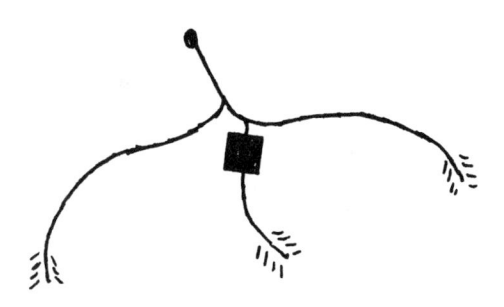

In the above example only the posterior (inferior) facile is blocked. This is a hemiblock (half-block). When only one of the fascicles of the left bundle branch is blocked it is a **hemiblock**. The above hemiblock is **left posterior hemiblock (LPH).**

QUESTION: Hemiblocks only occur in the left bundle.

A. True
B. False

ANSWER: A. True. Only the left bundle has two fascicles and blockage of one of these fascicles is a hemiblock. The right bundle branch does not have any fascicles and therefore cannot produce a hemiblock.

Chapter 6 -- Intraventricular Conduction Defects (IVCD)

Example:

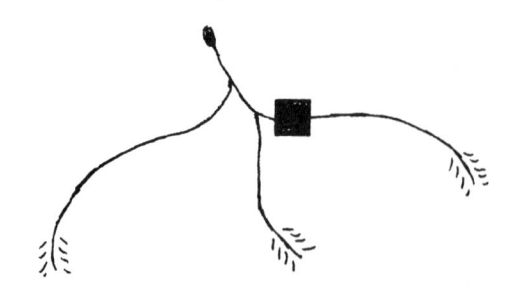

QUESTION: Which IVCD is depicted in the above example?

ANSWER: Left anterior descending hemiblock (LADH).

Recall the left anterior fascicle is also called the superior fascicle. Blockage of this fascicle is also referred to as LASH (Left Anterior Superior Hemiblock).

Chapter 6 -- Intraventricular Conduction Defects (IVCD)

In review, IVCDs include:

Right bundle branch block

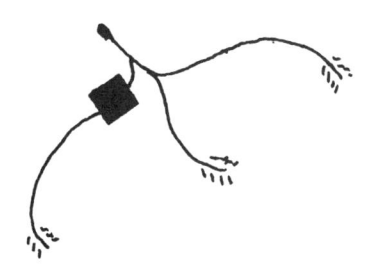

Left bundle branch block

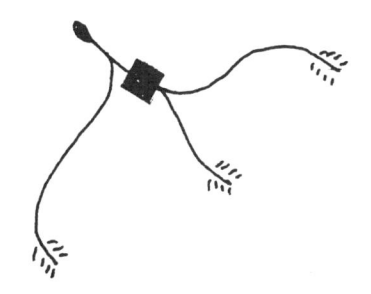

Left anterior descending hemiblock (LADH)

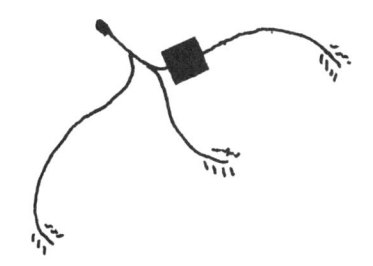

Left posterior hemiblock (LPH)

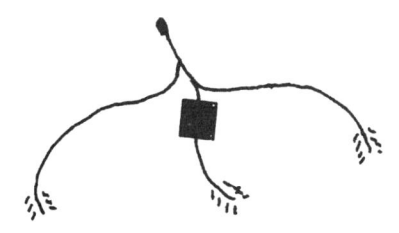

QUESTION: Are there other combinations of intraventricular conduction blocks?

ANSWER: Yes.

115

Chapter 6 — Intraventricular Conduction Defects (IVCD)

BIFASCICULAR BLOCKS

Example:

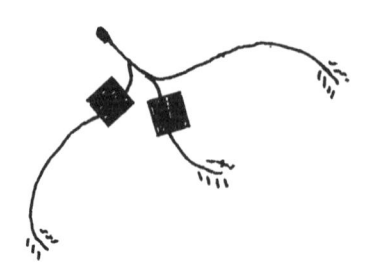

The above example depicts **RBBB with LPH**. The right bundle is blocked and one of the fascicles (left posterior) is also blocked. This is an example of a **bifascicular block**: two fascicles are blocked.

Example:

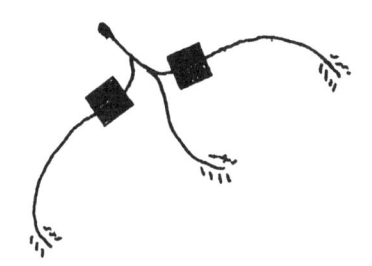

The above example depicts **RBBB with LADH** (left anterior descending hemiblock). This is another example of a **bifascicular block**.

In review, IVCDs include:

1. RBBB (right bundle branch block)
2. LBBB (left bundle branch block)
3. LADH (left anterior descending hemiblock)
4. LPH (left posterior hemiblock)
5. RBBB with LADH (a bifascicular block)
6. RBBB with LPH (a bifascicular block)

Chapter 6 — Intraventricular Conduction Defects (IVCD)

TYPES AND CAUSES OF IVCD

Clinically, the most common cause of

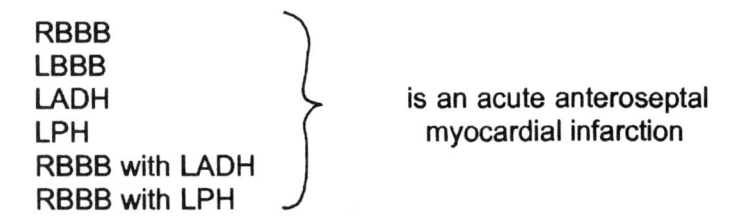

> RBBB
> LBBB
> LADH
> LPH
> RBBB with LADH
> RBBB with LPH

is an acute anteroseptal myocardial infarction

QUESTION: Why does acute anteroseptal myocardial infarction cause intraventricular conduction defects?

ANSWER: The coronary artery that supplies the anterior and septal wall is the same coronary artery that supplies the intraventricular conduction system (bundle of His, right bundle branch, and the left bundle branch including the two fascicles).

Right bundle branch block is also caused by myocarditis, valvular heart disease, and acute pulmonary embolus. Right bundle branch block may occur as a congenital condition with no underlying heart disease.

Left bundle branch block is most often associated with coronary artery disease. Left bundle branch block is seldom congenital.

Other causes of hemiblocks and bifascicular blocks will be discussed on page 140.

Chapter 6 -- Intraventricular Conduction Defects (IVCD)

NORMAL VENTRICULAR DEPOLARIZATION

In review:

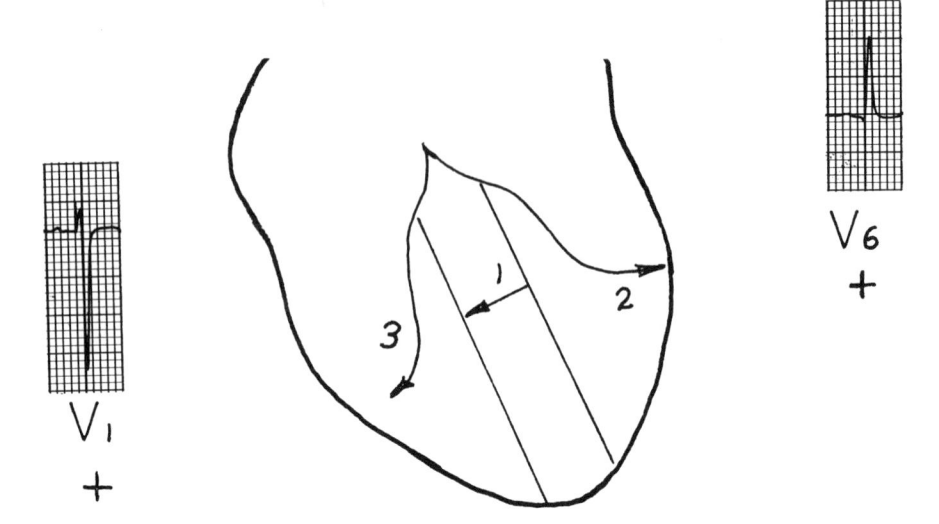

The picture above depicts normal ventricular depolarization, the position of the positive electrodes of V_1 and V_6, and the configuration of the complexes that result from normal ventricular depolarization in V_1 and V_6 (numbered 1, 2, 3).

1. **Septal depolarization** normally occurs via the left bundle branch and the wave of depolarization moves from left to right:

    V_1: An r is inscribed as ventricular septum depolarization moves towards the positive electrode.
    V_6: The physiological q wave is inscribed as ventricular septum depolarization moves away from the positive electrode.

2. **Left ventricular depolarization** occurs. The wave of depolarization moves from right to left on the frontal place and anterior to posterior on the precordial plane.

    V_1: An S is inscribed as left ventricular depolarization moves away from the positive electrode.
    V_6: An R is inscribed as the left ventricle depolarizes towards the positive electrode.

3. **Right ventricular depolarization** is usually overshadowed by the larger left ventricle.

    V_1: Right ventricular depolarization is not usually seen. Occasionally an rSr^1 will be seen in V_1 as a normal variant—when this occurs the r^1 is due to right ventricular depolarization. Remember when there is trouble in the right ventricle, changes will be seen in V_1 and V_2 due to their placement over the right ventricle.
    V_6: s waves are the result of right ventricular depolarization moving away from the positive electrode. If present, s waves normally are small in V_5 and V_6.

Chapter 6 — Intraventricular Conduction Defects (IVCD)

RIGHT BUNDLE BRANCH BLOCK

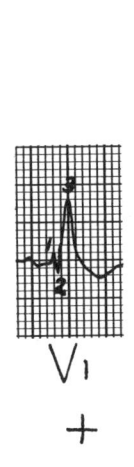

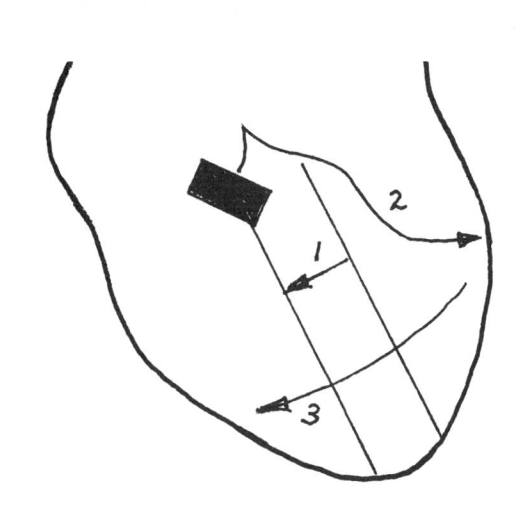

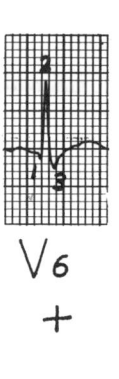

The picture above depicts ventricular depolarization when the right bundle branch is blocked. Note the positive electrodes of V_1 and V_6 and the waves of the complex that result (numbered 1, 2, 3).

1. **Septal depolarization** occurs via the intact left bundle branch and the wave of depolarization moves from left to right as it normally does.

    V_1: r wave
    V_6: q wave (the normal physiological q wave)

2. **Left ventricular depolarization** occurs normally via the intact left bundle branch.

    V_1: A downward deflection results from left (posterior) ventricular depolarization.
    V_6: R wave due to depolarization moving towards the positive electrode of V_6 as it normally does.

3. V_1: R' - an abnormal finding. The R' is inscribed as **delayed right ventricular depolarization** moves towards the positive electrode of V_1. Recall the right ventricle normally is silent on the ECG. Trouble in the right ventricle is inscribed in V_1 and V_2.
    V_6: Slurred s/S wave as the result of **delayed right ventricular depolarization** moving away from the positive electrode of V_6.

QUESTION: The rSR' pattern in V_1 and V_2 seen in right bundle branch block is frequently referred to as *rabbit ears*.

A. True
B. False

ANSWER: A. True.

Chapter 6 — Intraventricular Conduction Defects (IVCD)

Due to the delayed right ventricular depolarization, the duration of the complex will increase. **With complete right bundle branch block, the duration of the complex will be 0.12 seconds or greater.**

Secondary ST-T changes will be seen in V_1 and V_2 due to the abnormal repolarization, caused by the abnormal depolarization.

QUESTION: Abnormal depolarization causes abnormal repolarization.

A. True
B. False

ANSWER: A. True. Since depolarization is prolonged with bundle branch block, repolarization is abnormal.

The secondary ST-T changes in right bundle branch block will be seen in the right ventricular leads V_1 and V_2.

In summary, **RIGHT BUNDLE BRANCH BLOCK ECG CHARACTERISTICS:**

rSR' (rabbit ears) in V_1, V_2
Slurred s or S in V_5, V_6 (I, aVL)
Complex duration 0.12 seconds or greater
Secondary ST-T changes in the right precordial leads V_1 and V_2

NOTE: Practice 12 lead ECGs #8 and #9 on page 55 are examples of right bundle branch block.

Many people with RBBB have no evidence of underlying heart disease.

Figures 6 A and 6 B on the following pages are examples of right bundle branch block.

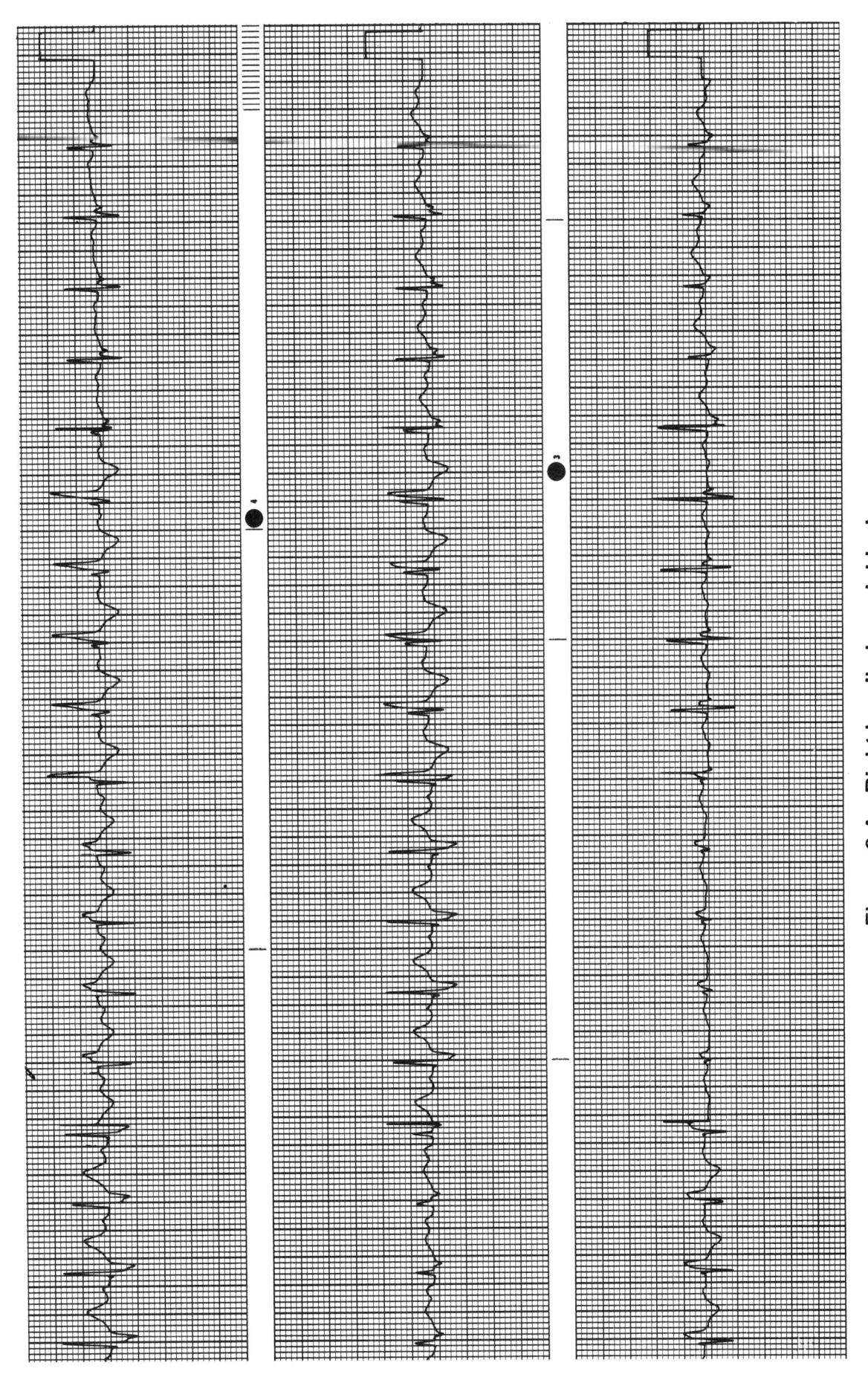

Figure 6 A. Right bundle branch block

Note that the rsR¹ in V_1, V_2; the secondary ST-T changes in V_1, V_2; the slurred s wave in V_5, V_6 (also in I and aVL); and the duration of the complex is 0.12 seconds.

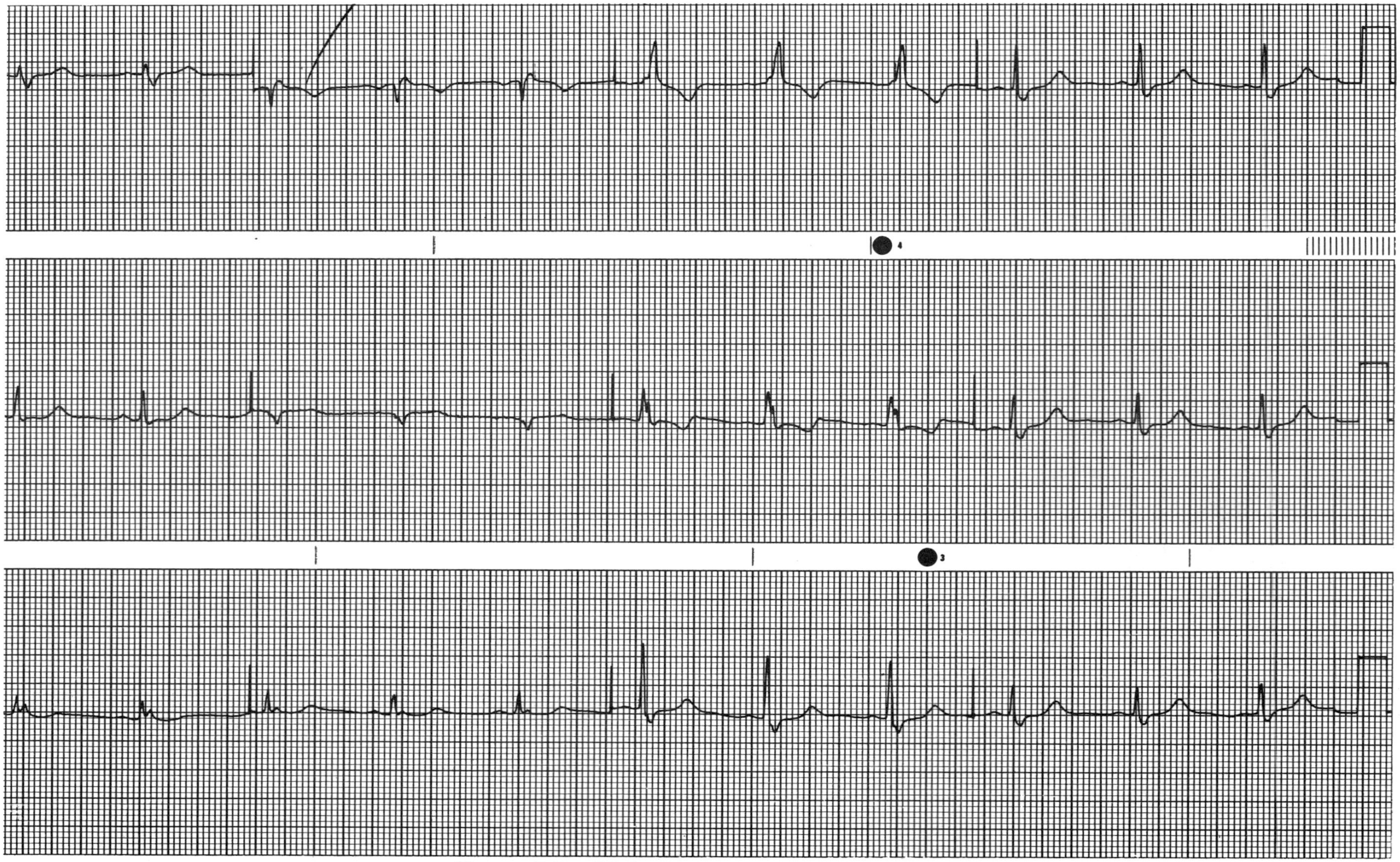

Figure 6 B. Right bundle branch block

Note that the rR¹ is more pronounced in V_2 than in V_1 in this example; secondary ST-T changes in V_1, V_2; the slurred s wave in V_5, V_6 (I, aVL); duration of the complex is 0.12 seconds.

Chapter 6 — Intraventricular Conduction Defects (IVCD)

LEFT BUNDLE BRANCH BLOCK

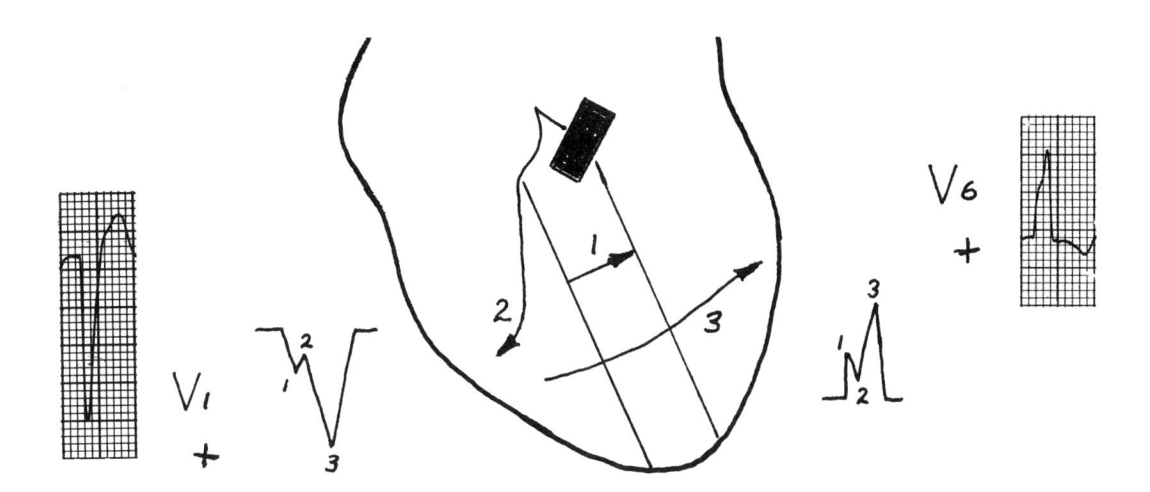

The picture above depicts ventricular depolarization when the left bundle branch is blocked. Note the positive electrodes of V_1 and V_6 and the waves of the complex that result (numbered 1, 2, 3).

1. **Ventricular septum depolarization** cannot occur via the left bundle because it is blocked. Ventricular septum depolarization occurs via the intact right bundle and moves abnormally from right to left.

    V_1: q or Q is inscribed as ventricular septum depolarization moves away from the positive electrode of V_1.

    V_6: r or R is inscribed as ventricular septum depolarization moves towards the positive electrode of V_6. The normal physiological q wave is absent.

2. **Right ventricular depolarization** occurs via the intact right bundle branch.

    V_1: An upward deflection which does not go above the isoelectric line may be inscribed. Usually this upward deflection is so small it is not seen. Recall that right ventricular depolarization is usually obscured on the ECG by the larger left ventricle. The left ventricle is now not only larger—it also has delayed depolarization which will further obscure right ventricular activity.

    V_6: A negative deflection which usually does not go below the isoelectric line.

3. **Delayed depolarization of the left ventricle** via the Purkinje network.

    V_1: Negative deflection resulting in a QS pattern.
    V_6: Positive deflection resulting in a monophasic pattern.

Chapter 6 — Intraventricular Conduction Defects (IVCD)

Sometimes an rS will be inscribed in V_1 and/or V_2 instead of the QS:

The waves inscribed as the result of right ventricular depolarization (2) usually do not reach the isoelectric line. So the LBBB complex in V_6 is usually monophasic, above the isoelectric line.

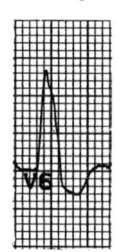

Due to the delayed left ventricular depolarization, the duration of the complex will increase. **In complete left bundle branch block the duration of the complex will be 0.12 seconds or greater.**

Secondary ST-T changes will also be seen due to the abnormal repolarization. **The secondary ST-T changes will be seen in the left lateral ventricular leads V_5 and V_6 (also I and aVL).**

In summary, **LEFT BUNDLE BRANCH BLOCK ECG CHARACTERISTICS:**

   QS or rS in V_1, V_2
   Loss of physiological q waves in V_5, V_6
   Monophasic R wave in V_5, V_6
   Complex duration 0.12 seconds or greater
   Secondary ST-T changes in the left precordial leads V_5 and V_6

| **Caution in interpretation:** | QS pattern in V_1 and V_2 mimics the QS pattern seen in these leads in the presence of anteroseptal myocardial infarction (Chapter 7). |

NOTE: Practice 12 leads #7, 10, and 11 on pages 54, 56, and 57 respectively, are examples of left bundle branch block.

Left bundle branch block without underlying heart disease is rare.

Figures 6 C and 6 D on the following pages are examples of left bundle branch block.

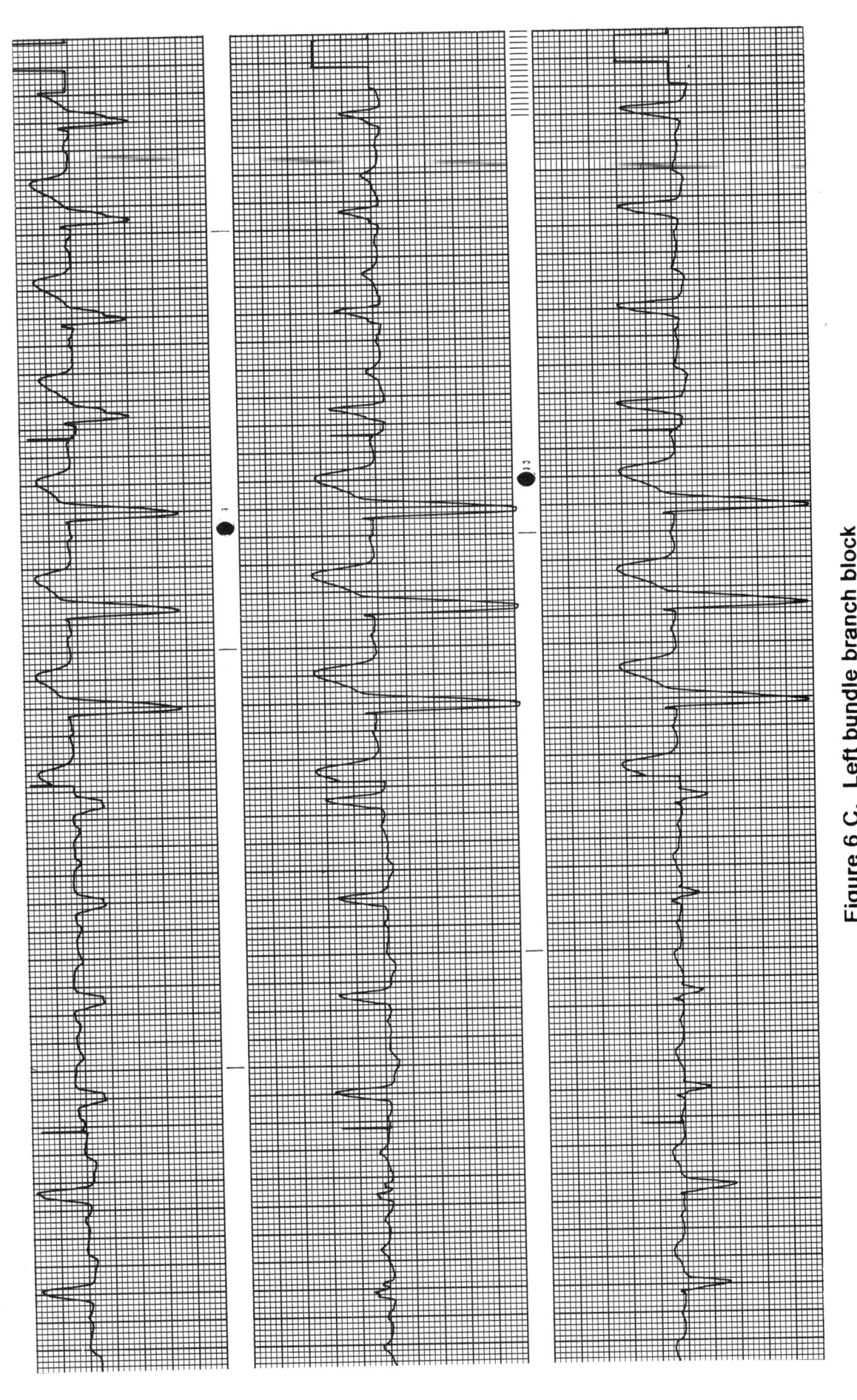

Figure 6 C. Left bundle branch block

Note the QS in V_1 and the abnormal rS in V_2, V_3, V_4; loss of septal q wave and the monophasic complex in V_5, V_6; secondary ST-T changes in V_6 (aVL); and the duration of the complex is 0.14 seconds.

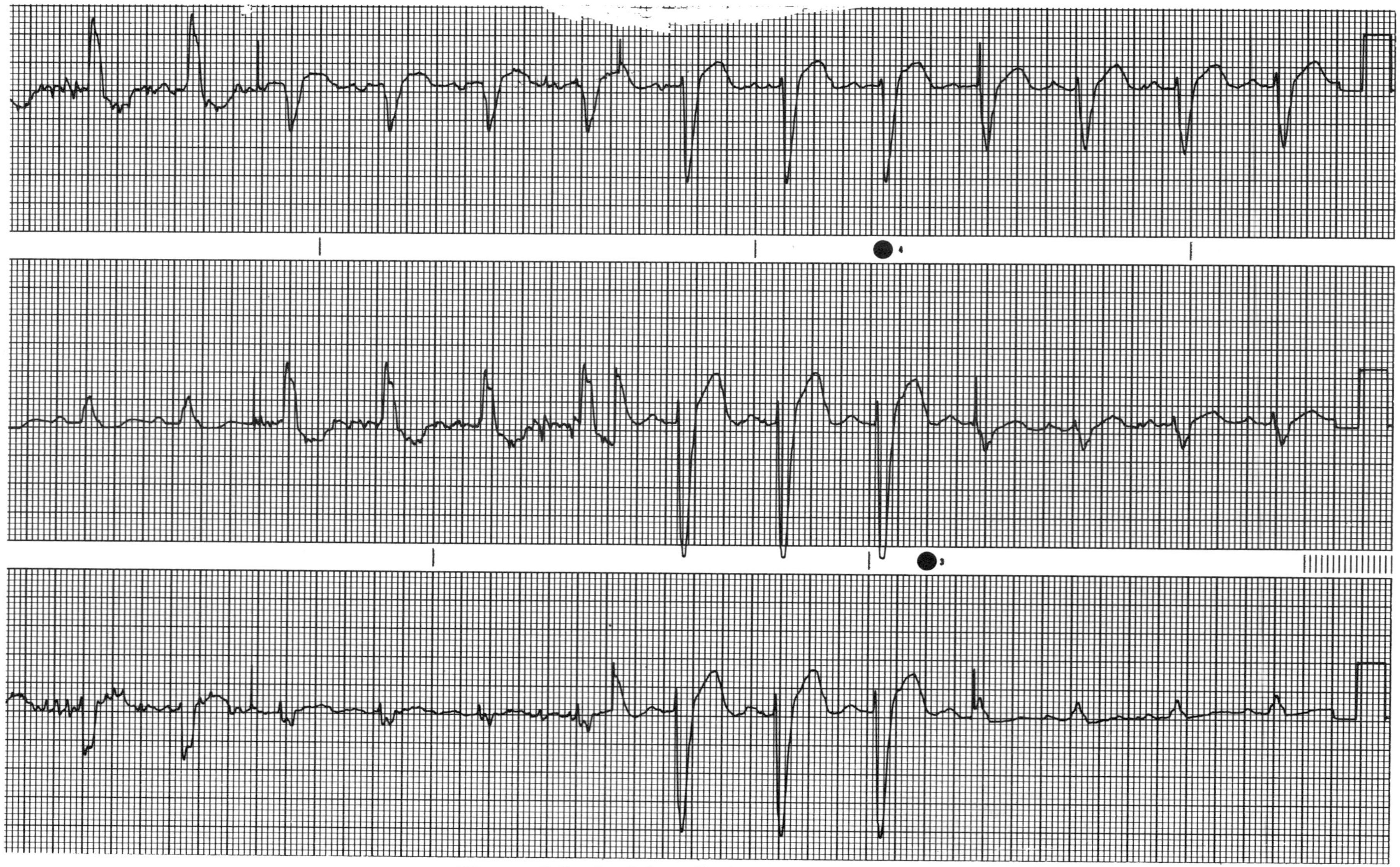

Figure 6 D. Left bundle branch block

Note the wide rS pattern in V_1, V_2 which is sometimes seen in left bundle branch block instead of the QS; the loss of septal q waves in V_5, V_6; monophasic R in V_6 (also I, aVL); secondary ST-T changes in V_6; the duration of the complex is 0.14 seconds.

Chapter 6 — Intraventricular Conduction Defects (IVCD)

AXIS DEVIATION WITH BUNDLE BRANCH BLOCK

The frontal plane axis in either right or left bundle branch block may be shifted towards the blocked bundle due to the delayed depolarization. Frontal plane axis deviation is not included as an ECG criteria for right or left bundle block because it may or may not occur.

Refer back to:

Figure 6 A, right bundle branch block: the axis is normal 0°

Figure 6 B, right bundle branch block: the axis is normal +90°

Figure 6 C, left bundle branch block: the axis is normal 0°

Figure 6 D, left bundle branch block: the axis is normal 0°

Note in both right and left bundle branch block, the progression of the R wave is abnormal.

PRACTICE 12 LEAD ECGs # 36-45

Assess the following 12 lead ECGs using these guidelines:

Basic rhythm:
Frontal plane axis:
R wave progression:
Complex configuration and duration:
P wave:
ST segment:
T wave:
Secondary ST-T changes:
12 Lead ECG Interpretation:

Interpret the 12 lead ECG as normal or abnormal and identify any bundle branch blocks that are present. Answers begin on page 137.

Chapter 6 – Intraventricular Conduction Defects (IVCD)

Practice 12 Lead ECG #36

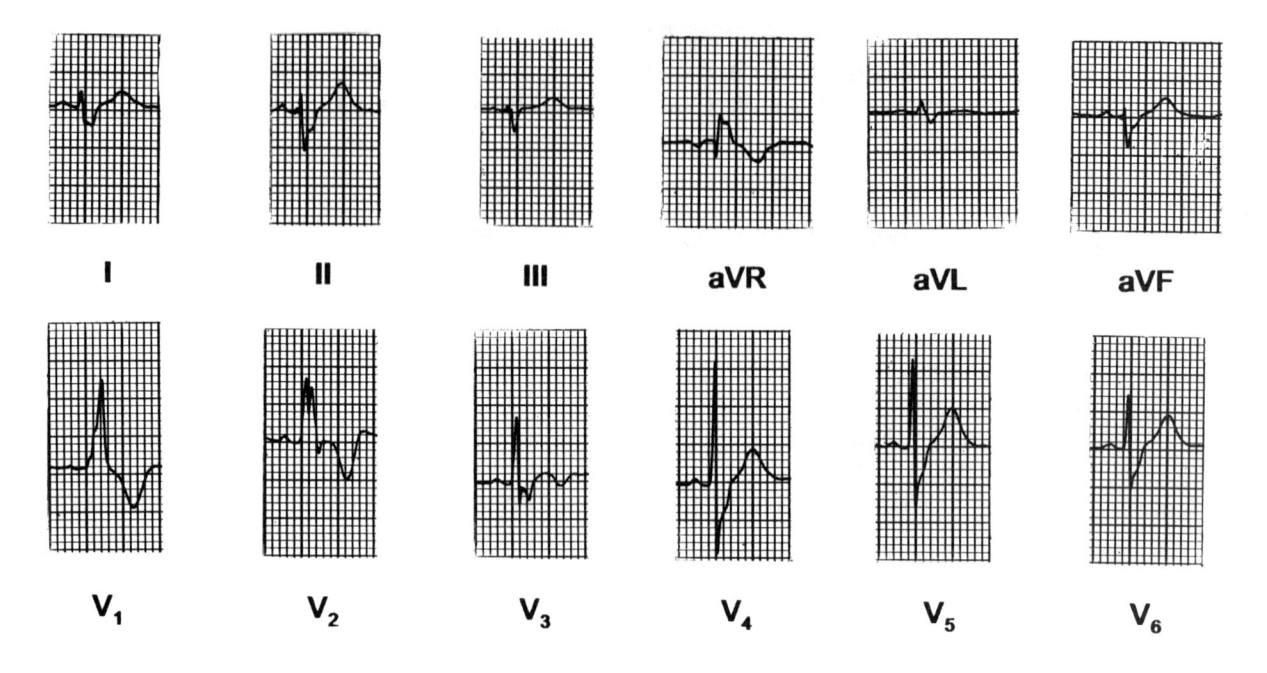

I   II   III   aVR   aVL   aVF

V₁   V₂   V₃   V₄   V₅   V₆

Practice 12 Lead ECG #37

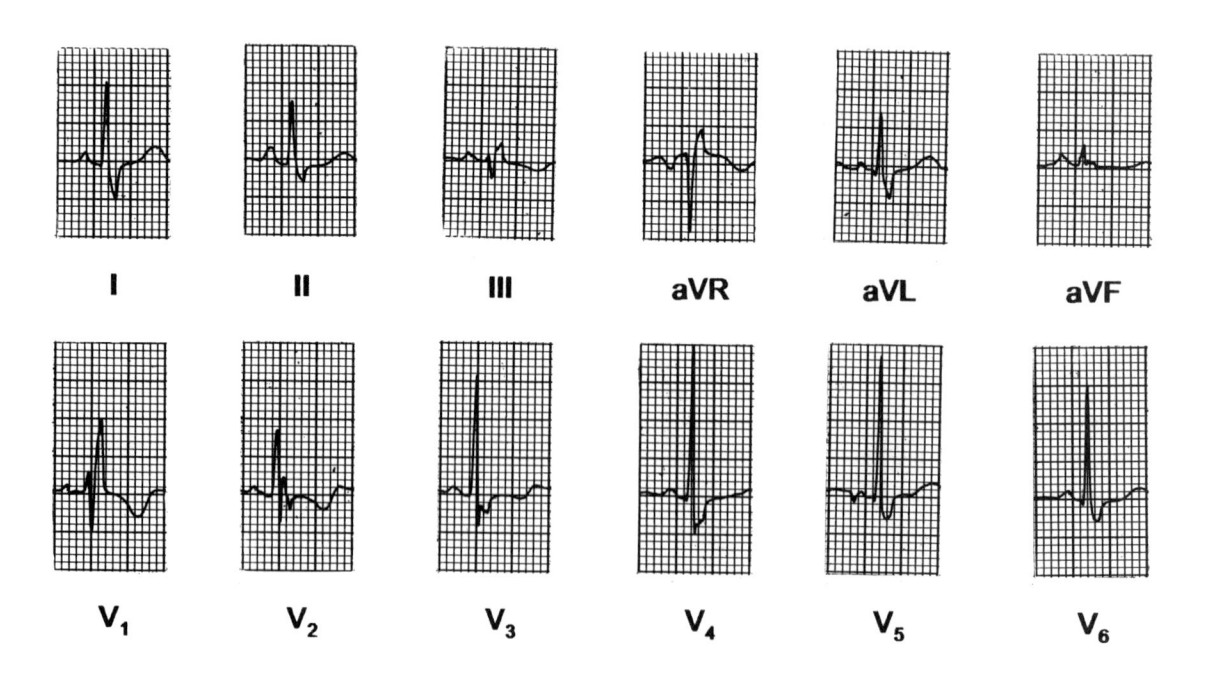

I   II   III   aVR   aVL   aVF

V₁   V₂   V₃   V₄   V₅   V₆

Practice 12 Lead ECG #38

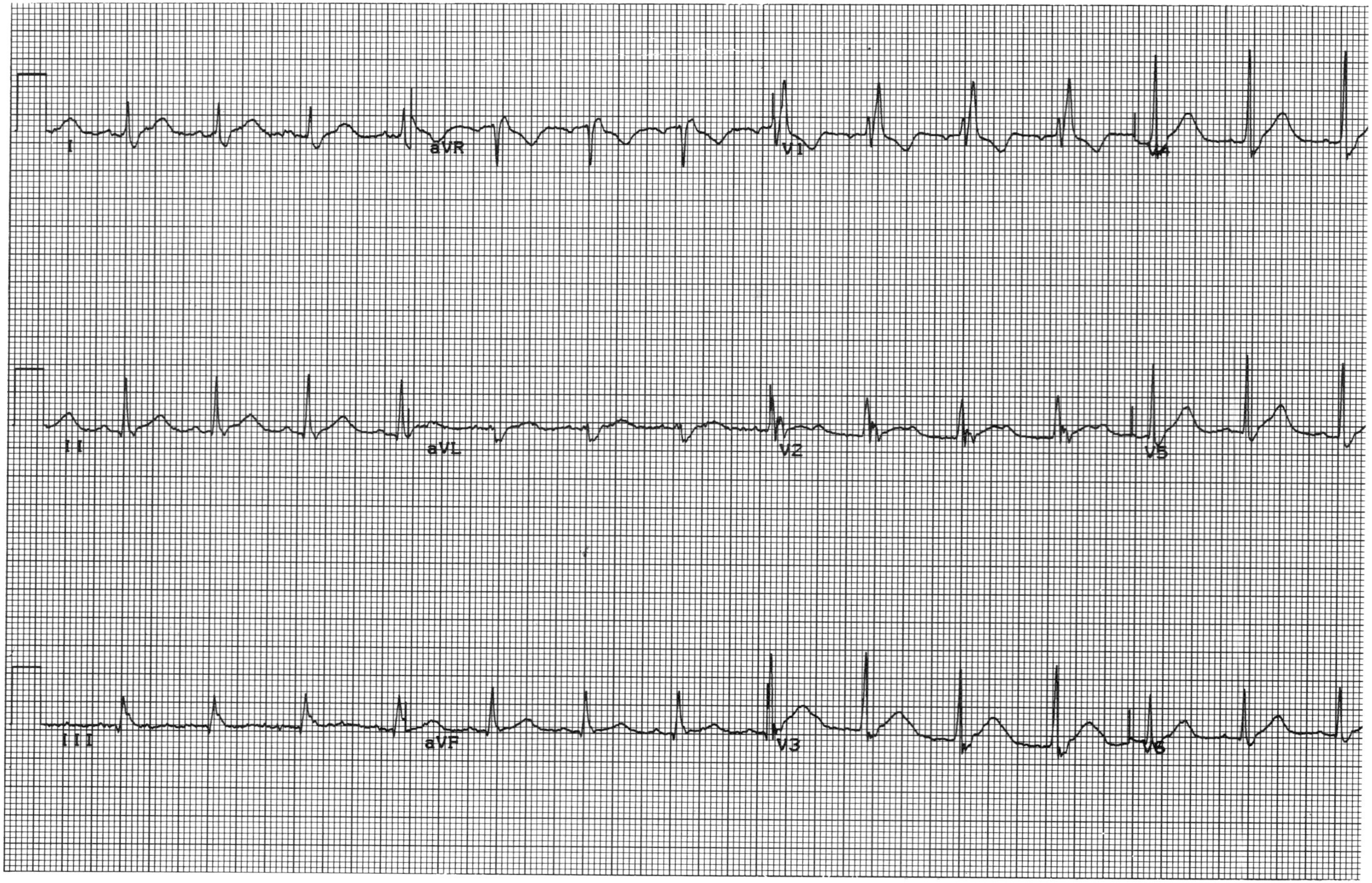

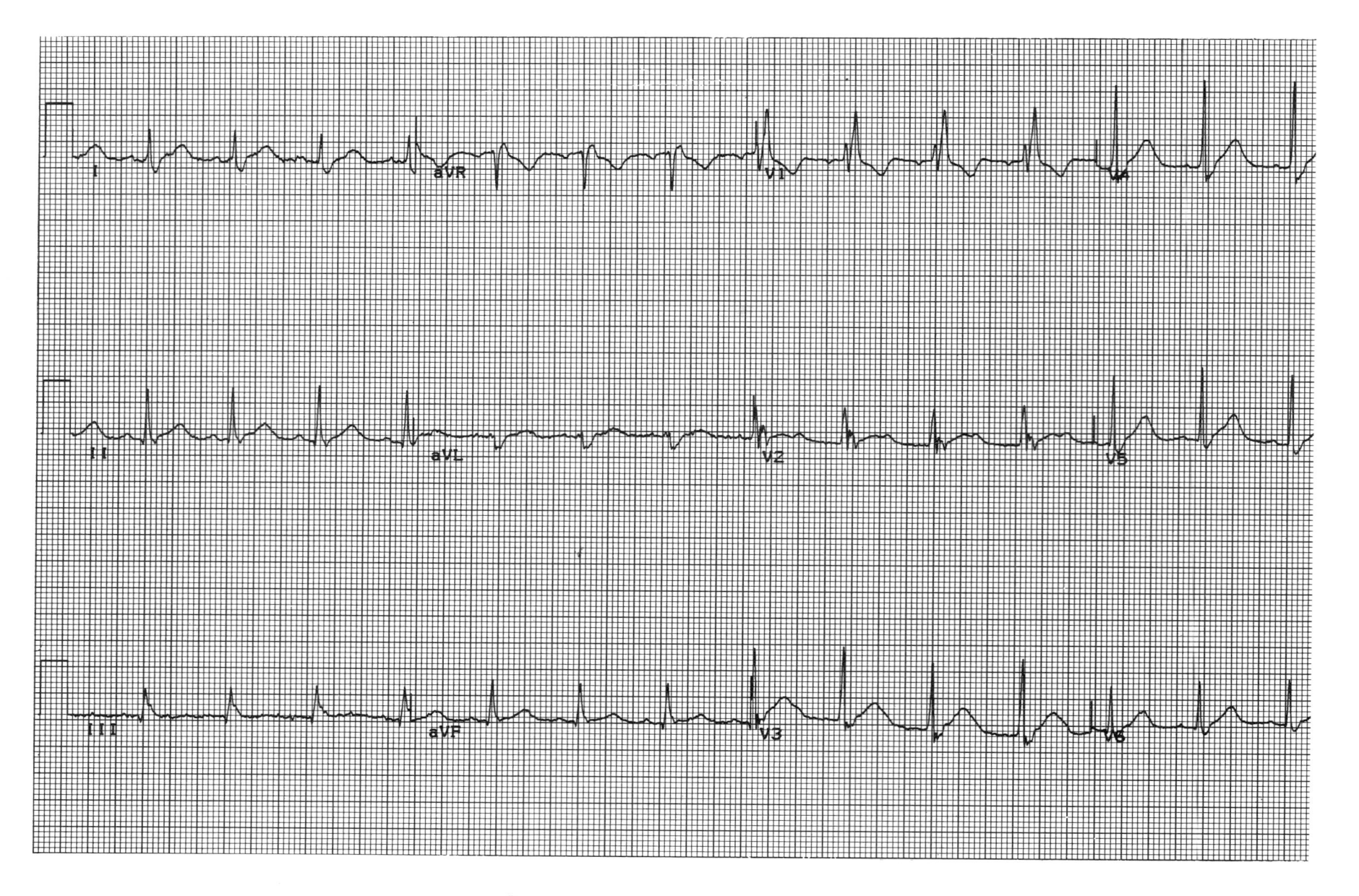

Practice 12 Lead ECG #39

Practice 12 Lead ECG #40

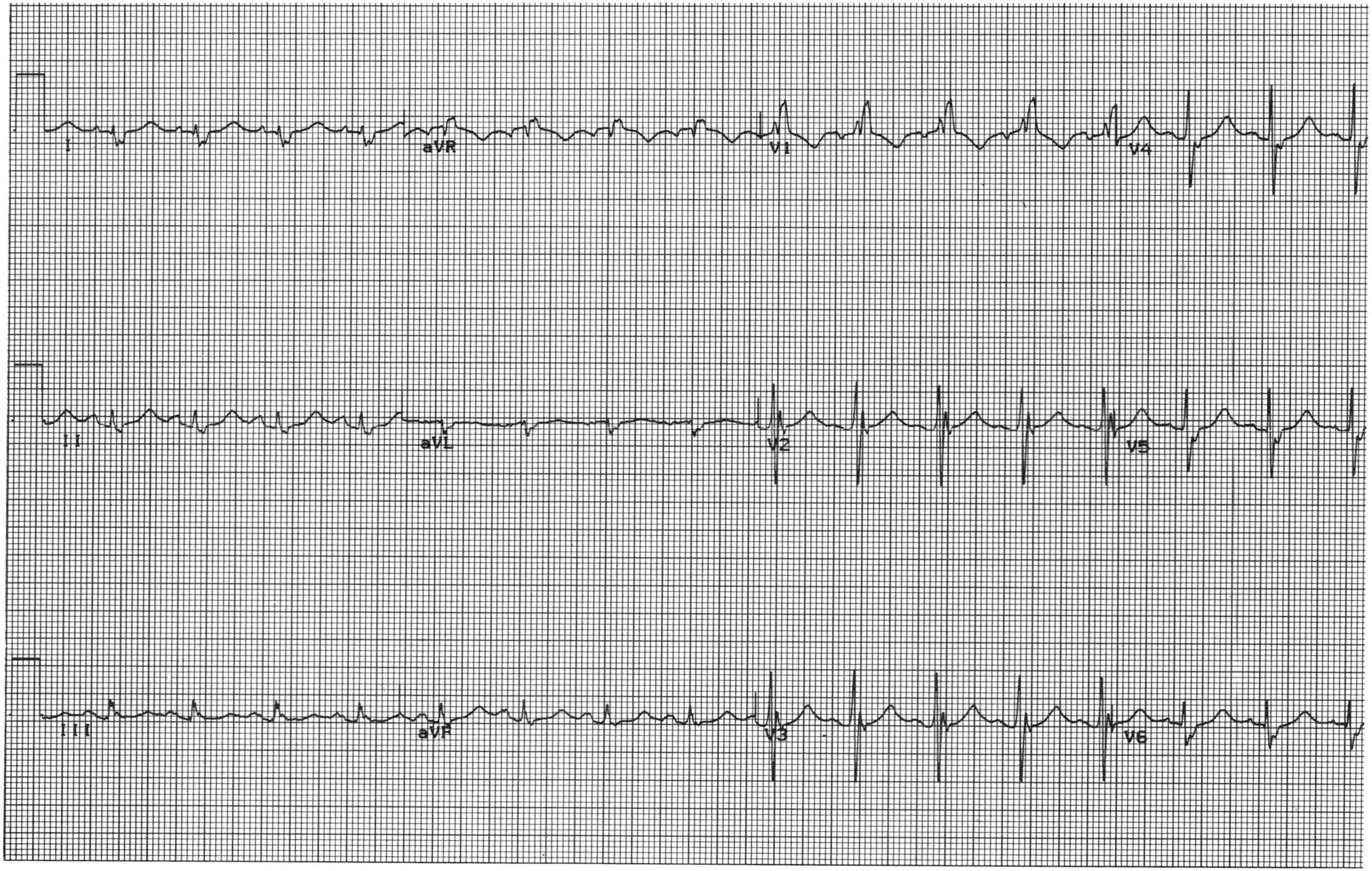

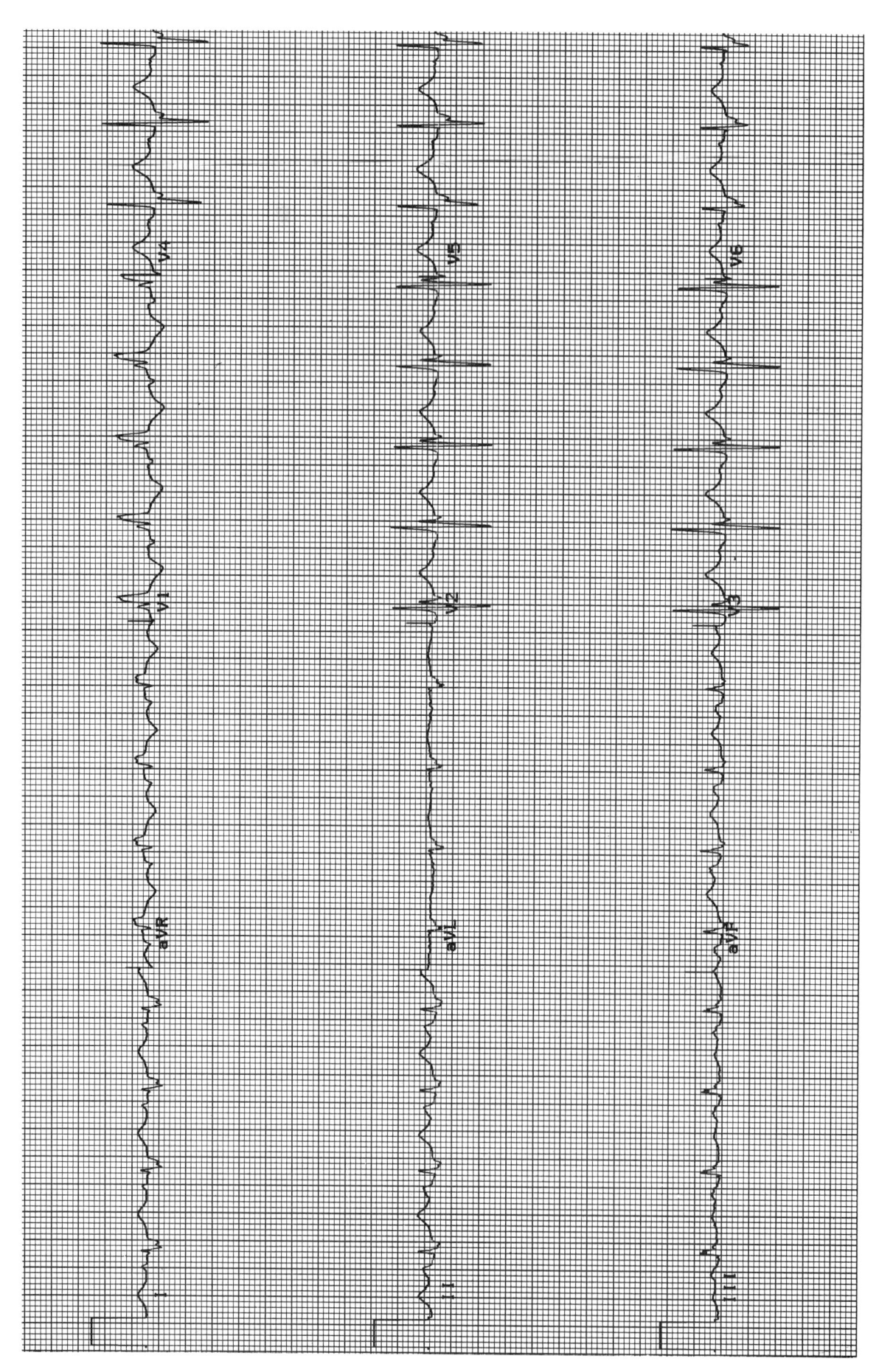

Practice 12 Lead ECG #41

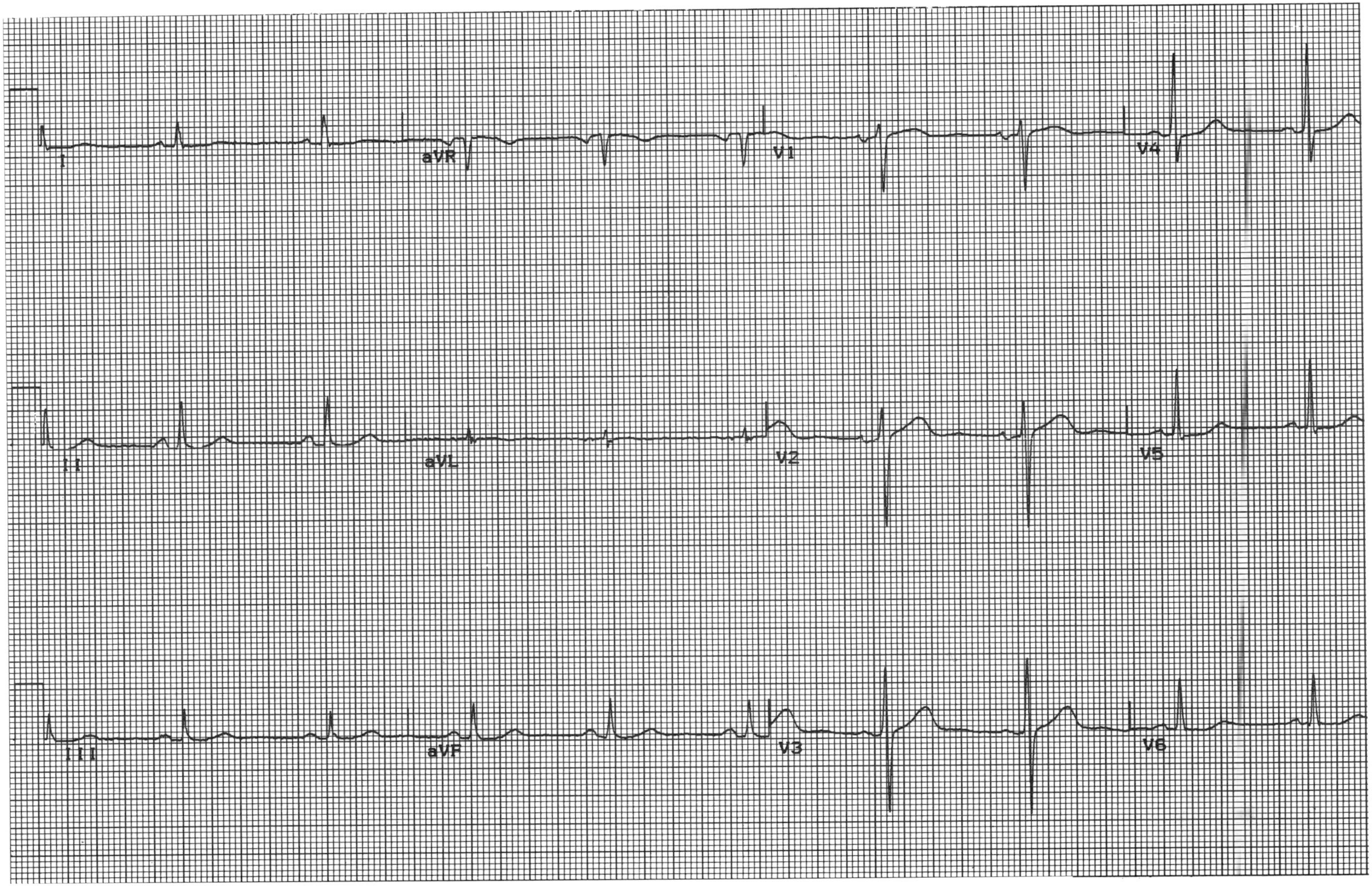

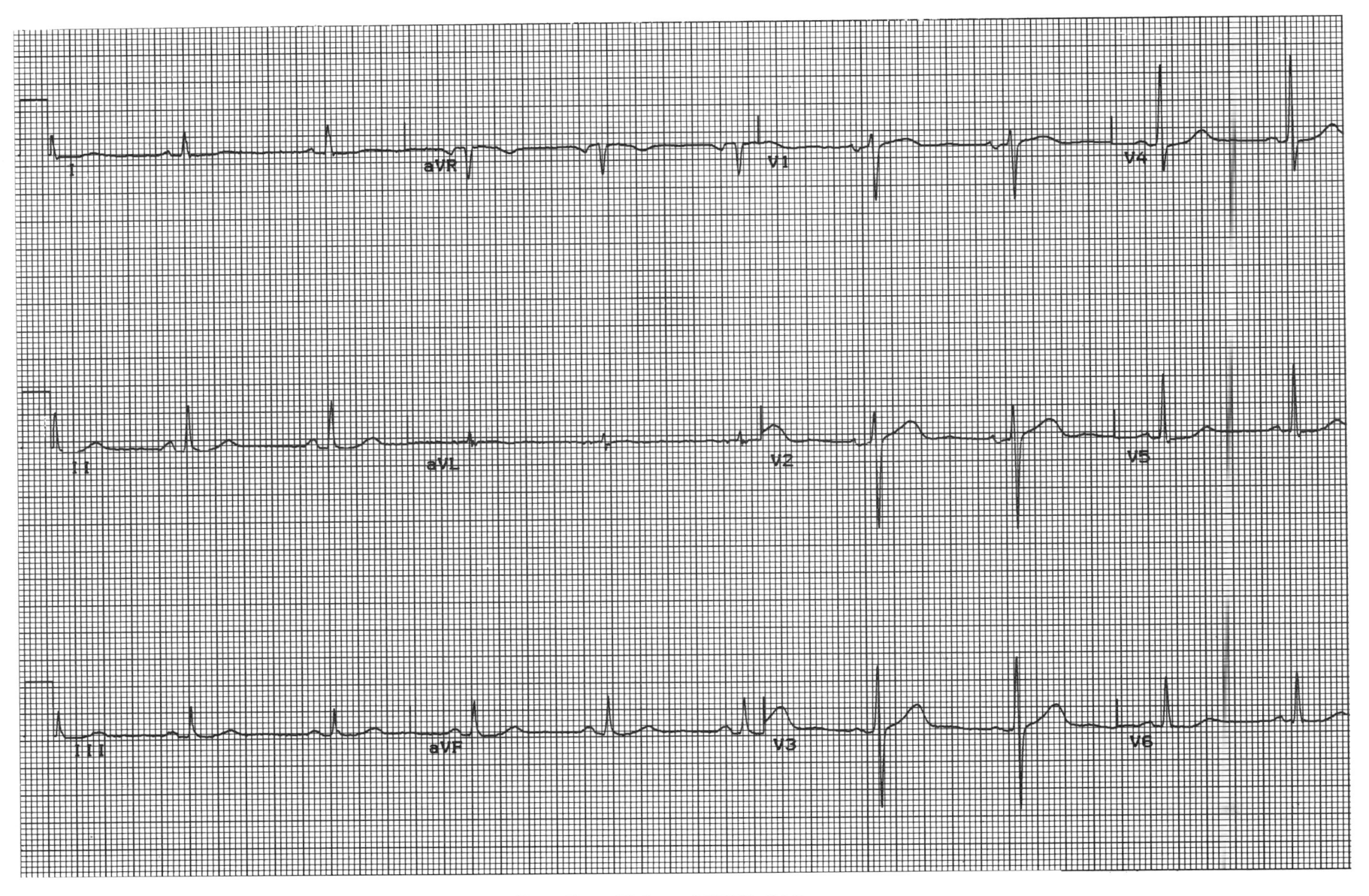

Practice 12 Lead ECG #42

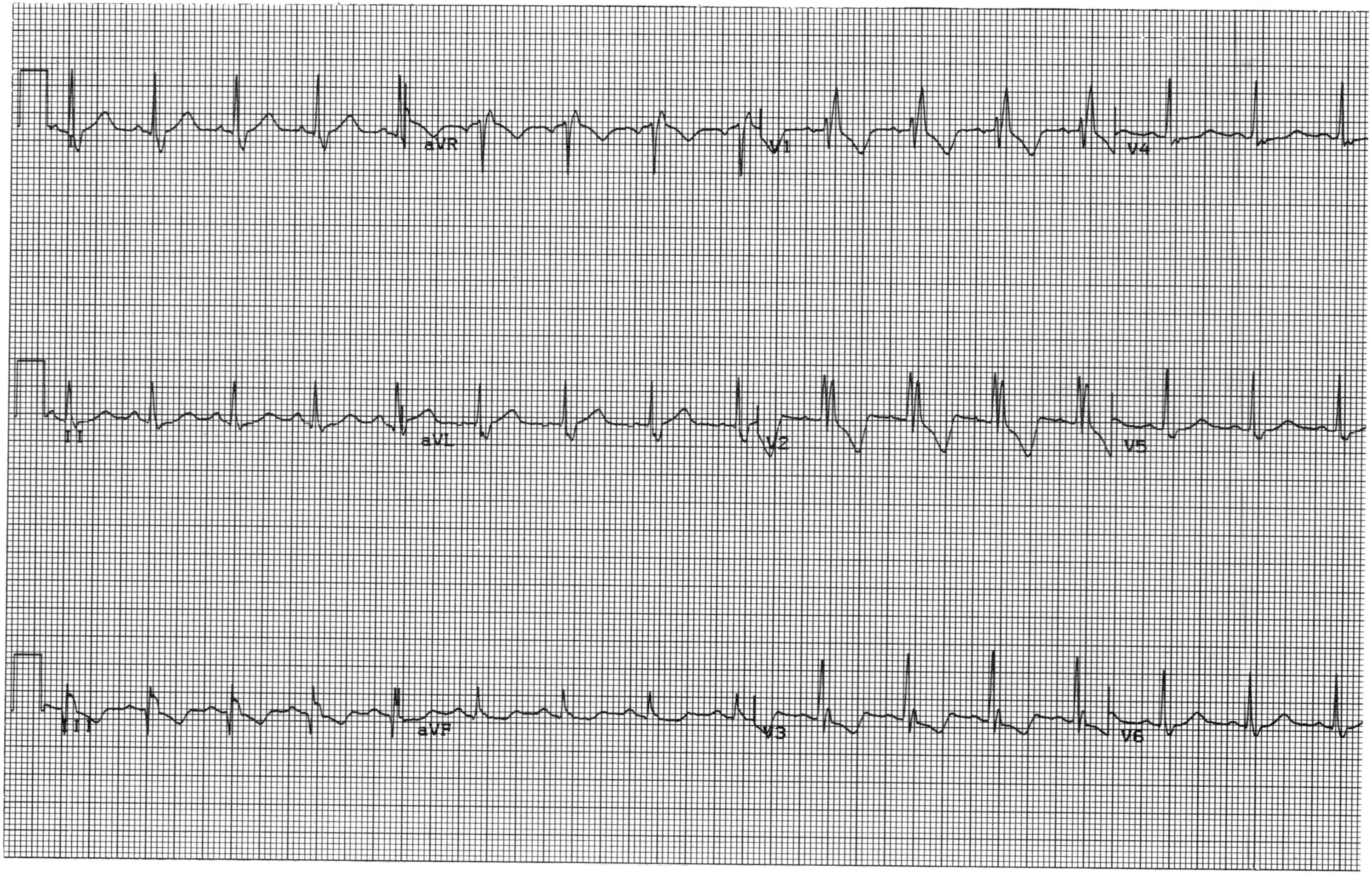

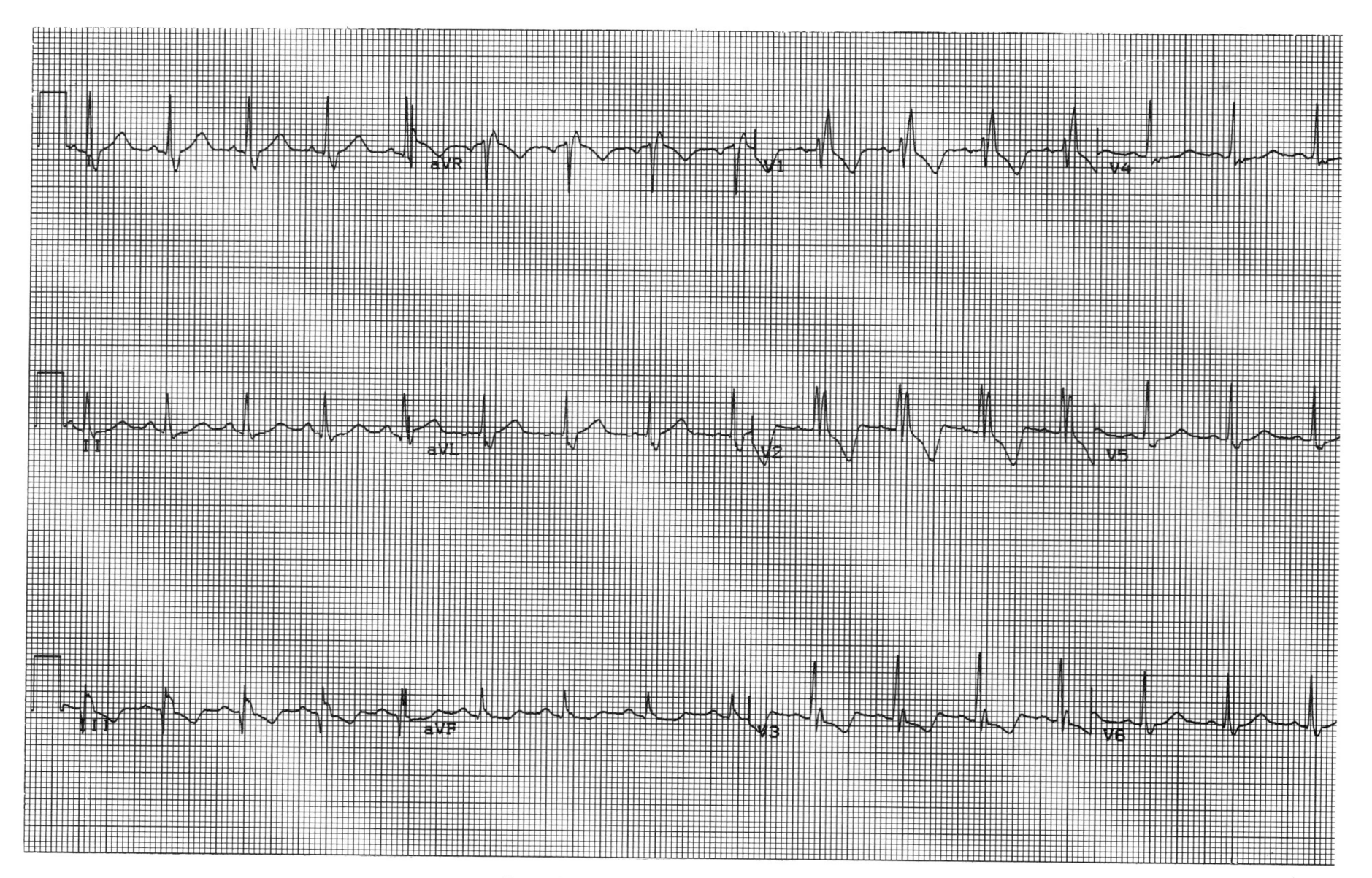

Practice 12 Lead ECG #43

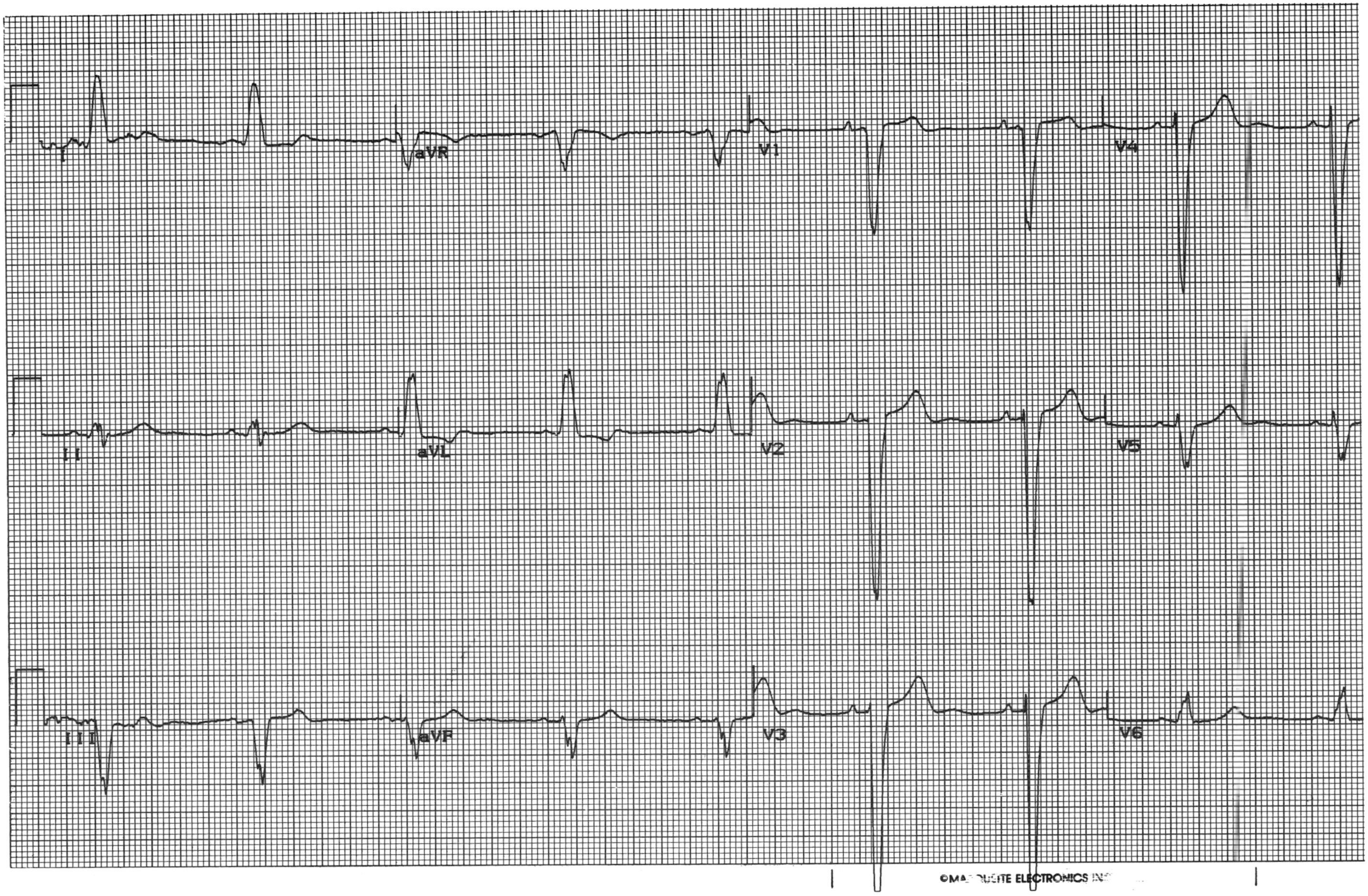

Practice 12 Lead ECG #44

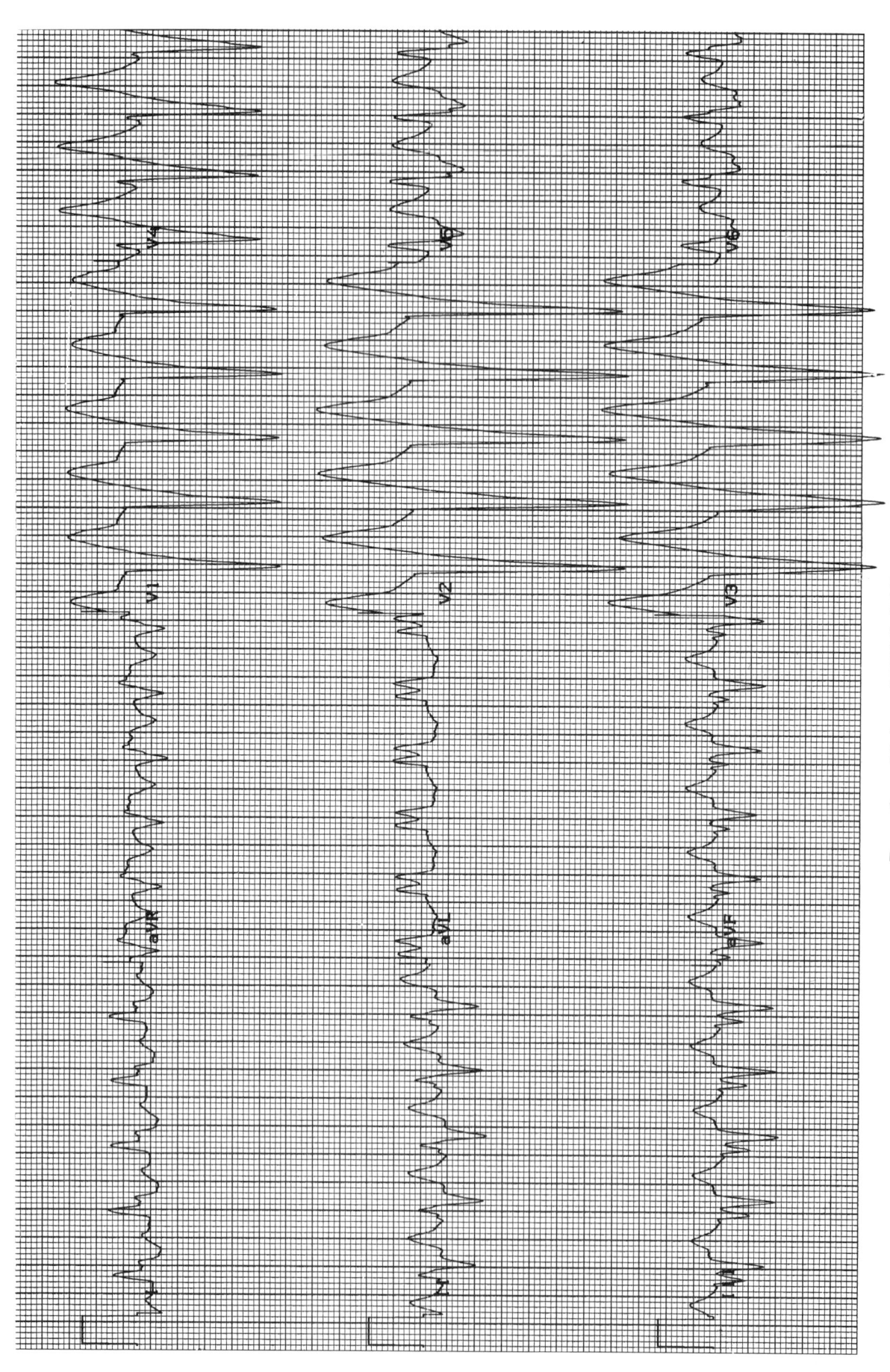

Practice 12 Lead ECG #45

Chapter 6 — Intraventricular Conduction Defects (IVCD)

ANSWERS TO PRACTICE 12 LEAD ECGs #36–45

36. **Basic rhythm:** Normal sinus rhythm
    Frontal plane axis: LAD quadrant -90° (lead I has the most equiphasic complex; aVF has a negative complex).
    R wave progression: Abnormal starting with RR^I in V_1; RR^Is in V_2; Rss^I in V_3
    Complex configuration: Abnormal configuration in many leads. Rabbit ear configuration in the right precordial leads alerts you to look for other characteristics of right bundle branch block. Also note the slurred and deep S waves in V_4, V_5, V_6.
    Complex duration: Abnormal: 0.12 seconds
    P wave: Normal
    Secondary ST-T changes: V_1, V_2
    12 Lead ECG Interpretation: Abnormal
      - Right bundle branch block

37. **Basic rhythm:** Normal sinus rhythm
    Frontal plane axis: Normal +30°
    R wave progression: Abnormal: rSR^I in V_1, Rsr^I in V_2; (look for RBBB)
      Complex duration: 0.12 seconds: Present
      Secondary ST-T changes: Present in V_1, V_2
    Slurred s waves: Present in V_5, V_6, I, aVL
    P wave: Normal
    12 Lead ECG Interpretation: Abnormal
      - Right bundle branch block

38. **Basic rhythm:** Normal sinus rhythm
    Frontal plane axis: Normal 0° (+10° corrected, see page 186)
    R wave progression: Abnormal: r in V_1 does not progress in V_2 or V_3 (loss of anterior forces); Rr^I in V_5
    Complex configuration: Abnormal as noted above and RR^I in other leads
    Complex duration: Abnormal: 0.12 seconds
    P wave: Normal
    ST segment: Elevated in V_1 and V_2
    Secondary ST-T changes: I, aVL, V_5, V_6
    12 Lead ECG Interpretation: Abnormal
      - Left bundle branch block

39. **Basic rhythm:** Normal sinus rhythm
    Frontal plane axis: Normal +60°
    R wave progression: Abnormal: rsR^I in V_1; Rsr^I in V_2
    Complex configuration: Abnormal as noted above and slurred s wave in I, aVL, V_5, V_6
    Complex duration: Abnormal: 0.12 seconds
    P wave: Normal
    Secondary ST-T changes: V_1, V_2
    12 Lead ECG Interpretation: Abnormal
      - Right bundle branch block

Chapter 6 – Intraventricular Conduction Defects (IVCD)

40. **Basic rhythm:** Normal sinus rhythm
    Frontal plane axis: LAD quadrant -60°
    R wave progression: Abnormal: Loss of anterior forces with transition in V_6
    Complex configuration: Abnormal as noted above and R^I/S^I in other leads
    Complex duration: Abnormal: 0.14 seconds
    P wave: Abnormal: Wide and notched in II with large P terminal in V_1
    Secondary ST-T changes: I, aVL, V_6
    12 Lead ECG Interpretation: Abnormal
    - P mitrale
    - Left bundle branch block

41. **Basic rhythm:** Sinus tachycardia
    Frontal plane axis: RAD quadrant +120° (aVR has the most equiphasic complex)
    R wave progression: Abnormal: rR^I in V_1; RSr^I in V_2, V_3
    Complex configuration: Abnormal as noted above and r^I/s^I in other leads
    Complex duration: Abnormal: 0.12 seconds
    P wave: Normal
    Secondary ST-T changes: V_1
    12 Lead ECG Interpretation: Abnormal
    - Sinus tachycardia
    - Right bundle branch block

    This 64-year-old woman developed sinus tachycardia and right bundle branch block shortly after coronary artery bypass surgery.

42. **Basic rhythm:** Normal sinus rhythm. This is the same patient seen in Practice 12 Lead ECG #41, 12 hours later.
    Frontal plane axis: Normal +60°
    R wave progression: Normal
    Complex configuration: Normal
    Complex duration: Normal
    P wave: Normal
    ST segment: Normal
    T wave: Normal
    Secondary ST-T changes: None
    12 Lead ECG Interpretation: Normal: Practice 12 lead ECG #41 is an example of transient intraventricular conduction defect due to the surgical trauma.

43. **Basic rhythm:** Normal sinus rhythm
    Frontal plane axis: Normal +30°
    R wave progression: Abnormal: rsR^I in V_1; RsR^I in V_2; Rsr^I in V_3
    Complex configuration: Abnormal as noted above and slurred s waves in V_5, V_6, I, aVL
    Complex duration: Abnormal: 0.12 seconds
    P wave: Normal
    Secondary ST-T changes: V_1, V_2, V_3
    12 Lead ECG Interpretation: Abnormal
    - Right bundle branch block

Chapter 6 — Intraventricular Conduction Defects (IVCD)

44. **Basic rhythm:** Sinus bradycardia
    Frontal plane axis: LAD quadrant -30°
    R wave progression: Abnormal: QS in V_1, V_2; rS in V_3, V_4, V_5
    Complex configuration: Abnormal as noted above and R^1/S^1 in other leads
    Complex duration: Abnormal: 0.14 seconds
    P wave: Normal
    Secondary ST-T changes: I, aVL
    ST segment: Slightly elevated in V_2, V_3
    12 Lead ECG Interpretation: Abnormal
    - Sinus bradycardia
    - Left bundle branch block

45. **Basic rhythm:** Sinus tachycardia (130 BPM)
    Frontal plane axis: LAD quadrant -30°
    R wave progression: Abnormal: Loss of anterior forces with transition in V_5.
    Complex configuration: Abnormal: QS in V_1, V_2, V_3; rS in V_4
    Complex duration: Abnormal: 0.16 seconds
    P wave: Difficult to see in most leads due to rapid rate. P waves are clearly seen in lead I.
    Secondary ST-T changes: I, aVL, V_5, V_6 (all of the left lateral leads)
    12 Lead ECG Interpretation: Abnormal
    - Sinus tachycardia
    - Left bundle branch block

Chapter 6 — Intraventricular Conduction Defects (IVCD)

HEMIBLOCKS

When only one of the fascicles of the left bundle branch is blocked it is called a hemiblock.

Hemiblocks may be congenital. An isolated hemiblock is not clinically significant. Clinically, the most common cause of a hemiblock is an acute myocardial infarction of the septum and/or the anterior wall. These patients need to be closely monitored for the development of a higher degree of block such as bifascicular block or complete heart block. Other causes of bifascicular block include hypertensive heart disease, aortic valve disease, and cardiomyopathies.

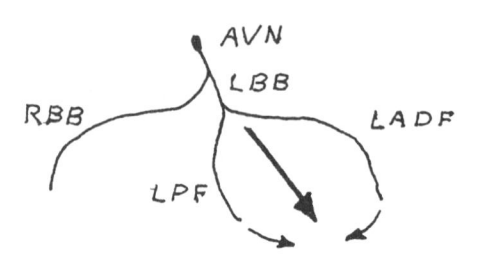

The above picture depicts part of the conduction system:

    AVN = AV Node
    RBB = Right Bundle Branch
    LBB = Left Bundle Branch
    LADF = Left Anterior Descending Fascicle
    LPF = Left Posterior Fascicle

The large arrow depicts the normal mean vector as it occurs from superior to inferior and from right-to-left in the frontal plane.

Chapter 6 -- Intraventricular Conduction Defects (IVCD)

LEFT ANTERIOR DESCENDING HEMIBLOCK

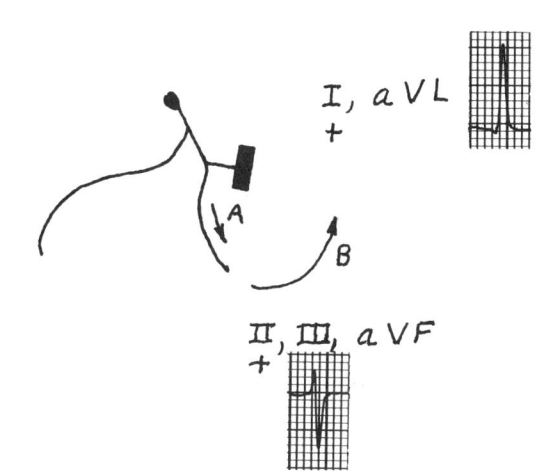

This picture depicts left anterior descending hemiblock (LADH). Initial depolarization (A) travels down the intact fascicle and inscribes a small r in II, III, and/or aVF and a small q wave in I and/or aVL. The terminal forces (B) swing around to depolarize the remainder of the left ventricle.

QUESTION: What kind of a frontal plane axis deviation will result from these terminal forces?

A. Right axis deviation
B. Left axis deviation

ANSWER: B. Left axis deviation

Left anterior descending hemiblock (LADH) causes a left axis deviation (LAD). LADH = LAD

Note the initials are the same: an easy way to remember that LADH causes an LAD.

In summary, **LEFT ANTERIOR DESCENDING HEMIBLOCK ECG CHARACTERISTICS**:

1. Left axis deviation (-30° or more leftward)
2. Small r wave in lead II, III, and/or aVF
3. Small q wave in lead I and/or aVL

LADH is seen more often than left posterior hemiblock (LPH).

An isolated left posterior hemiblock is rare. The posterior fascicle is less vulnerable because it is shorter and thicker than the anterior fascicle and is subject to less turbulence. The posterior fascicle also has a dual blood supply; the anterior fascicle has a single blood supply.

Figure 6 E on the following page is an example of LADH.

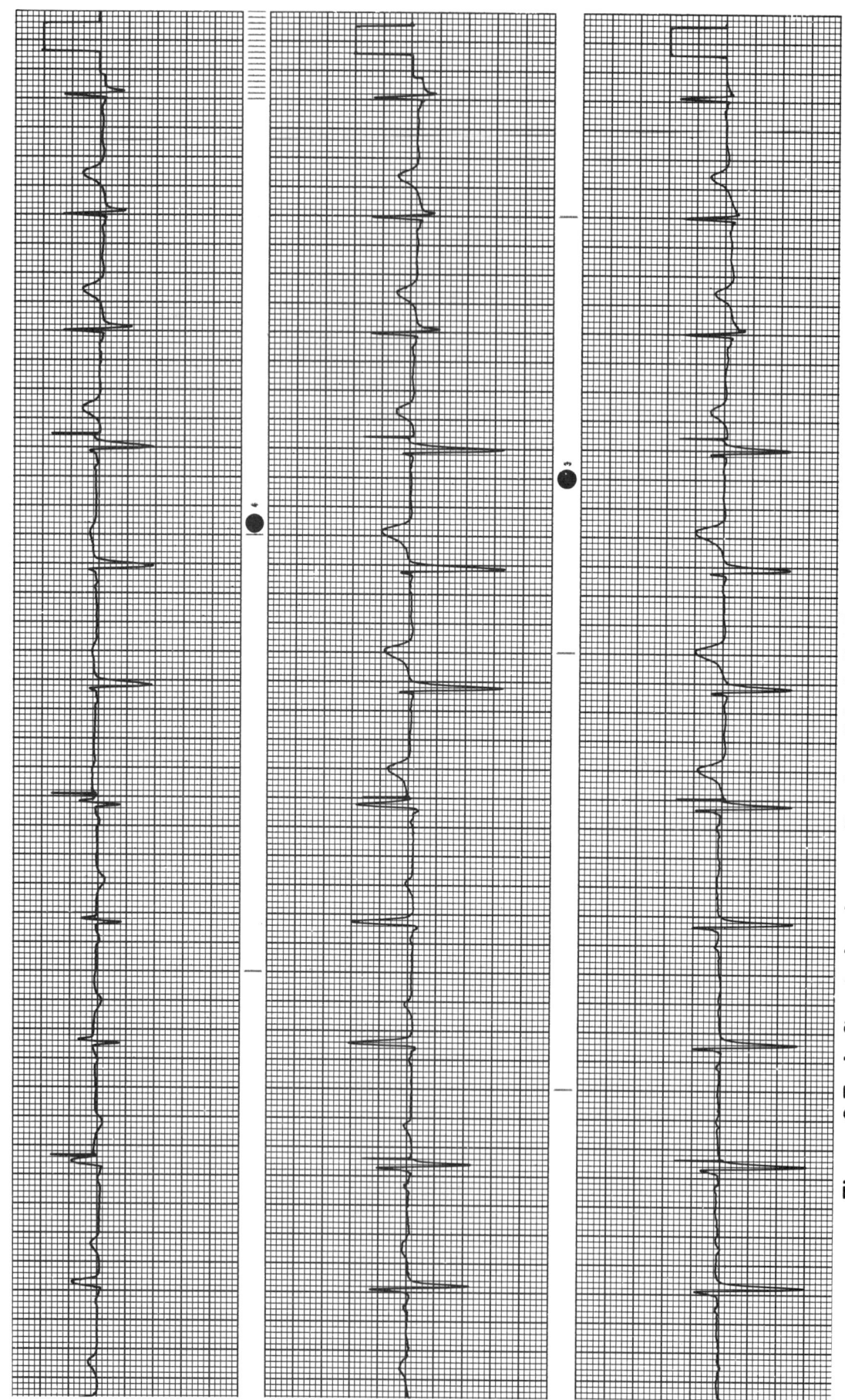

Figure 6 E. Left anterior descending hemiblock (LADH or LASH)
Note frontal plane axis is -60°; small r in II; small q in I.

Chapter 6 – Intraventricular Conduction Defects (IVCD)

LEFT POSTERIOR HEMIBLOCK (LPH)

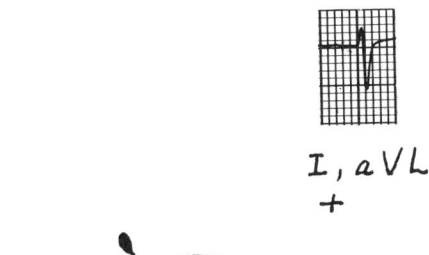

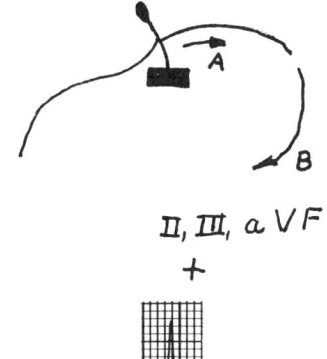

This picture depicts left posterior hemiblock (LPH). Initial depolarization (A) travels down the intact fascicle and inscribes a small r wave in I and/or aVL and a small q wave in II, III, and/or aVF. The terminal forces (B) swing around to depolarize the remainder of the left ventricle.

QUESTION: What kind of an axis deviation will result from these terminal forces?

ANSWER: Right axis deviation.

Left posterior hemiblock (LPH) causes a right axis deviation.

$$LPH = RAD$$

In summary, **LEFT POSTERIOR HEMIBLOCK ECG CHARACTERISTICS:**

1. **Right axis deviation (usually +110° or more rightward)**
2. **Small q wave in lead II, III, and/or aVF**
3. **Small r wave in lead I and/or aVL**
4. **No other evidence for right ventricular hypertrophy**

Figure 6 F on the following page is an example of left posterior hemiblock.

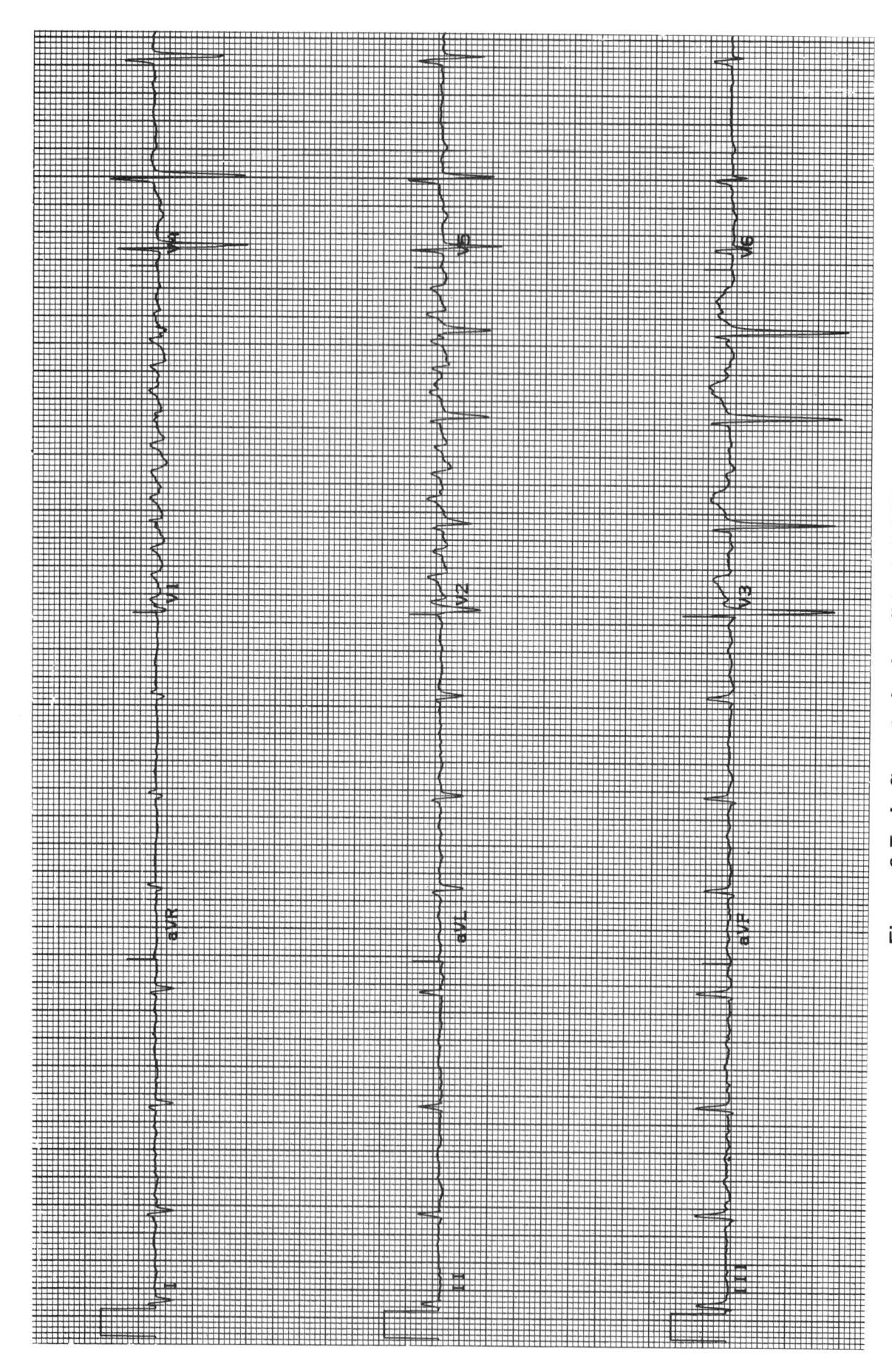

Figure 6 F. Left posterior hemiblock (LPH)
Note the frontal plane axis is +120°; small r in I; small q in III.

Chapter 6 — Intraventricular Conduction Defects (IVCD)

HEMIBLOCKS PRACTICE STRIPS

Identify hemiblock LADH or LPH on the following. Answers are on the following page.

1.

| I | II | III | aVR | aVL | aVF |

2.

| I | II | III | aVR | aVL | aVF |

3.

| I | II | III | aVR | aVL | aVF |

4.

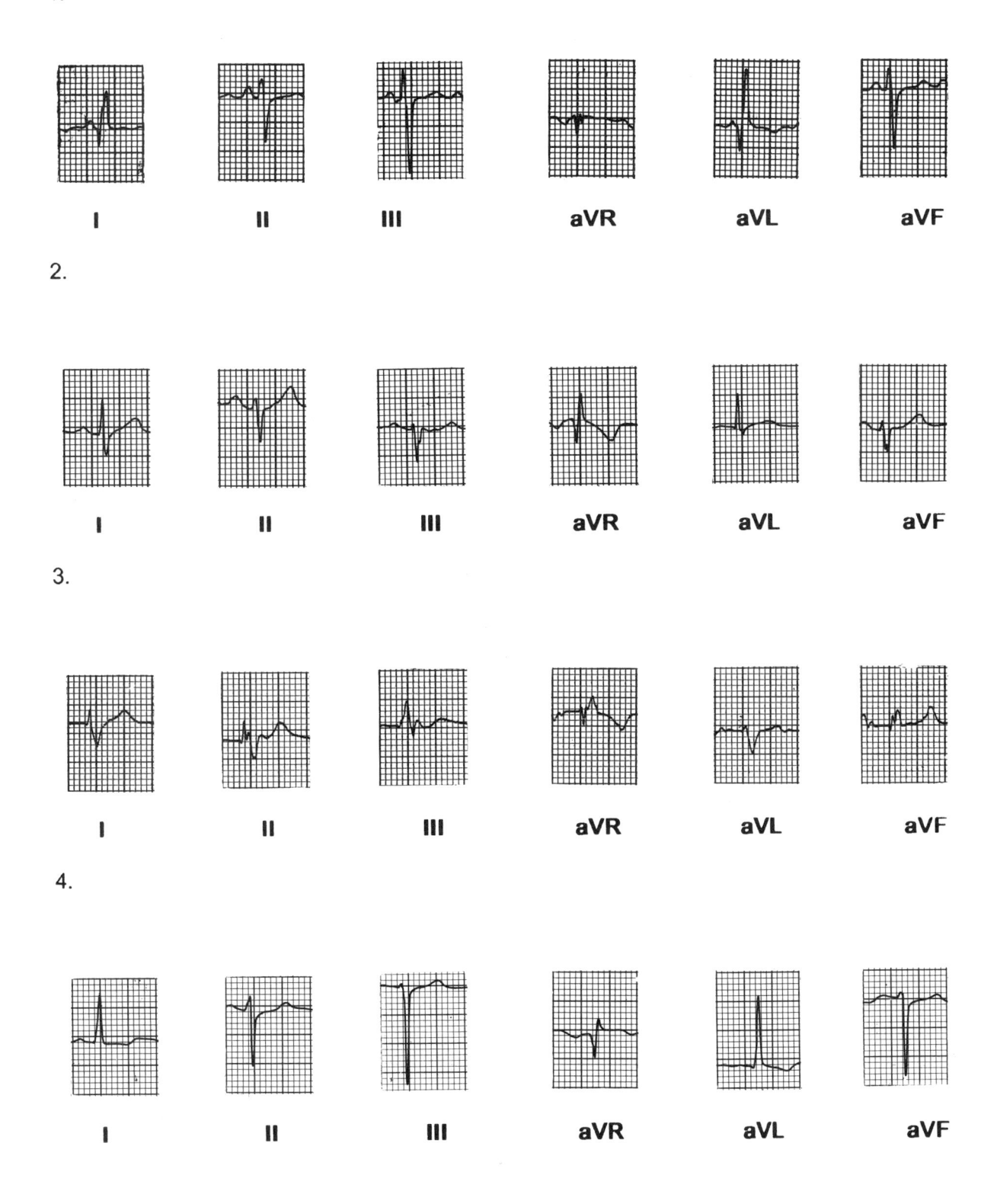

| I | II | III | aVR | aVL | aVF |

Chapter 6 — Intraventricular Conduction Defects (IVCD)

5.

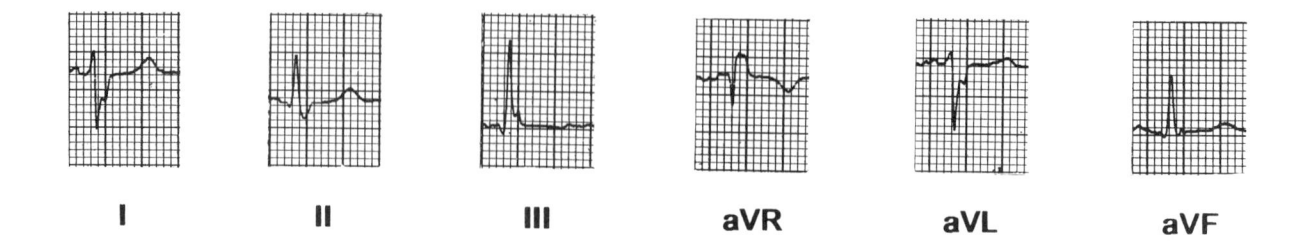

| I | II | III | aVR | aVL | aVF |

ANSWERS

1. **Frontal plane axis:** LAD quadrant -60°
    Small q in I
    Small r in II
   Interpretation: LADH

2. **Frontal plane axis:** LAD quadrant -60°
    Small q in aVL
    Small r in II
   Interpretation: LADH

3. **Frontal plane axis:** RAD quadrant +120°
    Small q in aVF
    Small r in I
    No other evidence for RVH
   Interpretation: LPH

4. **Frontal plane axis:** LAD quadrant -60°
    Small q in aVL
    Small r in II
   Interpretation: LADH

5. **Frontal plane axis:** RAD quadrant +120°
    Small q in aVF
    Small r in I
    No other evidence for RVH
   Interpretation: LPH

Notice in LADH the complex in lead I is mostly negative, and in LPH lead II has a mostly negative complex.

Finding the small wave in aVL is as good as finding it in lead I.

Finding the small wave in either III or aVF is as good as finding it in lead II.

Chapter 6 – Intraventricular Conduction Defects (IVCD)

BIFASCICULAR BLOCK

The ventricular conduction system has three fascicles – the right bundle branch plus the two fascicles on the left: the anterior and posterior fascicles. Complete blockage of all three fascicles is complete heart block (CHB). The definitive treatment of CHB is pacemaker insertion. A bifascicular block is the result of right bundle branch block plus blockage of one of the fascicles on the left. Bifascicular block is a serious condition with the same definitive treatment as complete heart block.

    RBBB + LADH   = bifascicular block

    RBBB + LPH   = bifascicular block

QUESTION: What is the definitive treatment of a bifascicular block?

ANSWER: Pacemaker insertion.

Figures 6 G and 6 H on the following two pages are examples of bifascicular blocks.

TRIFASCICULAR BLOCK

Trifascicular block is present when the patient has a bifascicular block plus some degree of AV heart block. For example, a right bundle branch block with a left anterior descending hemiblock and first degree AV heart block would be a trifascicular block.

QUESTION: What is the definitive treatment of a trifascicular block?

ANSWER: Pacemaker insertion.

Figure 6 I on page 150 is an example of trifascicular block.

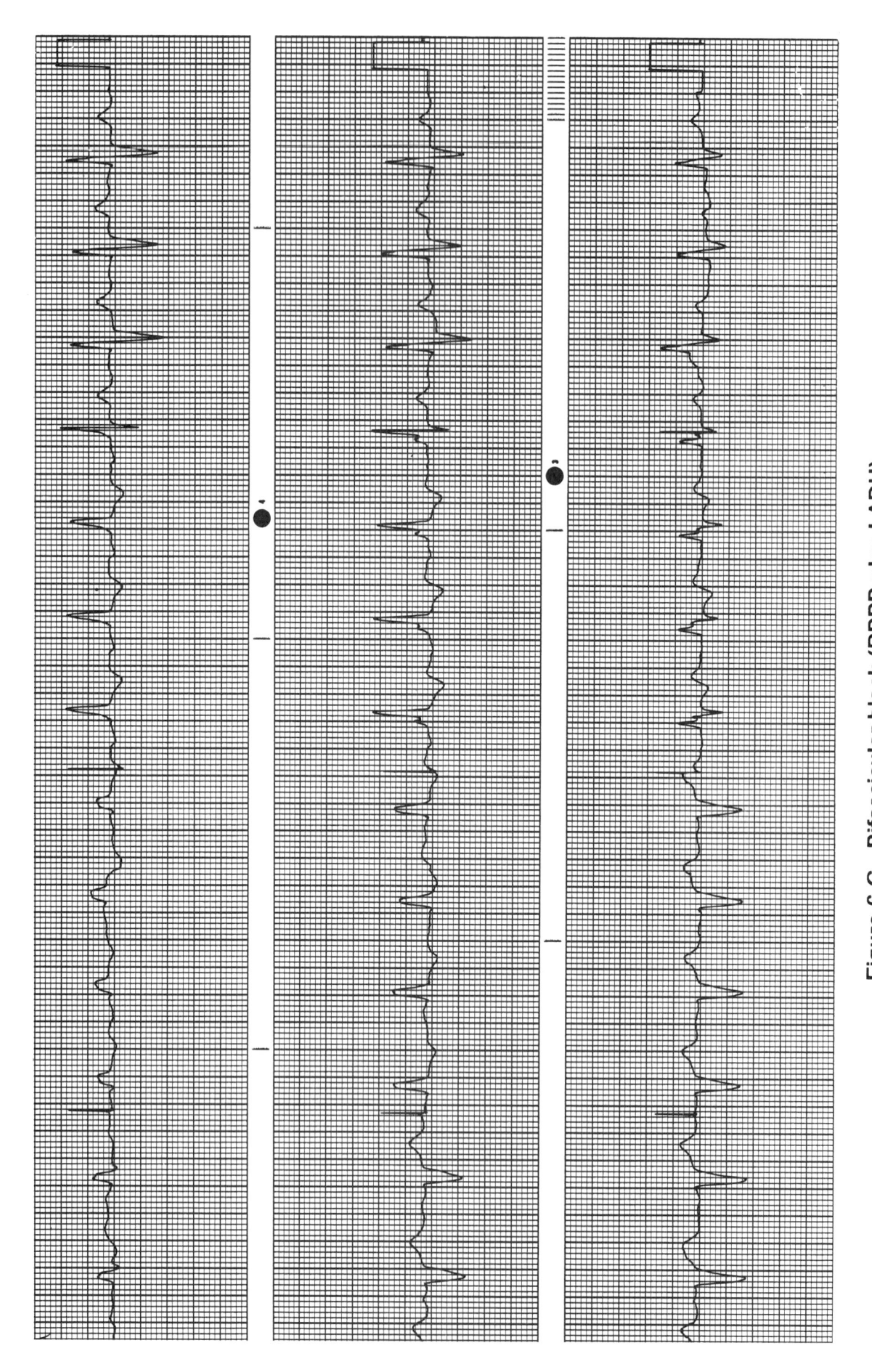

Figure 6 G. Bifascicular block (RBBB plus LADH)

Note the LADH and right bundle branch block characteristics: frontal plane axis -60°, small q in aVL, small r in II; rR' and secondary ST-T changes in V$_2$; slurred s in V$_6$; complex duration is 0.14 seconds.

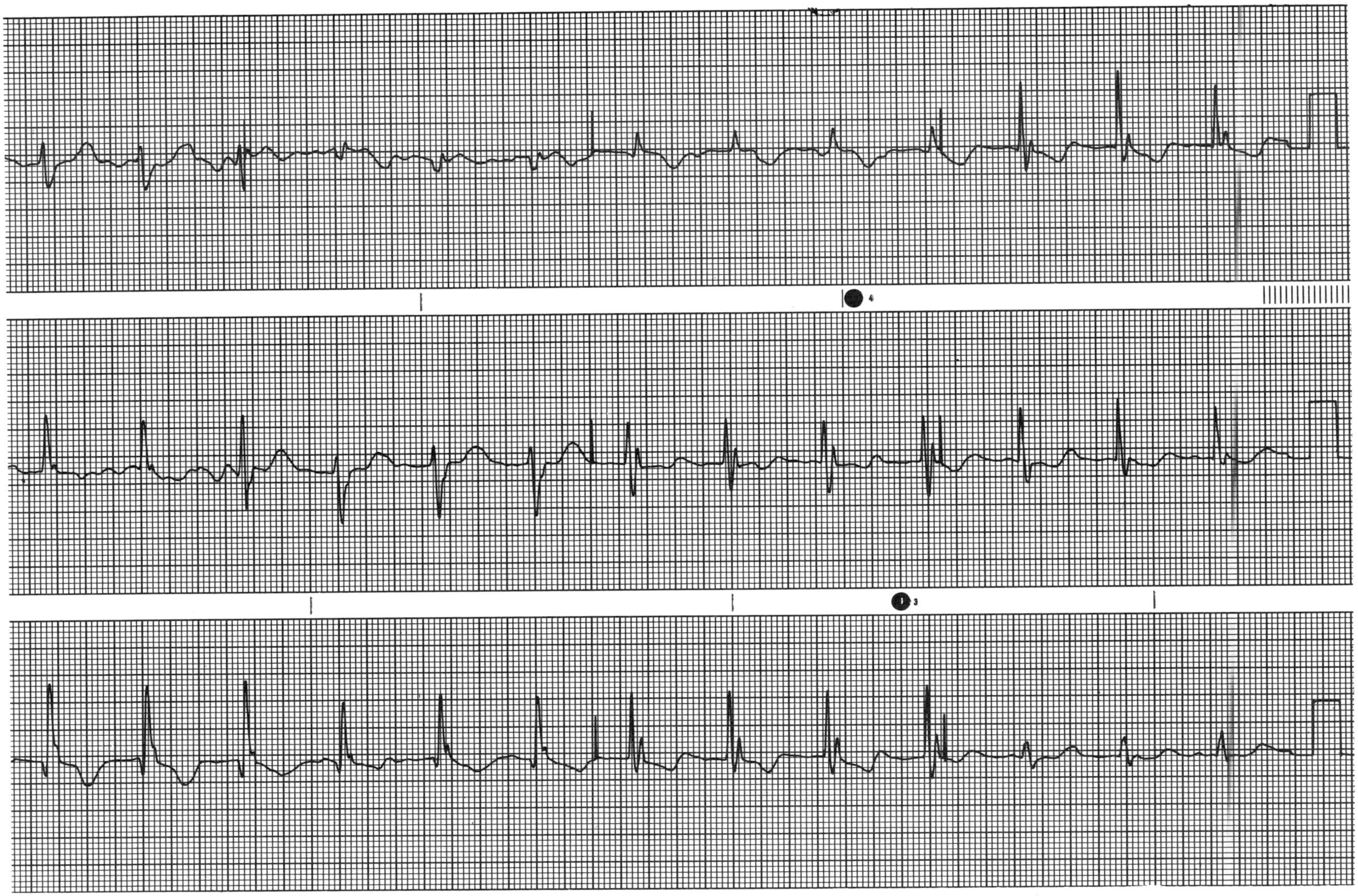

Figure 6 H. Bifascicular block (RBBB plus LPH)

Note the LPH and the RBBB characteristics: frontal plane axis is +120°; small r in aVL; small q in II; RSr' and secondary ST-T changes in V_2; slurred s in V_5; complex duration is 0.12 seconds.

Figure 61. Trifascicular block

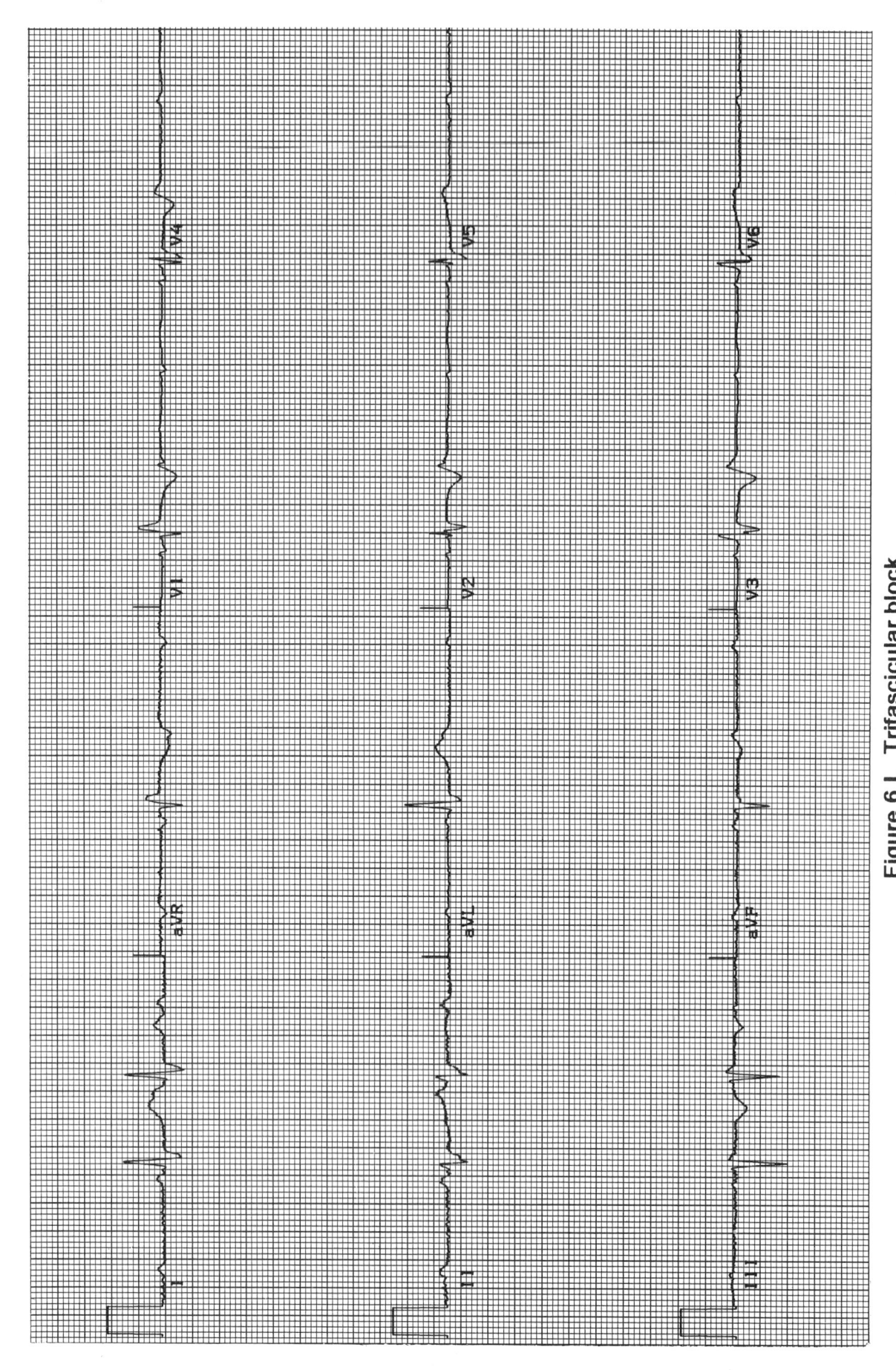

Note LADH and RBBB characteristics: frontal plane axis -30°; small r in II; rsR' in V_1 with secondary ST-T changes in V_1, V_2; slurred s waves in V_5 and V_6; small q in I; high degree of AV heart block.

Chapter 6 – Intraventricular Conduction Defects (IVCD)

PRACTICE 12 LEAD ECGs #46-70

Assess the following practice 12 lead ECGs using these guidelines:

Basic rhythm:
Frontal plane axis:
R wave progression:
Complex configuration and duration:
P wave:
ST segment:
T wave:
Secondary ST-T changes:
12 Lead ECG Interpretation:

Practice 12 lead ECGs #46-60 include the following intraventricular conduction defects:

RBBB
LBBB
LPH
LADH
RBBB with LPH
RBBB with LADH

Answers begin on page 167.

Practice 12 lead ECGs #61-70 will include the IVCDs plus chamber enlargements.

Answers begin on page 182.

Practice 12 Lead ECG #46

Practice 12 Lead ECG #47

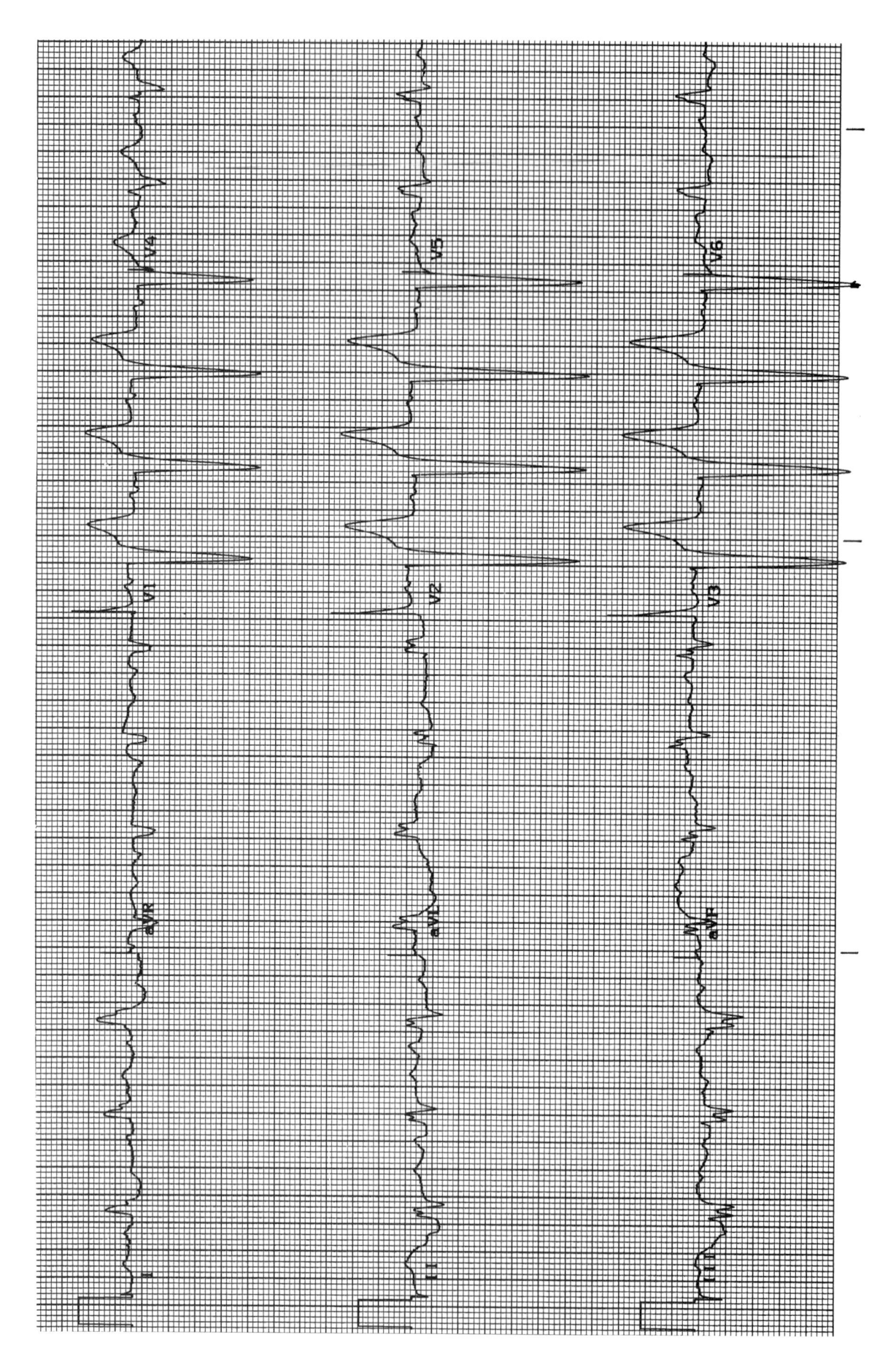

Practice 12 Lead ECG #48

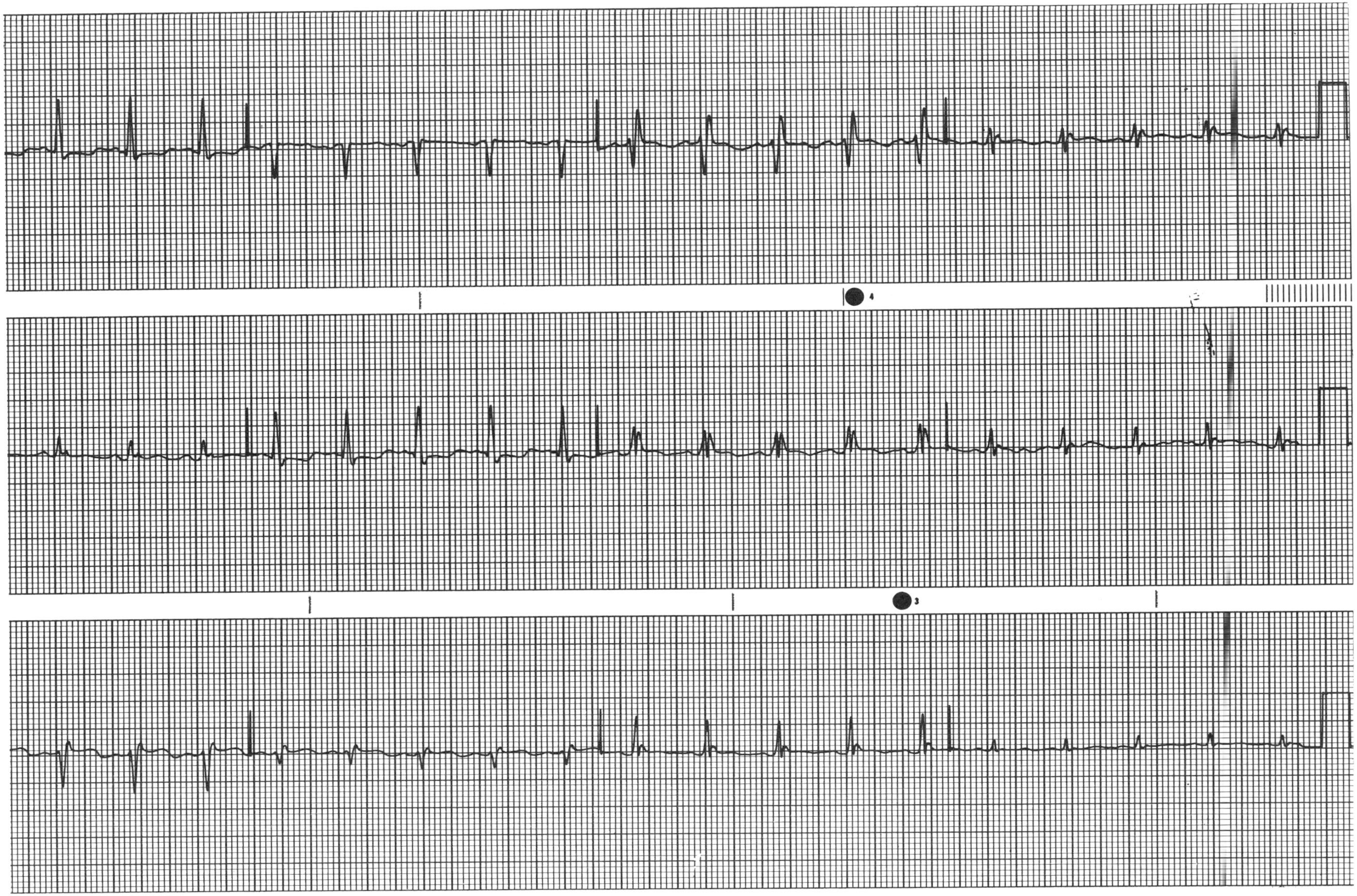

Practice 12 Lead ECG #49

Practice 12 Lead ECG #50

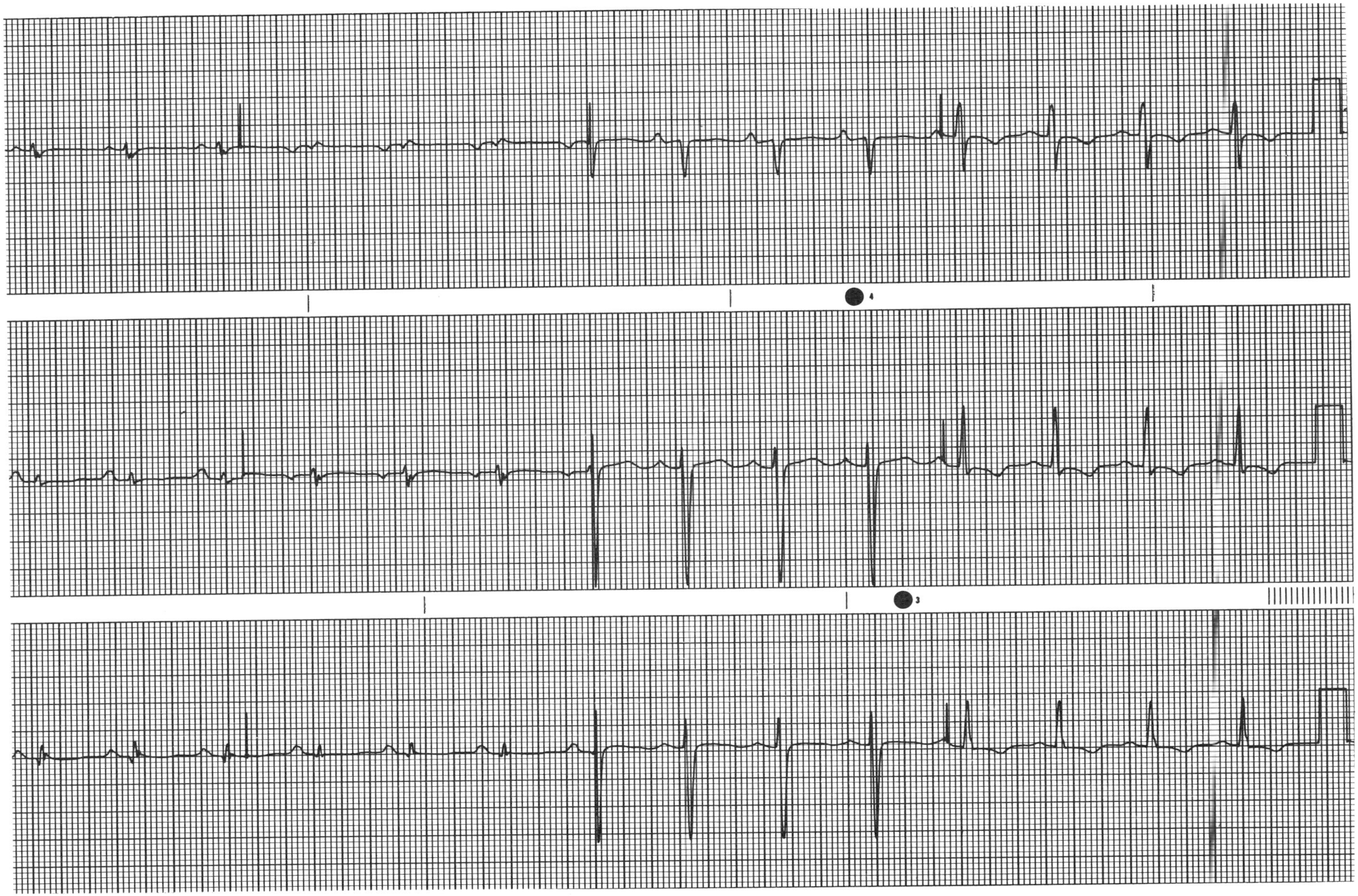

Practice 12 Lead ECG #51

Practice 12 Lead ECG #52

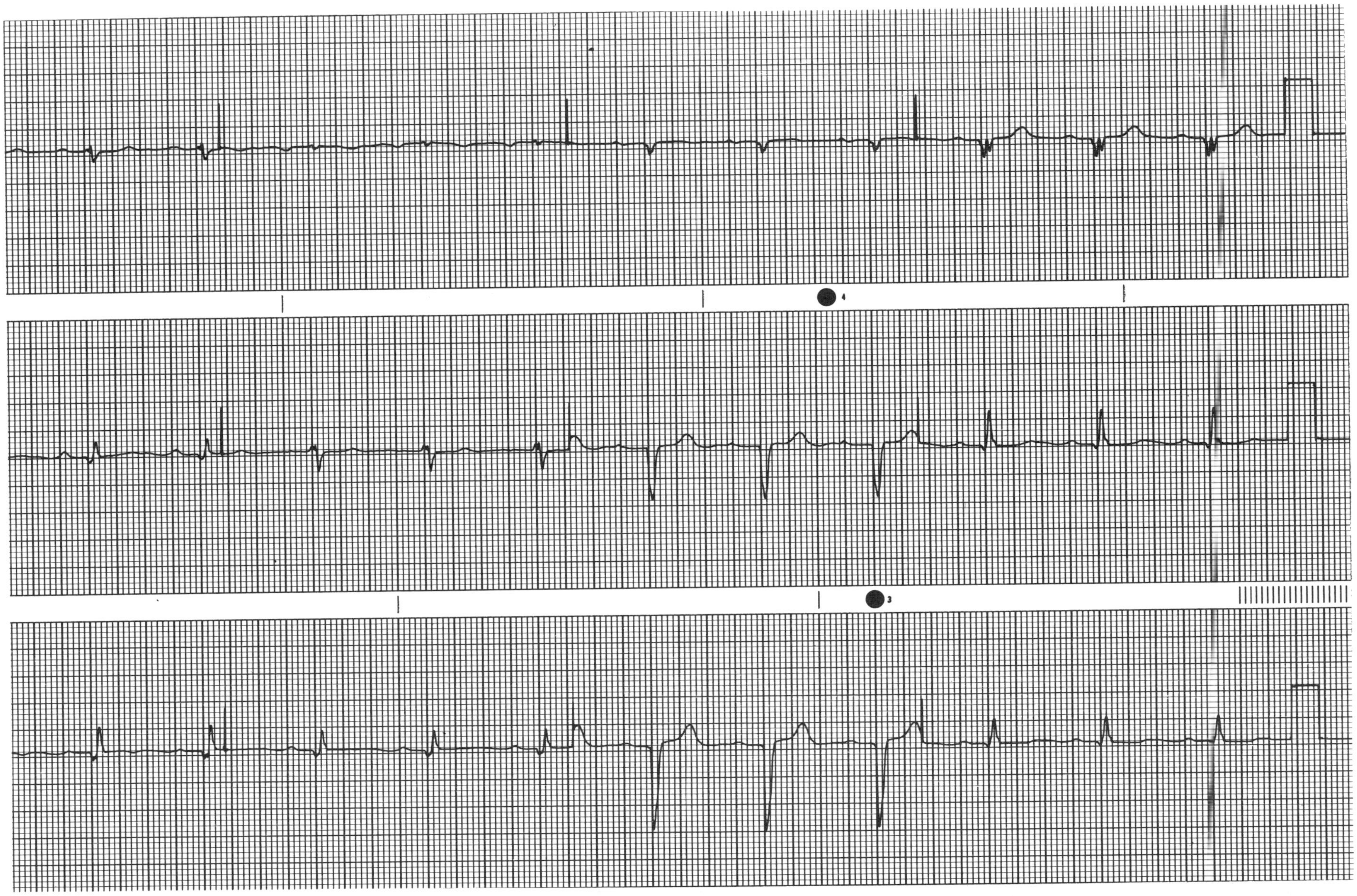

Practice 12 Lead ECG #53

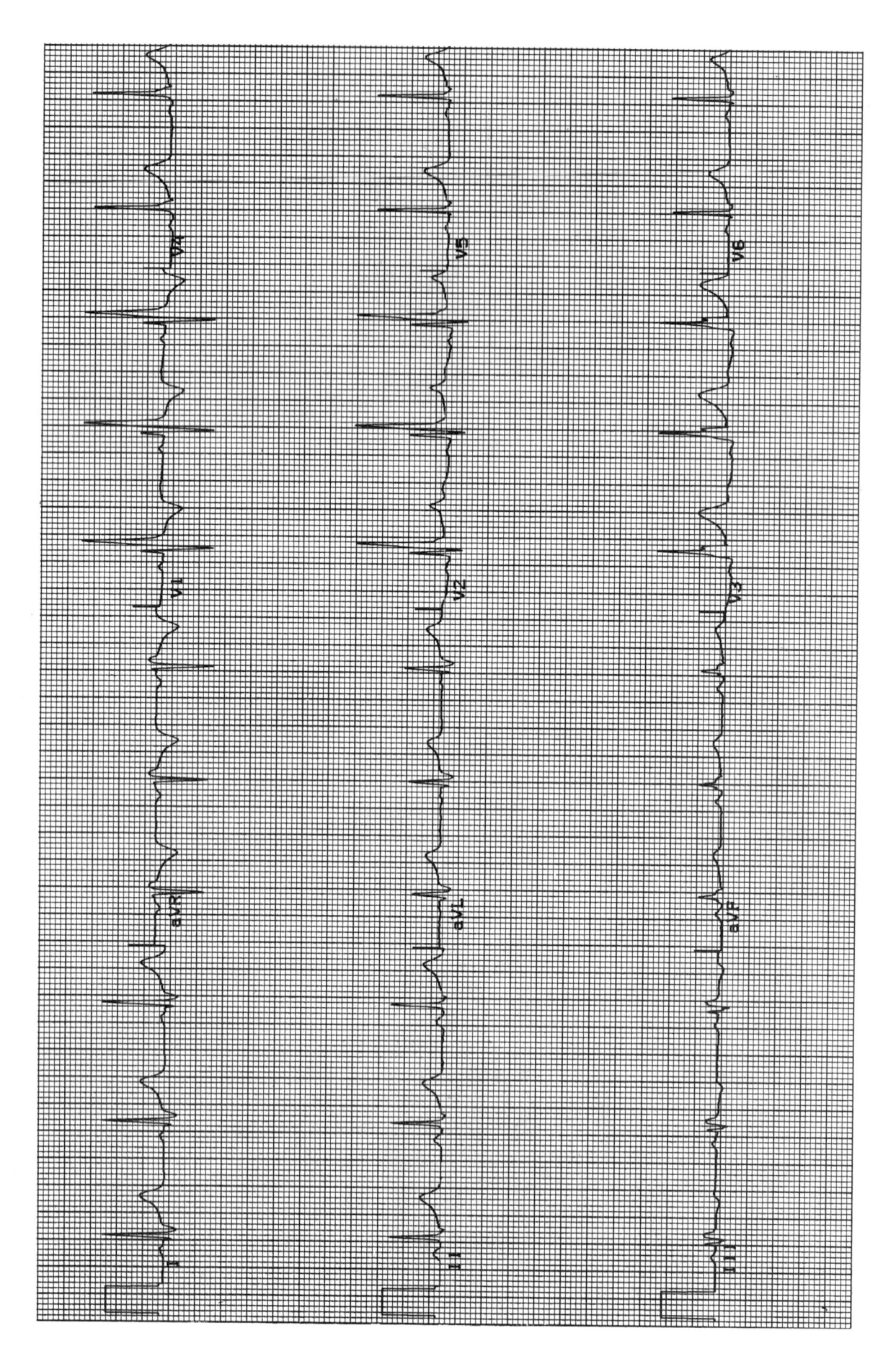

Practice 12 Lead ECG #54

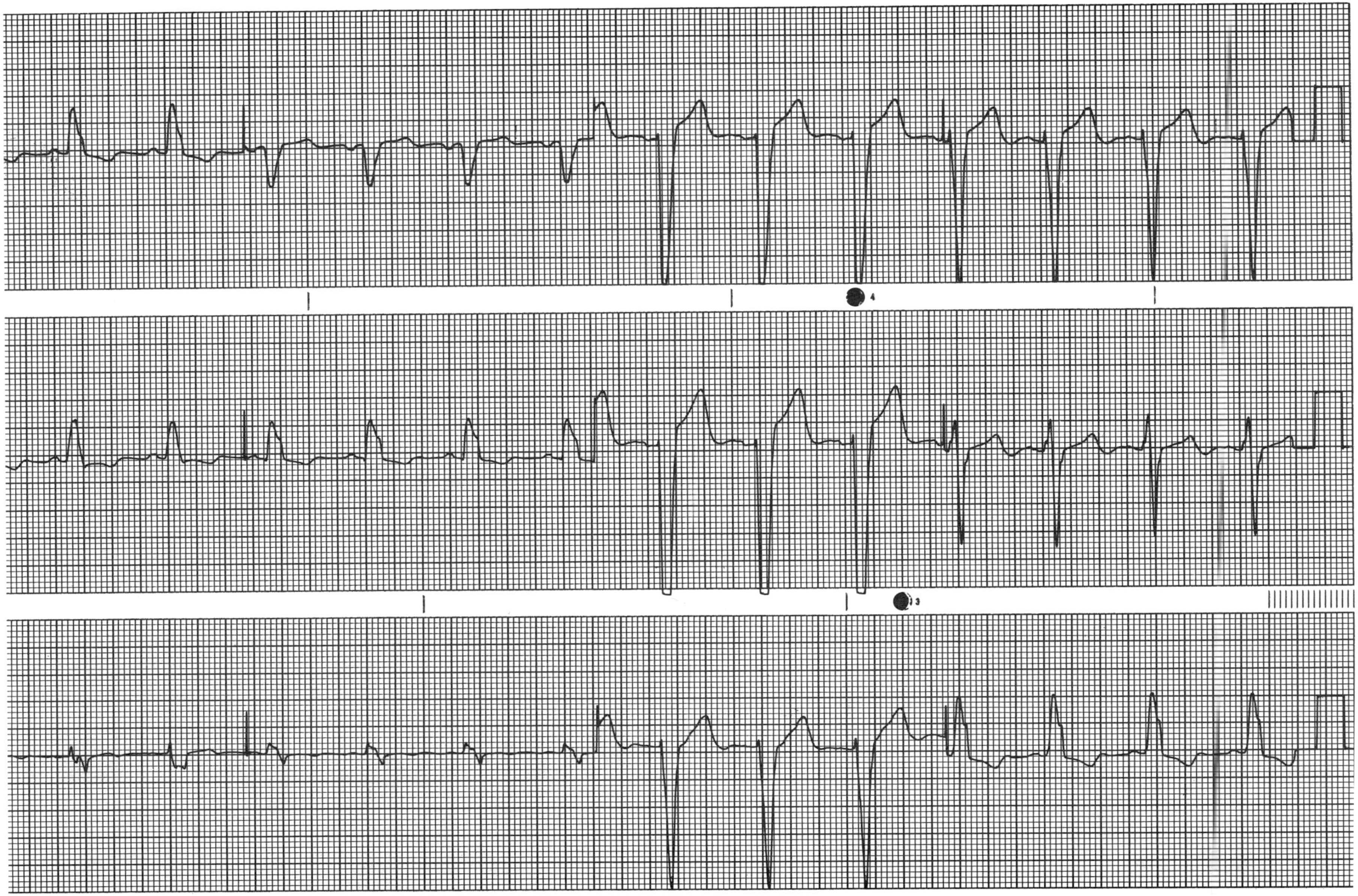

Practice 12 Lead ECG #55

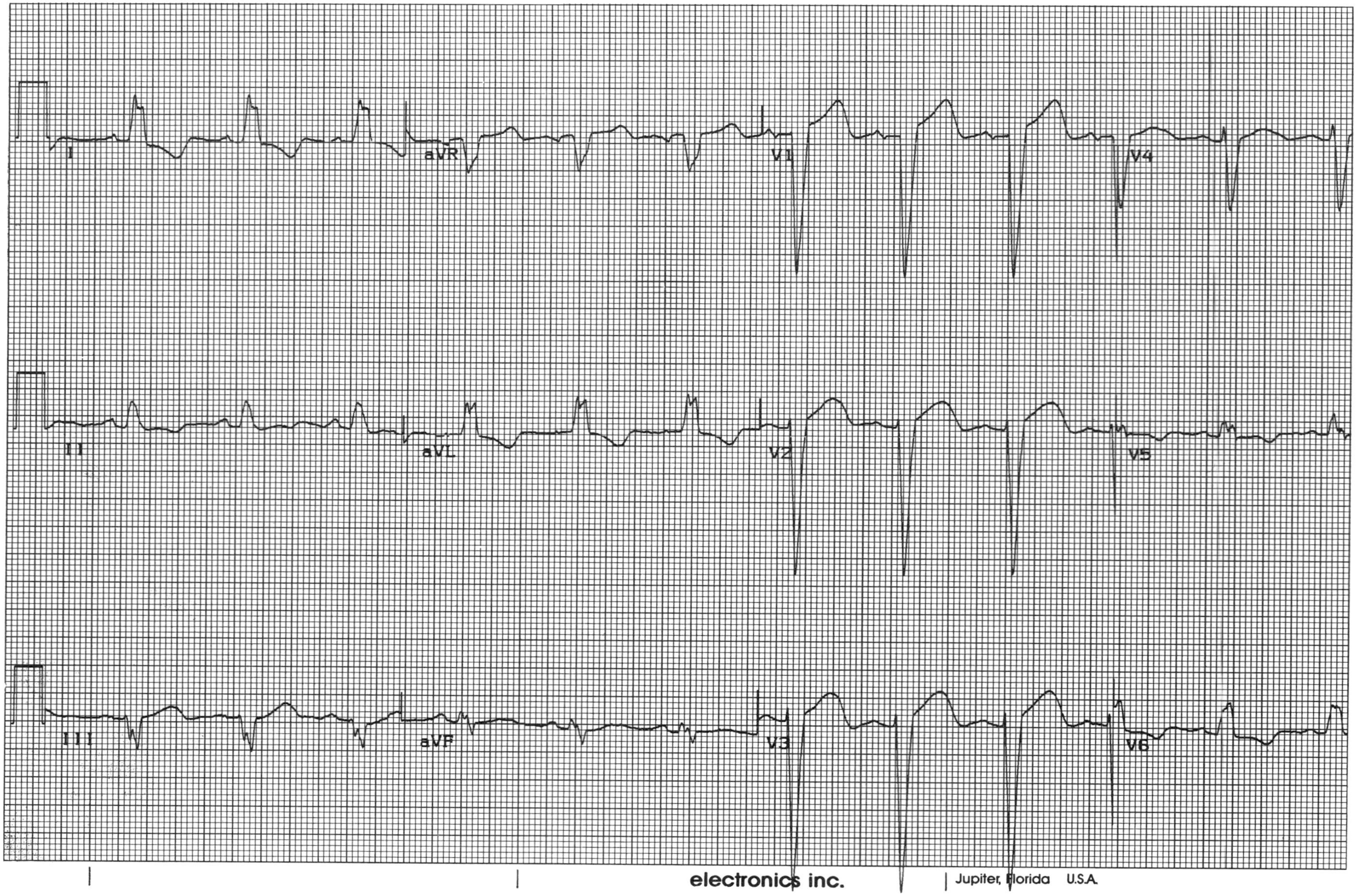

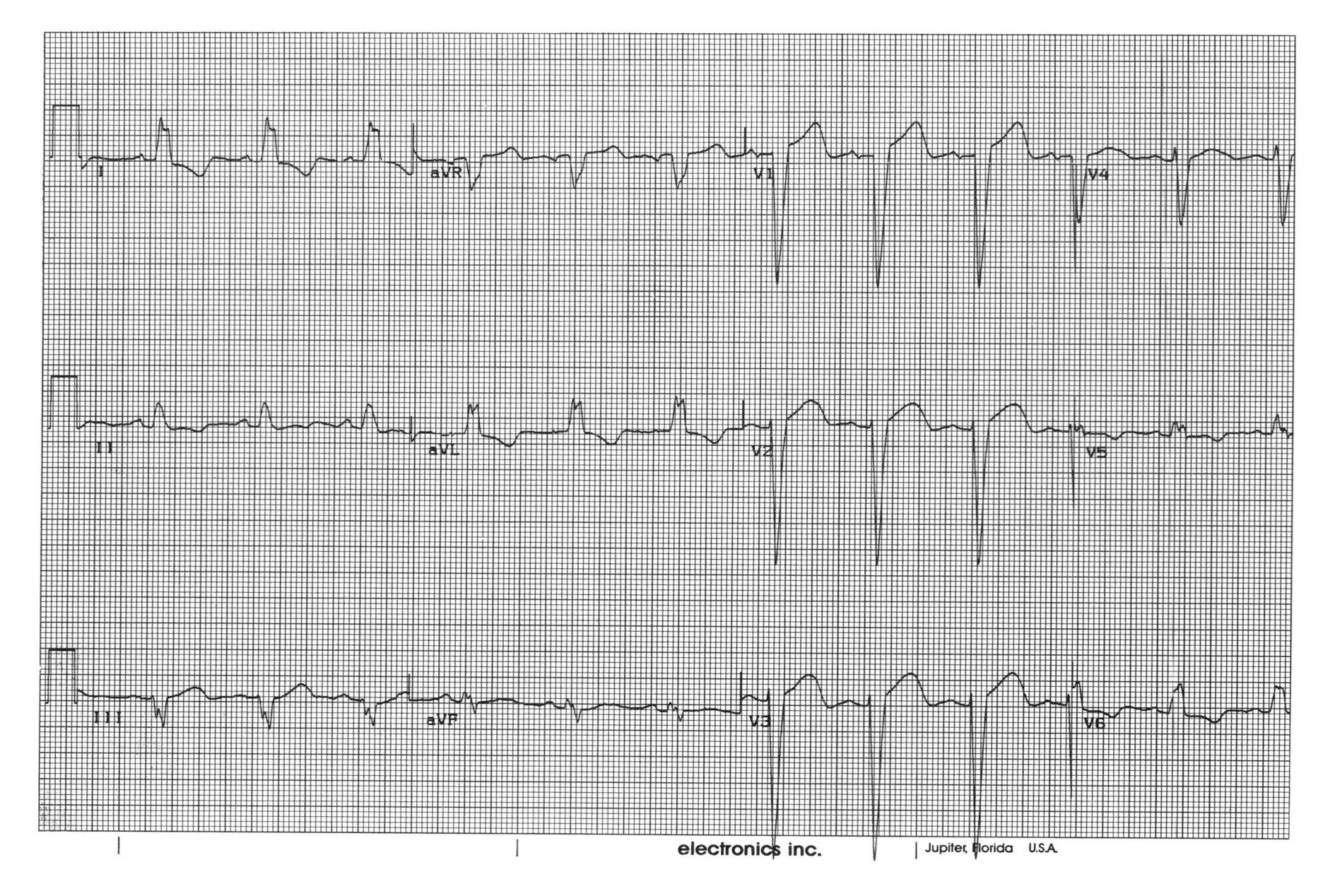

Practice 12 Lead ECG #56

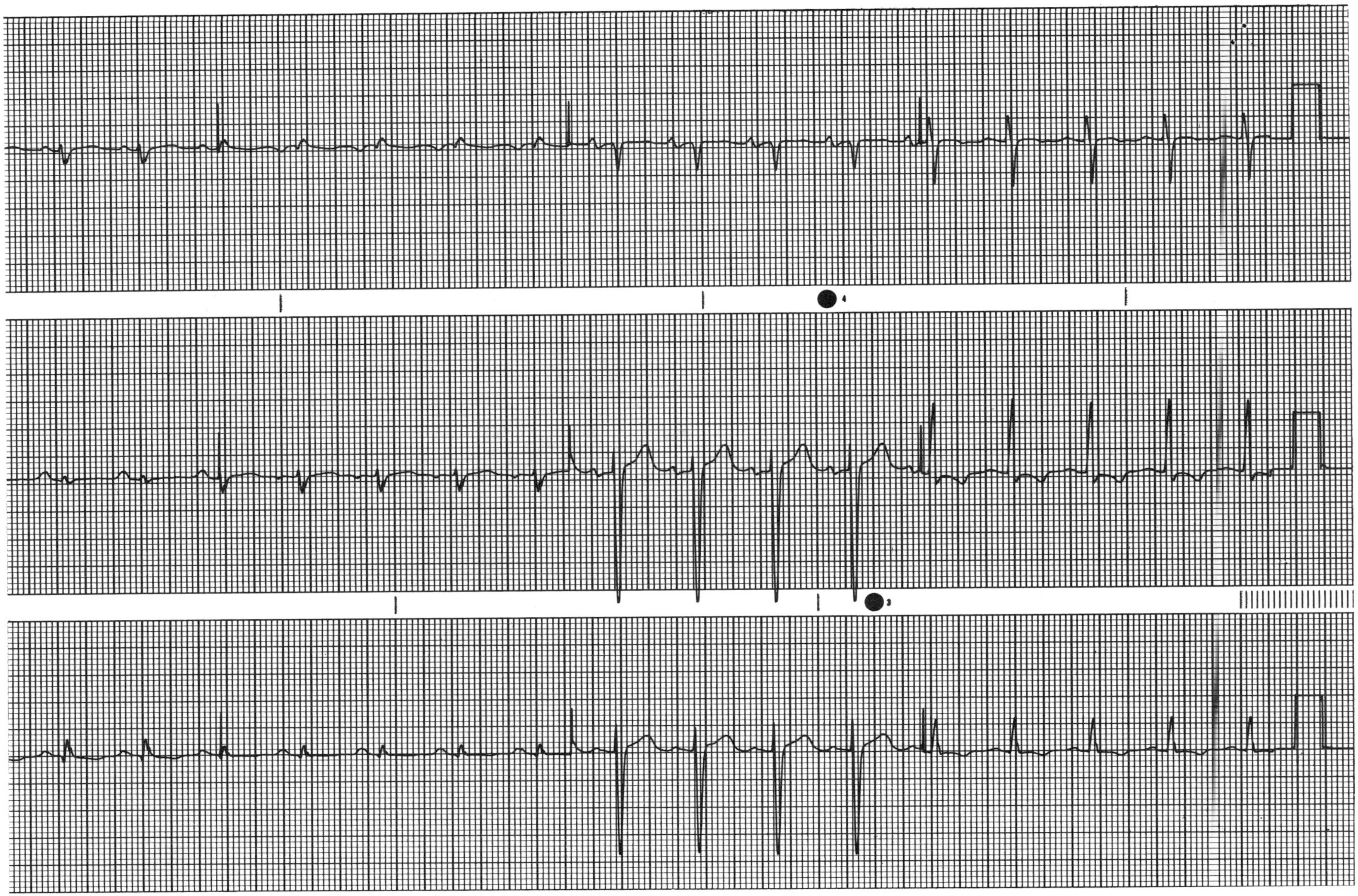

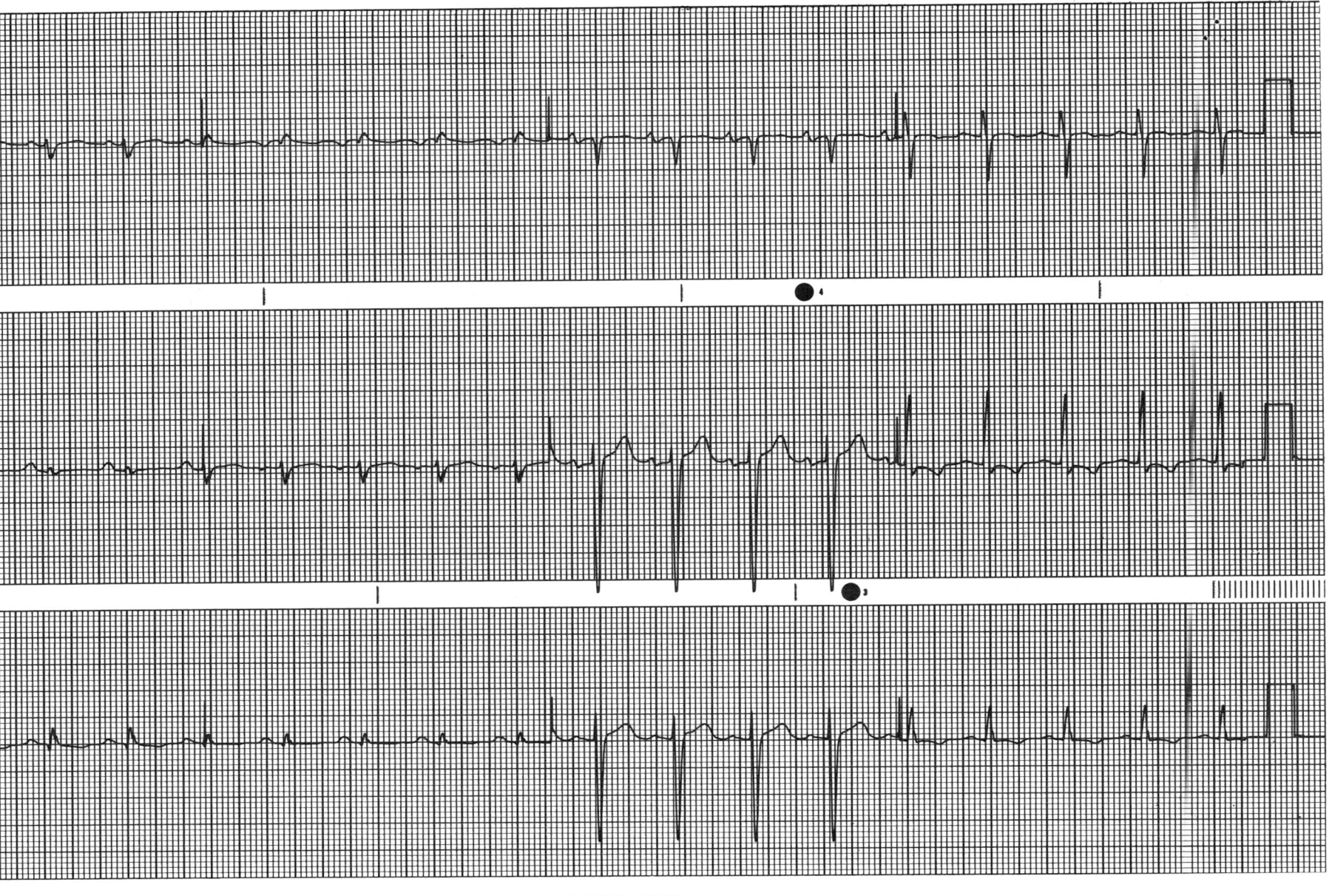

Practice 12 Lead ECG #57

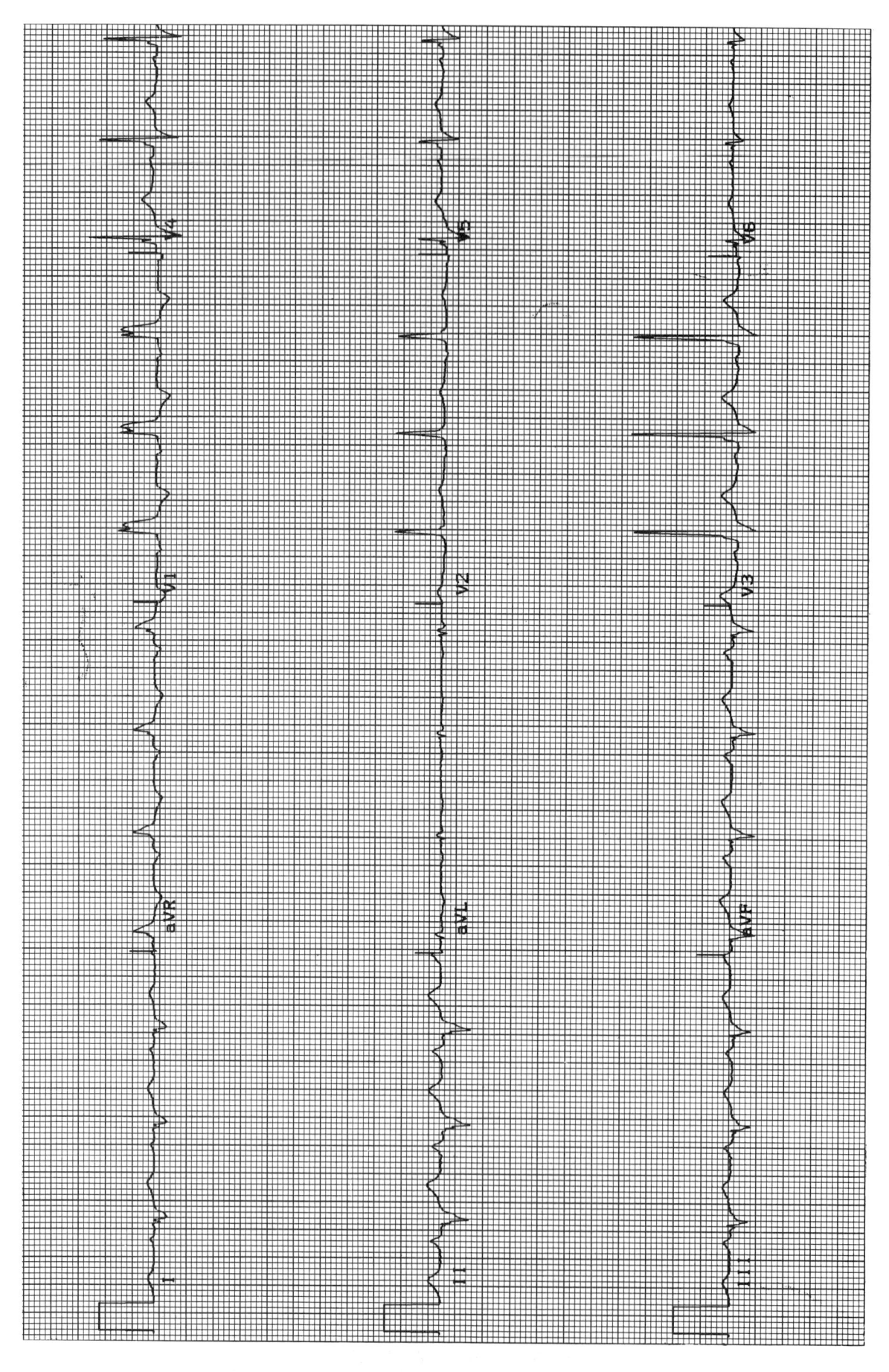

Practice 12 Lead ECG #58

Practice 12 Lead ECG #59

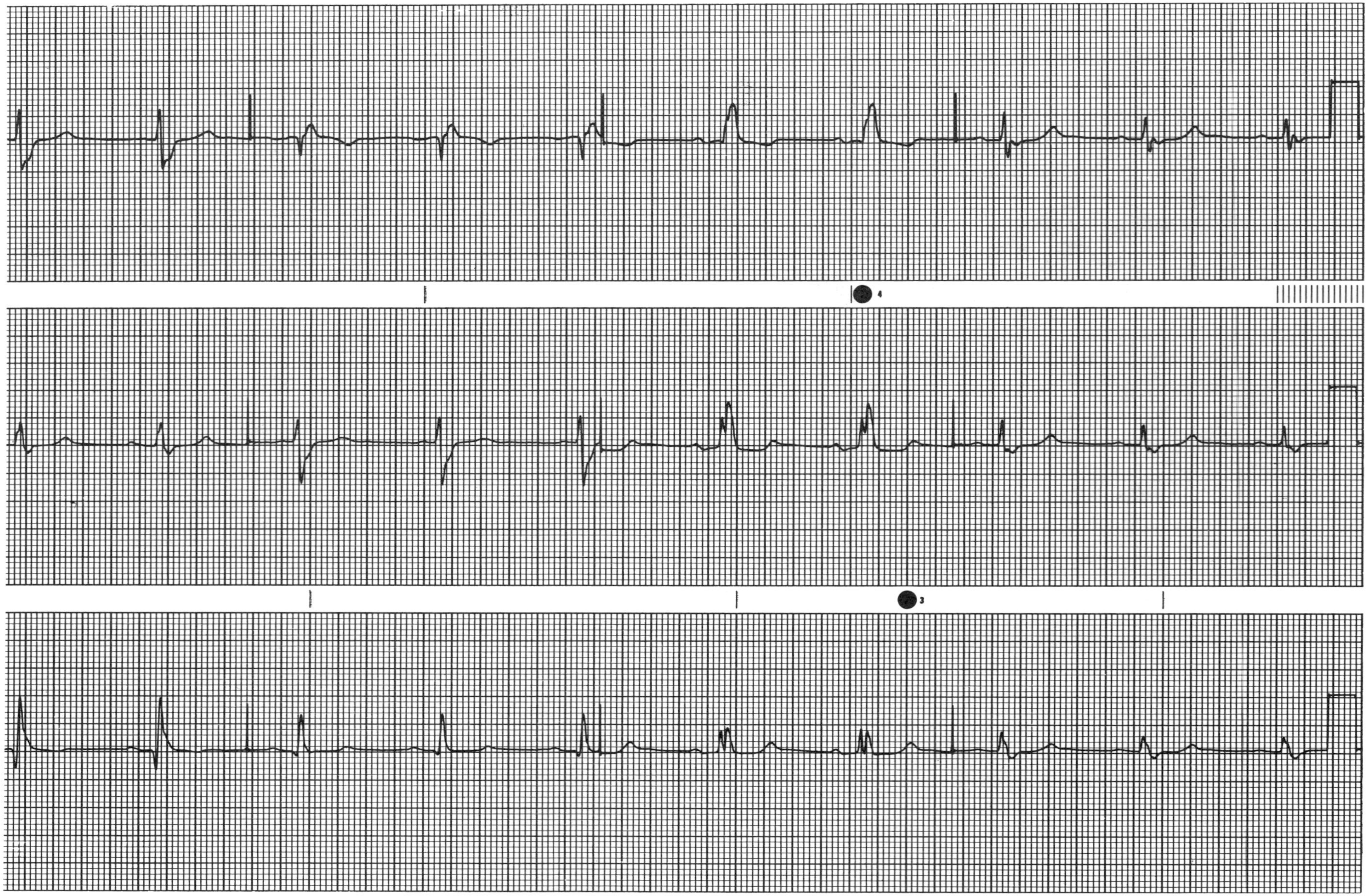

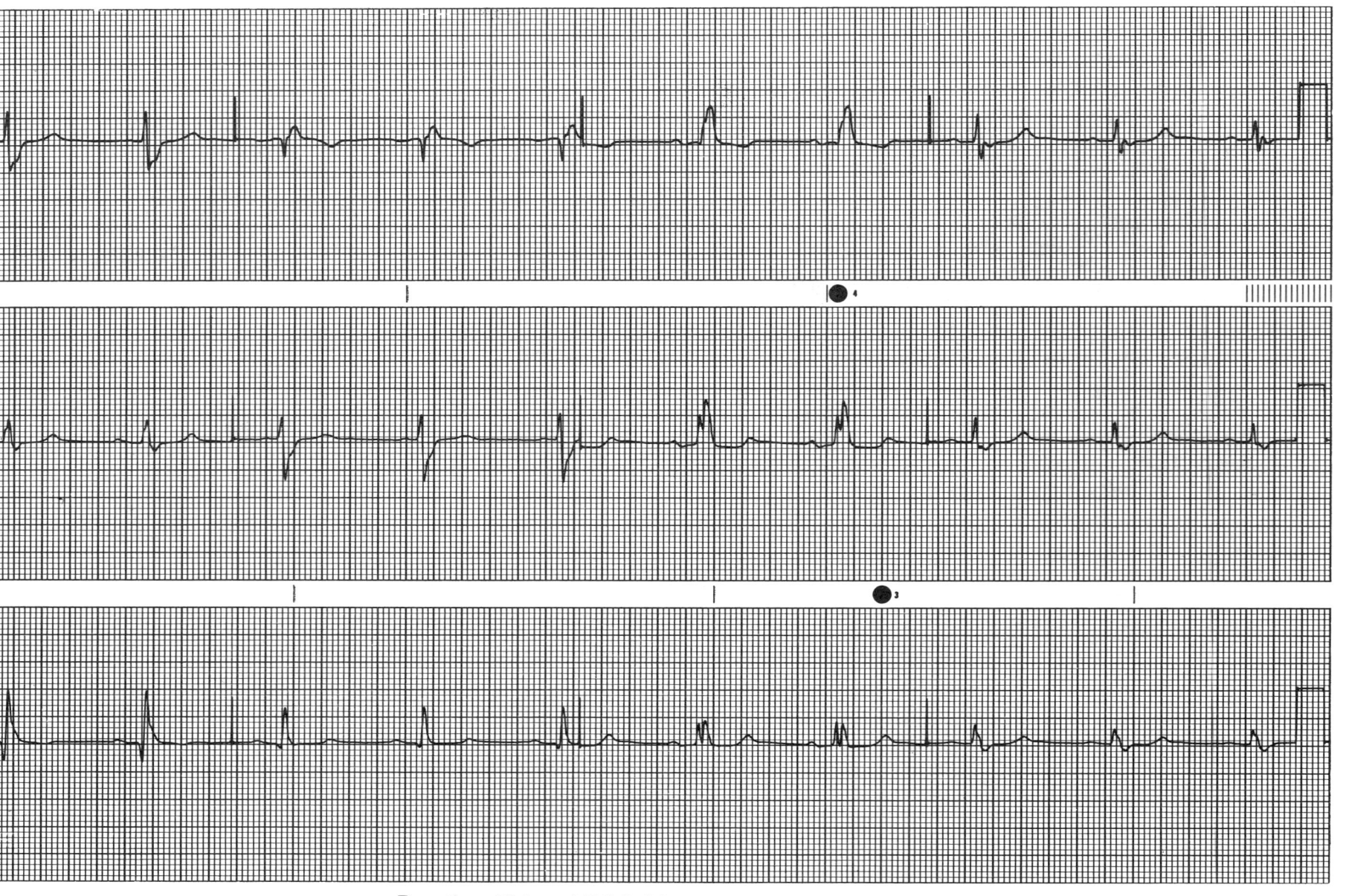

Practice 12 Lead ECG #60

Chapter 6 — Intraventricular Conduction Defects (IVCD)

ANSWERS TO PRACTICE 12 LEAD ECGs #46-60

46. **Basic rhythm:** Atrial fibrillation with rapid ventricular rate and PVCs (fifth beat in V_1, V_2, V_3)
    Frontal plane axis: LAD quadrant -60°
    R wave progression: Abnormal: qrR^1 in V_1; RR^1 in V_2, V_3
    Complex configuration: Abnormal as noted above and slurred s in V_5, V_6
    Complex duration: Abnormal: 0.12 seconds
    P wave: θ
    ST segment: Depressed in V_4, V_5, V_6
    Secondary ST-T changes: V_1, V_2, V_3
    12 Lead ECG Interpretation: Abnormal

    - Right bundle branch block ⎫ bifascicular block
    - Left anterior descending hemiblock ⎭

    - ST-T changes in V_4, V_5, V_6 may be due to lateral ischemia or digitalis effect (Chapters 7 and 9)
    - q wave in V_1 due to septal infarction (Chapter 7)

47. **Basic rhythm:** Second degree AV heart block type II. Patient is 81 years old and asymptomatic.
    Frontal plane axis: LAD quadrant -30°
    R wave progression: Normal
    Complex configuration: Small r in II, small q in I
    Complex duration: Normal
    P wave: Normal: PRi is constant and prolonged at 0.26 seconds. Every other P wave does not conduct. Some of the nonconducted P waves could easily be mistaken for U waves.
    ST segment: Normal
    T wave: Normal
    12 Lead ECG Interpretation: Abnormal
        - Second degree AV heart block type II
        - LADH

48. **Basic rhythm:** Normal sinus rhythm
    Frontal plane axis: Normal 0° (aVF has the most equiphasic complex)
    R wave progression: Abnormal: QS in V_1; rS in V_2, V_3, V_4 (loss of anterior forces) with transition in V_5 — too late!
    Complex configuration: Abnormal as noted above and RR^1/SS^1 in several leads
    Complex duration: Abnormal: 0.14 seconds
    P wave: Normal
    ST segment: Elevated in V_1, V_2, V_3
    Secondary ST-T changes: I, aVL, V_5, V_6
    12 Lead ECG Interpretation: Abnormal
        - Left bundle branch block

Chapter 6 — Intraventricular Conduction Defects (IVCD)

49. **Basic rhythm:** Sinus tachycardia
    Frontal plane axis: Normal 0°
    R wave progression: Abnormal starting with the rSR' in V_1; r r' in V_2; Rr' in V_3; rsr' in V_4, V_5
    Complex configuration: Abnormal as noted above and r' in several other leads
    Complex duration: Normal: 0.11 seconds
    P wave: Normal
    Secondary ST-T changes: V_1, V_2 (right precordial leads)
    12 Lead ECG Interpretation: Abnormal
    - Incomplete right bundle branch block. Bundle branch block is referred to as incomplete when the duration of the complex is less than 0.12 seconds.

50. **Basic rhythm:** Normal sinus rhythm
    Frontal plane axis: LAD quadrant -60° (-45° corrected. Correcting the frontal plane axis is discussed on page 186.)
    R wave progression: Normal
    Complex configuration: Small r in lead II, small q in lead I
    Duration of complex: Normal: 0.10 seconds
    P wave: Normal
    ST segment: Normal
    T wave: Normal
    Secondary ST-T changes: None
    12 Lead ECG Interpretation: Abnormal
    - Left anterior descending hemiblock

51. **Basic rhythm:** Normal sinus rhythm
    Frontal plane axis: RAD quadrant: +120°
    R wave progression: Normal
    Complex configuration: Small r in aVL, small q in III; low voltage in the frontal plane leads
    Complex duration: Normal: 0.08 seconds
    P wave: Normal
    ST segment: Normal
    T wave: Inverted in V_4, V_5, V_6 (consider lateral ischemia — Chapter 7)
    12 Lead ECG Interpretation: Abnormal
    - Left posterior hemiblock
    - Low voltage complex: consider pulmonary disease, pericardial effusion, or normal variant

Chapter 6 — Intraventricular Conduction Defects (IVCD)

52. **Basic rhythm:** Atrial fibrillation, controlled
    Frontal plane axis: Normal 0°
    R wave progression: Abnormal: loss of anterior forces and transition in V_6
    Complex configuration: Abnormal as noted above and RR^I in I, aVL, V_6; rSS^I in III; R^I in other leads
    Complex duration: Abnormal: 0.14 seconds
    P wave: θ
    ST-T segment: Elevated in V_1, V_2, V_3
    Secondary ST-T changes: I, aVL, V_5, V_6
    12 Lead ECG Interpretation: Abnormal
    - Atrial fibrillation
    - Left bundle branch block

53. **Basic rhythm:** Normal sinus rhythm with first degree AV heart block
    Frontal plane axis: RAD quadrant +120°
    R wave progression: Abnormal: Loss of anterior forces
    Complex configuration: Abnormal with qs in V_1 and V_4, QS in V_2, V_3; qR in II, III, aVF; small r in I; small q in II
    Complex duration: Normal: 0.10 seconds
    P wave: Normal
    ST segment: Normal with slight elevation in V_3
    T wave: Abnormally low/inverted in II, III, aVF
    12 Lead ECG Interpretation: Abnormal
    - First degree AV heart block
    - Left posterior hemiblock
    - Anteroseptal, inferior myocardial infarction (will be discussed in Chapter 8)

54. **Basic rhythm:** Normal sinus rhythm
    Frontal plane axis: Normal +30°
    R wave progression: Abnormal beginning with rSR^I in V_1
    Complex configuration: $r r^I$ in III; rSR^I in V_1; RsR^I in V_2; slurred s in I, aVL, V_5, V_6
    Complex duration: Abnormal: 0.12 seconds
    P wave: Normal
    Secondary ST-T changes: V_1
    12 Lead ECG Interpretation: Abnormal
    - Right bundle branch block

Note the width of the q waves in II, III, aVF, and V_1: These are pathological q waves which will be discussed in Chapter 8. Recall that q waves in V_1 are always pathological.

Recall that the most common clinical cause of the intraventricular conduction defects is anteroseptal myocardial infarction.

Chapter 6 — Intraventricular Conduction Defects (IVCD)

55. **Basic rhythm:** Normal sinus rhythm
    Frontal plane axis: Normal 0°
    R wave progression: Abnormal: r wave does not progress from V_1 to V_4 = loss of anterior forces.
    Complex configuration: Abnormal as noted above and RR' in several leads.
    Complex duration: Abnormal: 0.14 seconds
    P wave: Normal
    ST segment: Elevated in V_1, V_2
    Secondary ST-T changes: I, aVL, V_6
    12 Lead ECG Interpretation: Abnormal
    - Left bundle branch block

56. **Basic rhythm:** Normal sinus rhythm
    Frontal plane axis: Normal 0°
    R wave progression: Abnormal: Loss of anterior forces with transition in V_5
    Complex configuration: Abnormal as noted above and RR' or rr' in I, II, aVL, V_5, V_6; $rr's$ in aVF; rsS' in III.
    Duration of complex: Abnormal: 0.14 seconds
    P wave: Normal
    ST segment: Elevated in V_1, V_2, V_3
    Secondary ST-T changes: I, II, aVL, V_5, V_6
    12 Lead ECG Interpretation: Abnormal
    - Left bundle branch block

57. **Basic rhythm:** Sinus tachycardia
    Frontal plane axis: RAD quadrant +150°
    R wave progression: Abnormal: transition occurs in V_5
    Complex configuration: Small r in I, small q in III
    Complex duration: Normal
    P wave: Normal
    ST segment: Normal
    T wave: Inverted in III, V_4, V_5, V_6
    12 Lead ECG Interpretation: Abnormal
    - Left posterior hemiblock
    - Non-specific T wave abnormality (Chapter 9)

58. **Basic rhythm:** Normal sinus rhythm
    Frontal plane axis: No man's land quadrant -120°
    R wave progression: Abnormal: RR' in V_1
    Complex configuration: Abnormal as noted above and slurred s wave in V_5, V_6; r' or s' in most leads
    Complex duration: Abnormal: 0.12 seconds
    P wave: Normal
    Secondary ST-T changes: V_1
    12 Lead ECG Interpretation: Abnormal
    - Right bundle branch block

Chapter 6 — Intraventricular Conduction Defects (IVCD)

59. **Basic rhythm:** Sinus tachycardia
    Frontal plane axis: LAD quadrant -60°
    R wave progression: Abnormal: rR' in V_1, V_2; transition never occurs
    Complex configuration: Abnormal as noted above and slurred S waves in V_5, V_6; small q in I; small r in III
    Complex duration: Abnormal: 0.12 seconds
    P wave: Normal
    Secondary ST-T changes: V_1, V_2
    12 Lead ECG Interpretation: Abnormal
    - Sinus tachycardia
    - RBBB ⎫
    - LADH ⎬ bifascicular block

60. **Basic rhythm:** Normal sinus rhythm
    Frontal plane axis: RAD quadrant +120°
    R wave progression: Abnormal: RR' in V_1, V_2, V_3
    Complex configuration: Abnormal as noted above with small r in aVL; small q in aVF
    Complex duration: Abnormal: 0.14 seconds
    P wave: Normal
    Secondary ST-T changes: V_1, V_2
    12 Lead ECG Interpretation: Abnormal
    - Right bundle branch block ⎫
    - Left posterior hemiblock   ⎬ bifascicular block

Practice 12 lead ECGs #61-70 follow, with answers beginning on page 182.

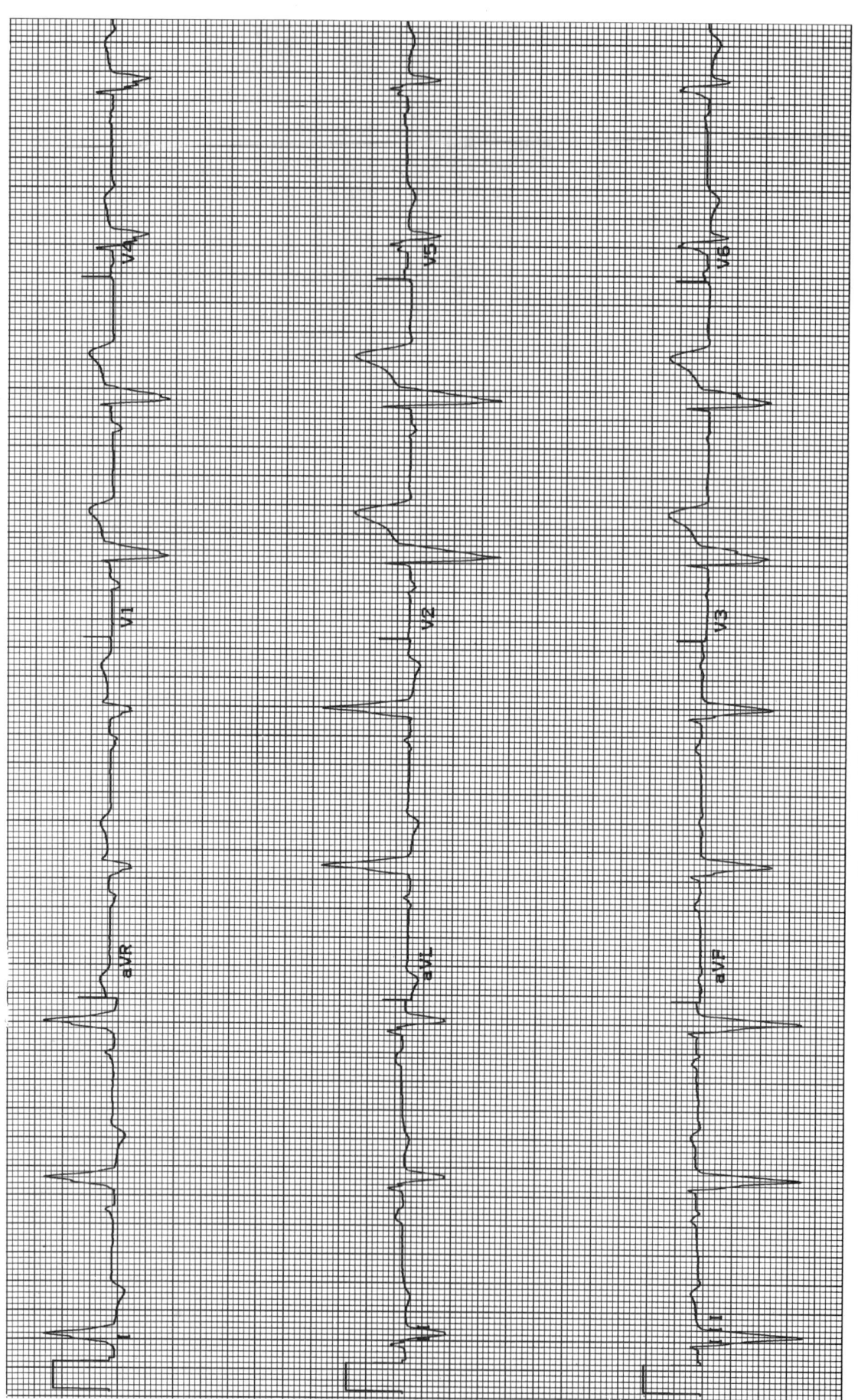

Practice 12 Lead ECG #61

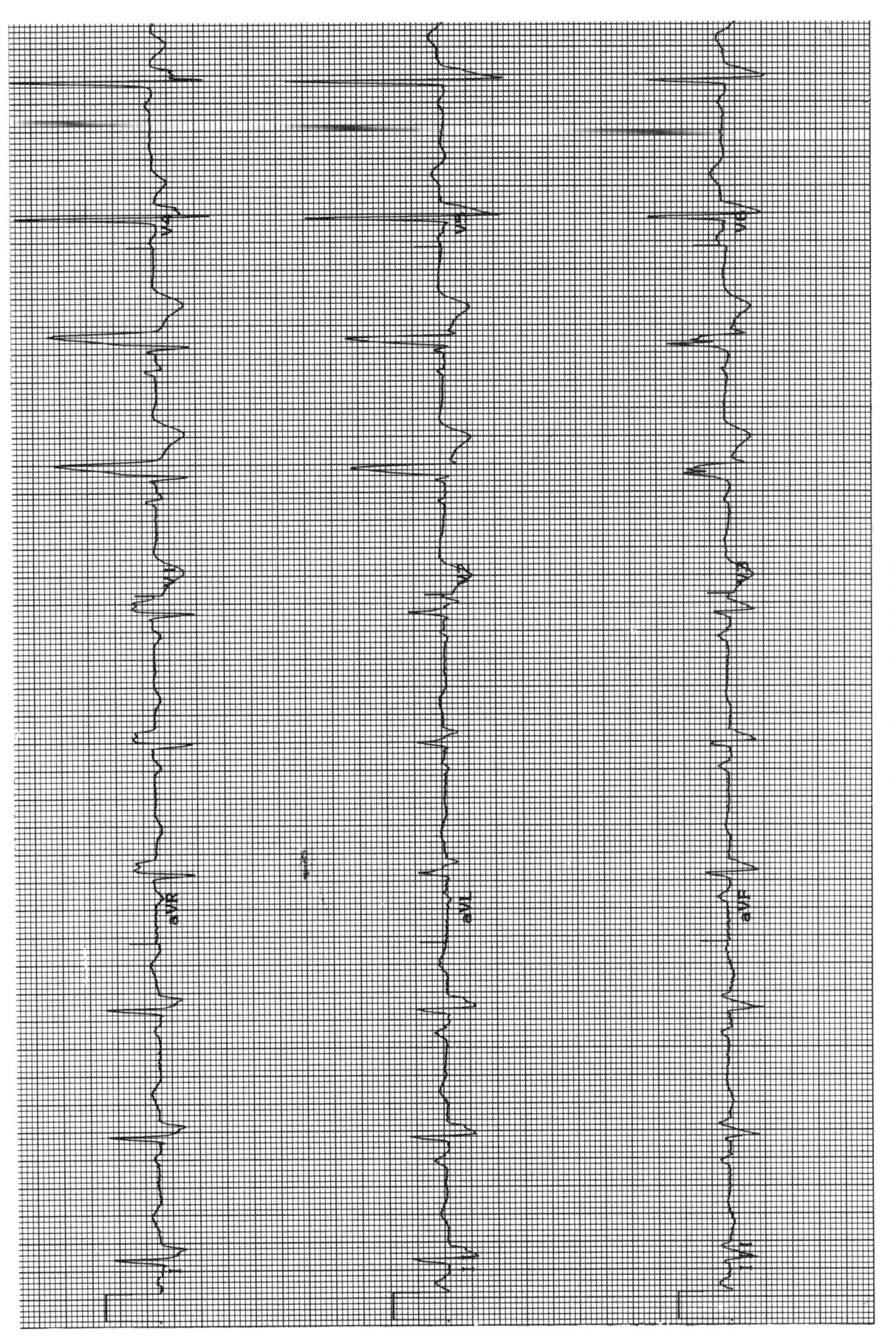

Practice 12 Lead ECG #62

Practice 12 Lead ECG #63

Practice 12 Lead ECG #64

Practice 12 Lead ECG #65

Practice 12 Lead ECG #66

Practice 12 Lead ECG #67

Practice 12 Lead ECG #68

Practice 12 Lead ECG #69

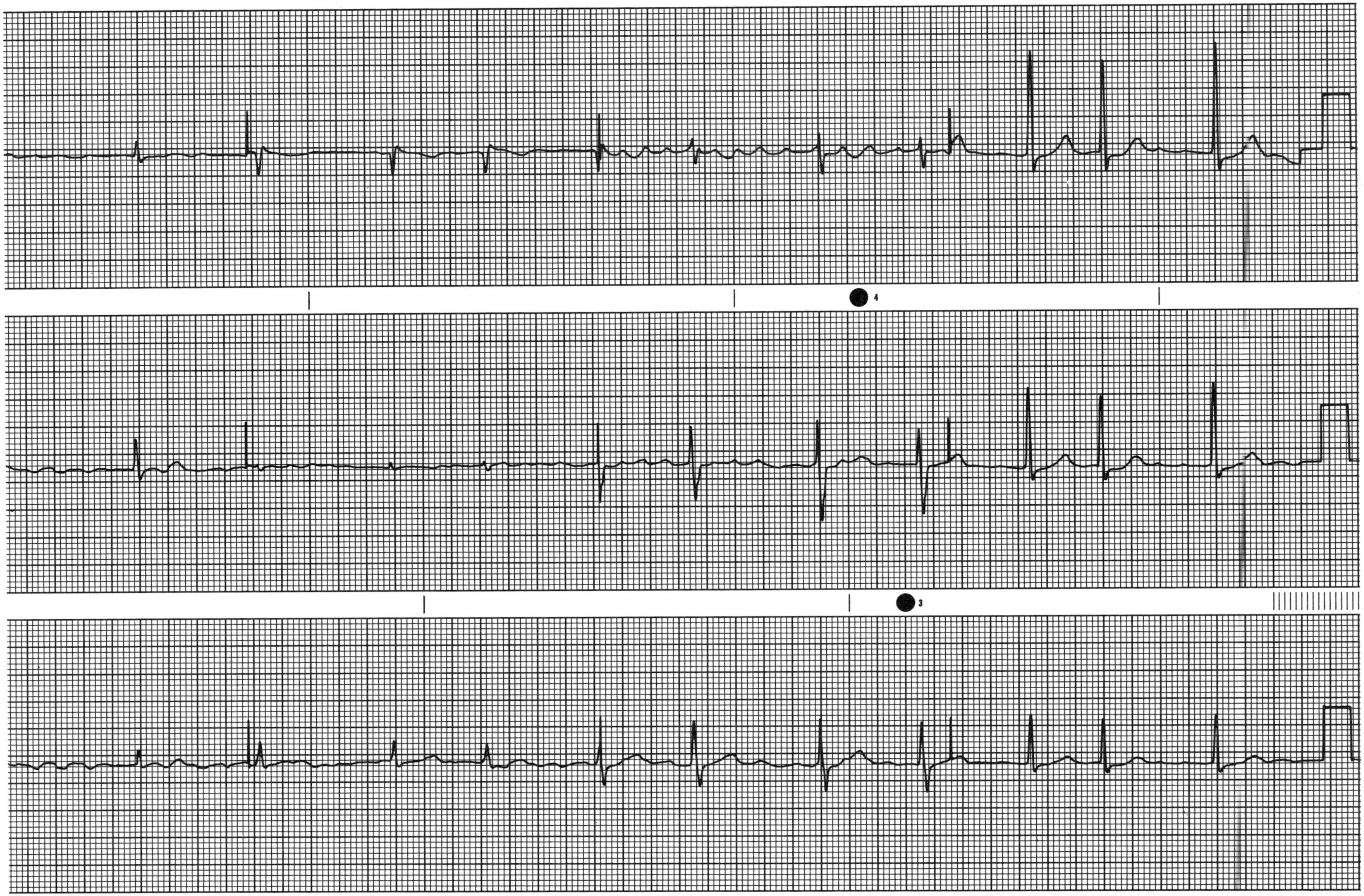

Practice 12 Lead ECG #70

Chapter 6 — Intraventricular Conduction Defects (IVCD)

ANSWERS TO PRACTICE 12 LEAD ECGs #61-70

61. **Basic rhythm:** Sinus bradycardia with first degree AV heart block (PRi 0.22 seconds)
    Frontal plane axis: LAD quadrant -30°
    R wave progression: Abnormal: Loss of anterior forces in V_3, V_4; transition occurs in V_6 — too late!
    Complex configuration: Abnormal as noted above and R' in other leads
    Complex duration: Abnormal: 0.16 seconds
    P wave: Wide and notched in II, III; abnormal P terminal in V_1
    ST segment: Elevated in V_1, V_2, V_3
    Secondary ST-T changes: I, aVL, V_5, V_6
    T wave: Inverted in II
    12 Lead ECG Interpretation: Abnormal
    - Sinus bradycardia with first degree AV heart block
    - Left bundle branch block
    - P mitrale

62. **Basic rhythm:** Normal sinus rhythm
    Frontal plane axis: Normal 0°
    R wave progression: Abnormal: rSR' in V_1; $rR's$ in V_2; $RR's$ in V_3; RSs' in V_4 and V_5
    Complex configuration: Abnormal as noted above and R'/S' in other leads; deep slurred S waves in V_5, V_6; R wave in V_5 = 27 mm
    Complex duration: Abnormal: 0.16 seconds
    P wave: Wide and notched in II, III; large P terminal (greater than 1 mm deep and wide) in V_1
    Secondary ST-T changes: V_1, V_2, V_3, V_4
    Other: VAT in V_5 is 0.05 seconds
    12 Lead ECG Interpretation: Abnormal
    - P mitrale
    - Right bundle branch block
    - Left ventricular hypertrophy
    LVH Estes score for this patient:

Voltage criteria	3
Secondary ST-T changes (patient not on digitalis)	3
qRs interval increased (due to RBBB)	0
VAT in V_5 = 0.05 seconds	1
Abnormal P terminal in V_1	3
TOTAL	10 points

Chapter 6 — Intraventricular Conduction Defects (IVCD)

63. **Basic rhythm:** Sinus tachycardia
    Frontal plane axis: LAD quadrant -30°
    R wave progression: Normal
    Complex configuration: R in V_5, $V_6 \geq 25$ millimeters
    Complex duration: Normal: 0.08 seconds
    P wave: Wide in II, III, aVF (also notched in III, aVF if you look closely); abnormal P terminal in V_1, V_2
    Secondary ST-T changes: V_4, V_5, V_6
    12 Lead ECG Interpretation: Abnormal
      - Sinus tachycardia
      - P mitrale
      - Left ventricular hypertrophy
    Estes score for this patient (on digitalis)
Voltage criteria	3
Secondary ST-T changes	2
Left axis deviation -30°	2
Abnormal P terminal in V_1	3
TOTAL	10 points

64. **Basic rhythm:** Normal sinus rhythm
    Frontal plane axis: LAD quadrant -60°
    R wave progression: Abnormal with rsR' in V_1 and RR's in V_2
    Complex configuration: Abnormal as noted above and large, slurred S in V_5, V_6; small r in II; small q in I
    Complex duration: Abnormal: 0.14 seconds
    P wave: Wide and notched in II, III, aVF; abnormal P terminal in V_1
    Secondary ST-T changes: V_1, V_2
    12 Lead ECG Interpretation: Abnormal
      - P mitrale
      - Right bundle branch block   } bifascicular block
      - Left anterior descending hemiblock

65. **Basic rhythm:** Normal sinus rhythm
    Frontal plane axis: Normal 0°
    R wave progression: Abnormal: r in V_1 fails to progress and persists across the precordium as an r wave
    Complex configuration: Abnormal as noted above and RR' in I, II, aVL, aVF; loss of septal q wave in V_5, V_6
    Complex duration: Abnormal: 0.14 seconds
    P wave: Normal
    ST segment: Elevated in V_1, V_2, V_3
    Secondary ST-T changes: I, aVL
    12 Lead ECG Interpretation: Abnormal
      - Left bundle branch block

Chapter 6 — Intraventricular Conduction Defects (IVCD)

66. **Basic rhythm:** Normal sinus rhythm
    Frontal plane axis: LAD quadrant -30°
    R wave progression: Abnormal: Loss of anterior forces
    Complex configuration: Abnormal as noted above and R' in several leads.
    Complex duration: Abnormal: 0.14 seconds
    P wave: Normal
    ST segment: Slightly elevated in V_1, V_2
    Secondary ST-T changes: I, aVL, V_5, V_6
    12 Lead ECG Interpretation: Abnormal
    - Left bundle branch block

67. **Basic rhythm:** Normal sinus rhythm
    Frontal plane axis: Normal +30°
    R wave progression: Normal
    Complex configuration: Normal
    Complex duration: Normal
    P wave: Normal
    ST segment: Normal
    T wave: Normal
    Secondary ST-T changes: None
    12 Lead ECG Interpretation: Normal

68. **Basic rhythm:** Atrial fibrillation, controlled
    Frontal plane axis: RAD quadrant +120°
    R wave progression: Normal with transition in V_4
    Complex configuration: Small r in I; small q in III
    Complex duration: Normal: 0.08 seconds
    P wave: Normal
    ST segment: Normal
    T wave: Difficult to see because of fibrillatory waves
    12 Lead ECG Interpretation: Abnormal
    - Atrial fibrillation, controlled
    - Left posterior hemiblock
    - Nonspecific T wave abnormality (Chapter 9)

69. **Basic rhythm:** Sinus tachycardia
    Frontal plane axis: Normal 0°
    R wave progression: Normal
    Complex configuration: Normal
    Complex duration: Normal
    P wave: Normal
    ST segment: Normal
    T wave: Normal
    Secondary ST-T changes: None
    12 Lead ECG Interpretation: Normal except for sinus tachycardia

Chapter 6 — Intraventricular Conduction Defects (IVCD)

70. **Basic rhythm:** Atrial fibrillation, controlled
    Frontal plane axis: Normal +60°
    R wave progression: Normal
    Complex configuration: Normal
    Complex duration: Normal
    P wave: θ
    ST segment: Normal
    T wave: Difficult to see due to fibrillatory waves
    Secondary ST-T changes: θ
    12 Lead ECG Interpretation: Normal except for atrial fibrillation

Chapter 6 – Intraventricular Conduction Defects (IVCD)

CORRECTING THE FRONTAL PLANE AXIS

To correct the axis, i.e., increase its accuracy, the rule is 5° for every 1 millimeter difference:

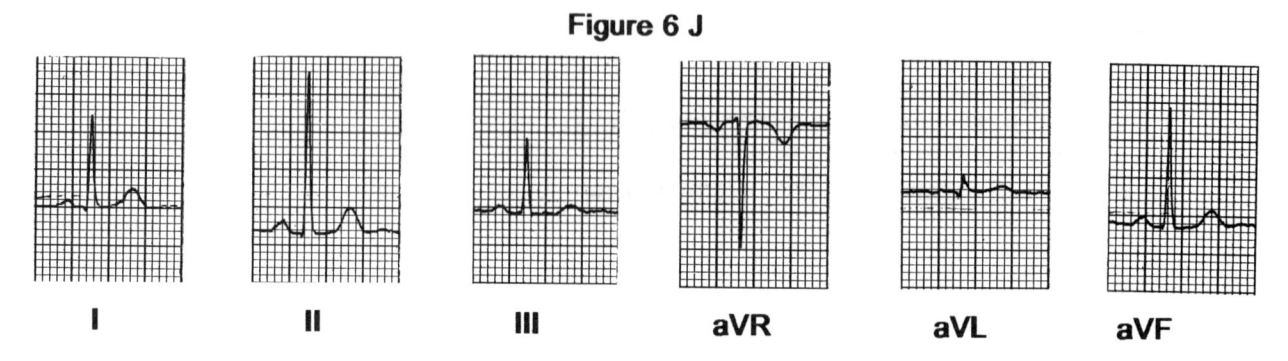

Figure 6 J

| I | II | III | aVR | aVL | aVF |

In Figure 6 J, aVL is 1 millimeter more positive than negative, so the axis of +60° is corrected by swinging it 5° towards aVL on the hexaxial figure.

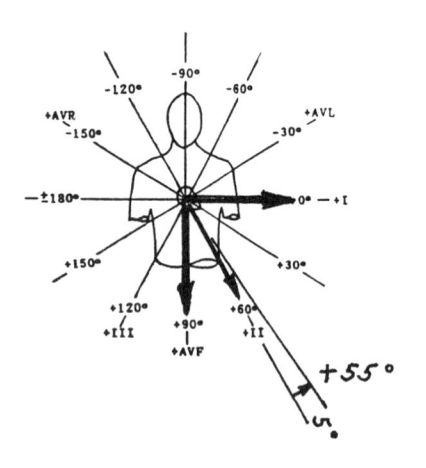

5° towards aVL (the complex is more positive than negative so we know it is going more towards aVL than away from aVL).

Reconsider practice tracing #62 on page 173. The axis was identified as 0°. However, the complex in aVF is more negative than positive. The complex in aVF is 4 millimeters positive but 6 millimeters negative – a difference of 2 millimeters. The rule is 5° for each millimeter. In tracing # 62 the difference is 2 millimeters or 10°. Starting at the plotted axis of 0°, swing the axis 10° away from aVF: the corrected axis is RAD quadrant -10°.

You swing away from aVF because in this case aVF is more negative. You would swing towards aVF if aVF were more positive. It is not necessary to correct the axis but it is discussed because people wonder why the axis is not always a number divisible by 30. And it is fun to know how to do it!

Correcting the axis is putting the icing on the cake. It is not necessary to correct a normal axis of +30° or +60°. Correcting a normal axis of 0° or +90°, however, may swing the axis into the left axis deviation or the right axis deviation quadrant, respectively.

CHAPTER 7
MYOCARDIAL ISCHEMIA, INJURY, AND INFARCTION

We will be looking at myocardial ischemia, injury, and infarction of the left ventricle. The left ventricle is larger than the right and it works harder. Myocardial infarctions usually occur in the left ventricle and that will be the focus of our discussion.

CORONARY ARTERY DISTRIBUTION

There are two main coronary arteries, the right and the left. The left coronary artery divides into two main branches: the left circumflex and the left anterior descending coronary arteries. Consider the coronary artery distribution to the left ventricle and the conduction system of the heart:

1. The **right coronary artery** supplies the right heart; in the left ventricle it supplies the inferior surface, 2/3 of the posterior, and part of the left lateral wall. The right coronary artery also supplies the SA node in 55 percent of the population and the AV node in 90 percent of the population.

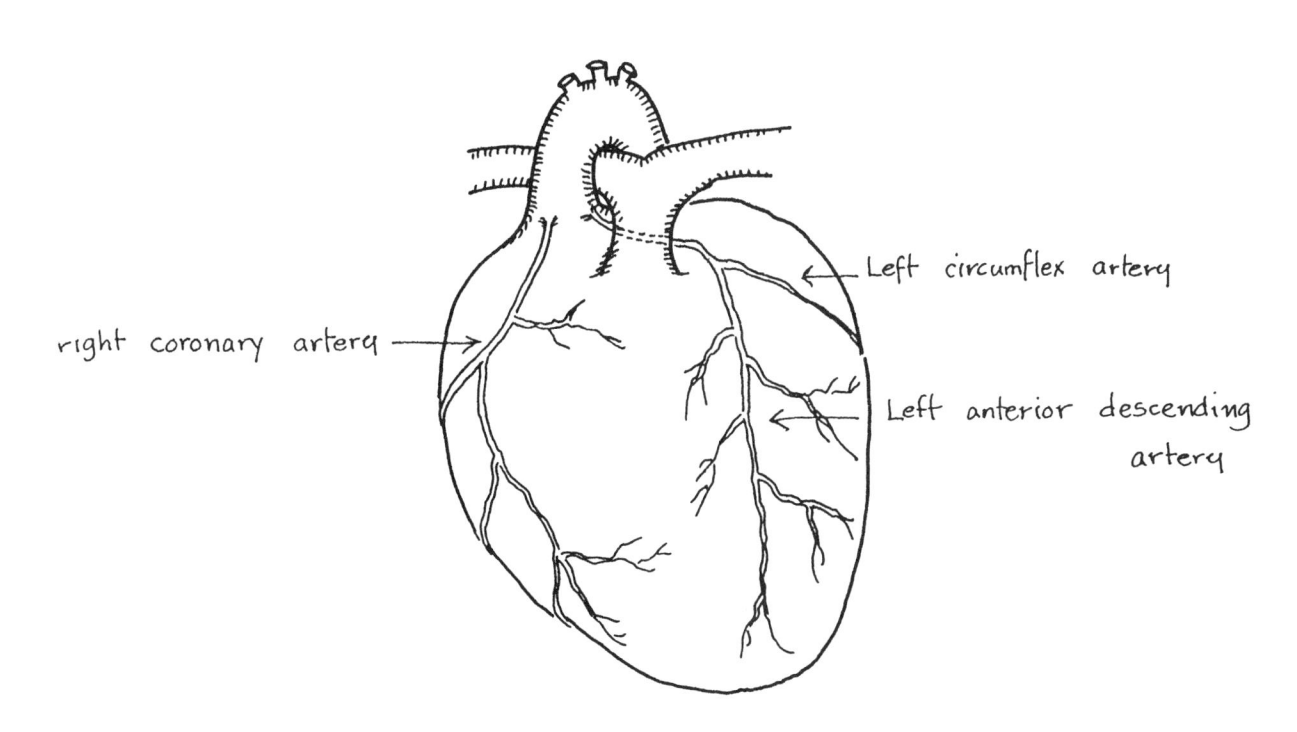

QUESTION: While monitoring the ECG of your patient with an acute inferior infarction, you would be especially alert for conduction problems with the SA node and the AV node.

A. True
B. False

ANSWER: A. True, because the coronary artery that supplies the inferior wall also supplies the SA and AV nodes. AV heart blocks such as first degree, second degree (Mobitz I and Mobitz II), and third degree may occur. Problems with the SA node include sinus bradycardia, sinus tachycardia, sinus arrest, and sick sinus syndrome.

Chapter 7 — Myocardial Ischemia, Injury, and Infarction

2. The **left coronary artery** bifurcates into two main branches: the left circumflex and the left anterior descending arteries.

   a. The **left circumflex coronary artery** supplies the lateral wall of the left ventricle and part of the posterior wall. It also supplies the remaining 45 percent of the population's SA node and 10 percent of the population's AV node.

QUESTION: While monitoring the ECG of your patient with an acute lateral wall infarction, you would be especially alert for conduction problems with the SA node and the AV node.

A. True
B. False

ANSWER: A. True. Because the left circumflex also supplies the AV node and the SA node in a small percentage of the population – first degree, second degree, and third degree AV heart block may be present. Problems with the SA node include sinus bradycardia, sinus tachycardia, sinus arrest, and sick sinus syndrome.

   b. The **left anterior descending coronary artery** supplies the anterior wall of the left ventricle, the intraventricular septum, and part of the lateral wall of the left ventricle. This artery supplies the conduction system of the ventricle and is called *the artery of sudden death* by some less optimistic people. Blockage of this artery impedes oxygen to the ventricular conduction system which can lead to sudden, unexpected death.

QUESTION: While monitoring the ECG of your patient who has an acute septal and/or anterior myocardial infarction, you would be especially alert for conduction problems with the right and left bundle branches.

A. True
B. False

ANSWER: A. True. Because this artery supplies the conduction system of the ventricle (bundle of His, the right and left bundle branches), intraventricular conduction defects are likely to occur with acute septal and/or anterior myocardial infarction.

Recall that the most common cause of all of the intraventricular conduction defects is an acute myocardial infarction of the septum and/or anterior wall.

Chapter 7 — Myocardial Ischemia, Injury, and Infarction

REVIEW OF THE LEADS

INFERIOR LEADS

IN THE FRONTAL PLANE:

In the frontal plane, leads II, III, aVF look at the inferior wall of the ventricle.

QUESTION: Which coronary artery supplies the inferior surface of the heart?

ANSWER: The right coronary artery.

QUESTION: Myocardial infarctions involving the inferior surface of the heart will be seen in which leads?

ANSWER: The inferior leads: II, III, aVF

LEFT LATERAL LEADS

Leads I and aVL are left lateral leads.

QUESTION: What other two leads in the precordial plane are also left lateral leads?

ANSWER: V_5 and V_6.

ECG changes of myocardial ischemia, injury, and infarction of the left lateral wall will be evident in the left lateral leads I, aVL, V_5, and V_6.

It is not necessary to see changes in all four leads. However, to be considered significant, changes should be seen in at least two leads.

IN THE PRECORDIAL PLANE:

SEPTUM AND ANTERIOR LEADS

V_1 (V_2) looks at the intraventricular septum
(V_2), V_3, V_4 looks at the anterior wall

V_5, V_6 looks at left lateral wall as noted above

NOTE: V_2 is in parentheses above because sometimes it covers the septum and sometimes it covers the anterior wall.

Chapter 7 — Myocardial Ischemia, Injury, and Infarction

Pictorial Review of the 12 Leads and the Walls They Face

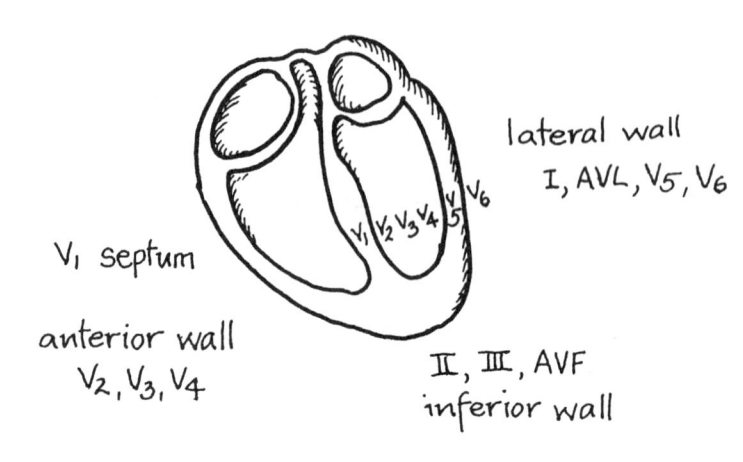

I, aVL, V$_5$, V$_6$: These four left lateral leads see changes in the lateral wall of the left ventricle.

V$_1$ (V$_2$) will see changes in the intraventricular septum – a wall of the left ventricle.

(V$_2$), V$_3$, V$_4$ will see changes in the anterior wall of the left ventricle.

I, aVL, V$_5$, V$_6$ will see changes in the left lateral wall.

The three inferior leads **II, III, aVF** will see changes in the inferior wall.

QUESTION: There are 12 leads in the 12 lead ECG. Which lead is not represented in the above picture?

ANSWER: aVR. The positive electrode of aVR is on the right shoulder. It is looking at the base of the heart. aVR is not useful in the interpretation of myocardial infarction.

The left ventricle is composed of five walls: the septum, anterior, lateral, posterior, and inferior walls.

QUESTION: Which wall is not represented in the above picture?

ANSWER: The posterior wall.

There is no positive electrode beyond V$_6$ so no lead covers the posterior wall. V$_1$ and V$_2$ must do double duty and report changes in posterior wall infarctions.

Now that you know where to look – what are you looking for?

Chapter 7 — Myocardial Ischemia, Injury, and Infarction

MYOCARDIAL ISCHEMIA, INJURY, AND INFARCTION ECG CRITERIA

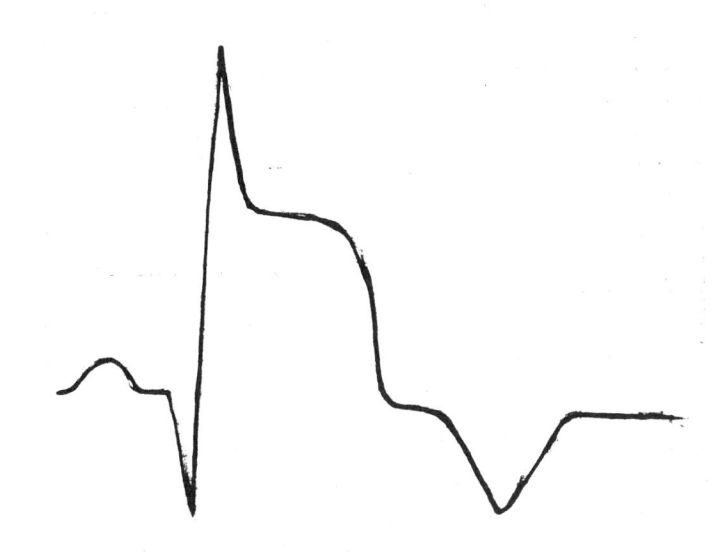

Q wave

Elevated ST segment

Inverted T wave

The three ECG changes are pathological Q waves, elevated ST segments, and inverted T waves.

Transmural infarction is characterized by ischemia, injury, and death of a part of the entire thickness of the ventricular wall. This causes changes in both ventricular depolarization and ventricular repolarization which are seen on the ECG.

ST SEGMENT ELEVATION

The earliest ECG indication of transmural myocardial infarction is elevation of the ST segment in the leads facing the affected area of the ventricle.

QUESTION: What is the normal position of the ST segment on the ECG?

ANSWER: The normal ST segment is on the isoelectric line or no more than one millimeter above or below it.

Elevated ST segments are produced by an abnormal electrical charge on the membrane of the myocardial cell. As a result, an abnormal current flow causes elevation of the ST segment.

The amount of ST segment elevation is variable. Sometimes it may only elevate one or two millimeters above the isoelectric line and is difficult to assess without a baseline ECG or a later tracing to compare with. Other times, ST segment elevation may be several millimeters tall and obscure the downstroke of the R wave.

Chapter 7 -- Myocardial Ischemia, Injury, and Infarction

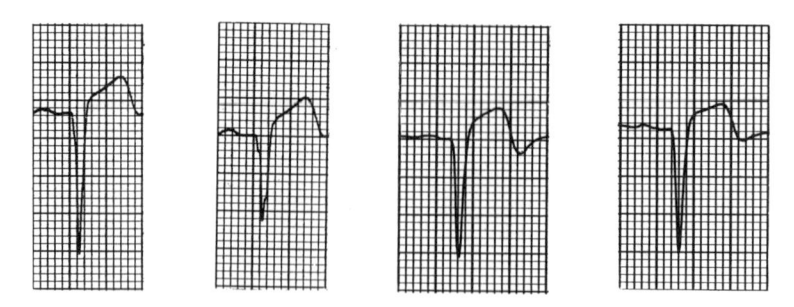

Elevated ST Segments

The elevated ST segments may last for only a few hours or a few days. The ST segments should return to the isoelectric line within two weeks.

Tall, peaked T waves may be seen in the early stages of myocardial infarction. These are sometimes referred to as hyperacute T waves. Hyperacute T waves may be seen before the ST segment elevates or with ST segment elevation. These hyperacute T waves are believed to be due to subendocardial ischemia. In any case, they do not persist very long and usually are not seen.

PATHOLOGICAL Q WAVES

Abnormal Q waves begin to appear several hours or days after the clinical manifestations of the infarction. Q waves usually develop when the ST segments are elevated.

QUESTION: What is the appearance of a normal, physiological q wave?

ANSWER: Normal physiological q waves are small, usually less than 1 millimeter deep or wide. Normal q waves are less than one-fourth the height of their R wave.

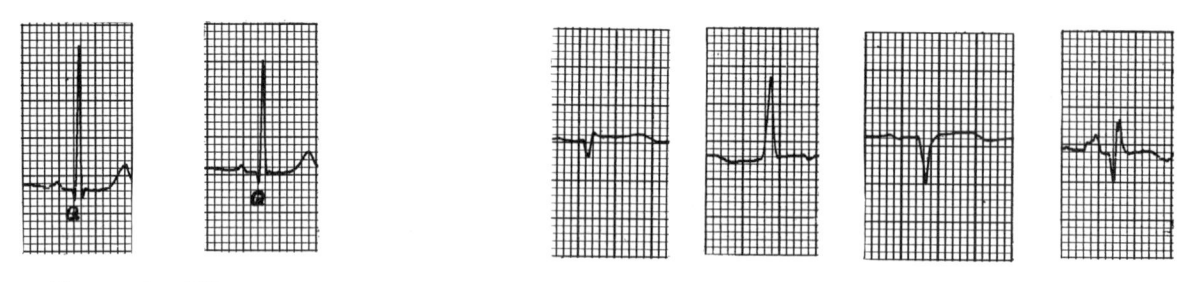

Normal q Waves   **Pathological Q Waves**

Chapter 7 — Myocardial Ischemia, Injury, and Infarction

Recall the principle:

Infarction means death. Electrical forces do not move towards dead cells, but away. As depolarization moves away from the positive electrode of the affected lead, pathological Q waves are inscribed.

T WAVE INVERSION

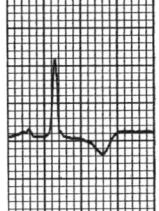

Myocardial ischemia causes symmetrical inversion of the T wave. These are primary T wave abnormalities reflecting an actual change in ventricular repolarization. As the ST segment begins to return to the isoelectric line, the symmetrical inversion of the T wave appears. The inverted T waves become progressively deeper as the ST segment elevation returns to the isoelectric line.

Figure 7 A on the following page is an example of an acute myocardial infarction of the anterolateral wall. Before looking at 7 A answer the following three questions:

QUESTION: Which leads will show an infarction of the anterior and lateral walls?

ANSWER: The anterior wall leads are V_2, V_3, V_4. The lateral wall leads are V_5, V_6, I, aVL.

QUESTION: Do you need to see changes in all of the above leads to be significant?

ANSWER: No. However, to be significant you should see changes in two or more of the leads.

QUESTION: What ECG changes do you expect to see with an acute myocardial infarction?

ANSWER: ST segment elevation and pathological Q waves. Inverted T waves may be present.

With an acute anterolateral myocardial infarction you will see elevated ST segments within a few minutes to hours, followed by the development of pathological Q waves.

Review Figure 7 A on the following page. There are pathological Q waves in V_2, V_3, V_4 (anterior wall), and I, aVL, V_5, V_6 (lateral wall). The ST segments are also elevated in all of the aforementioned leads. This indicates an acute myocardial infarction of the anterior and the lateral walls—an anterolateral infarction.

Figure 7 A also has inverted T waves in leads II, III, aVF (inferior wall), which indicates ischemia.

The interpretation of Figure 7 A is acute anterolateral infarction with inferior ischemia.

Figure 7 A. Acute anterolateral infarction with inferior ischemia

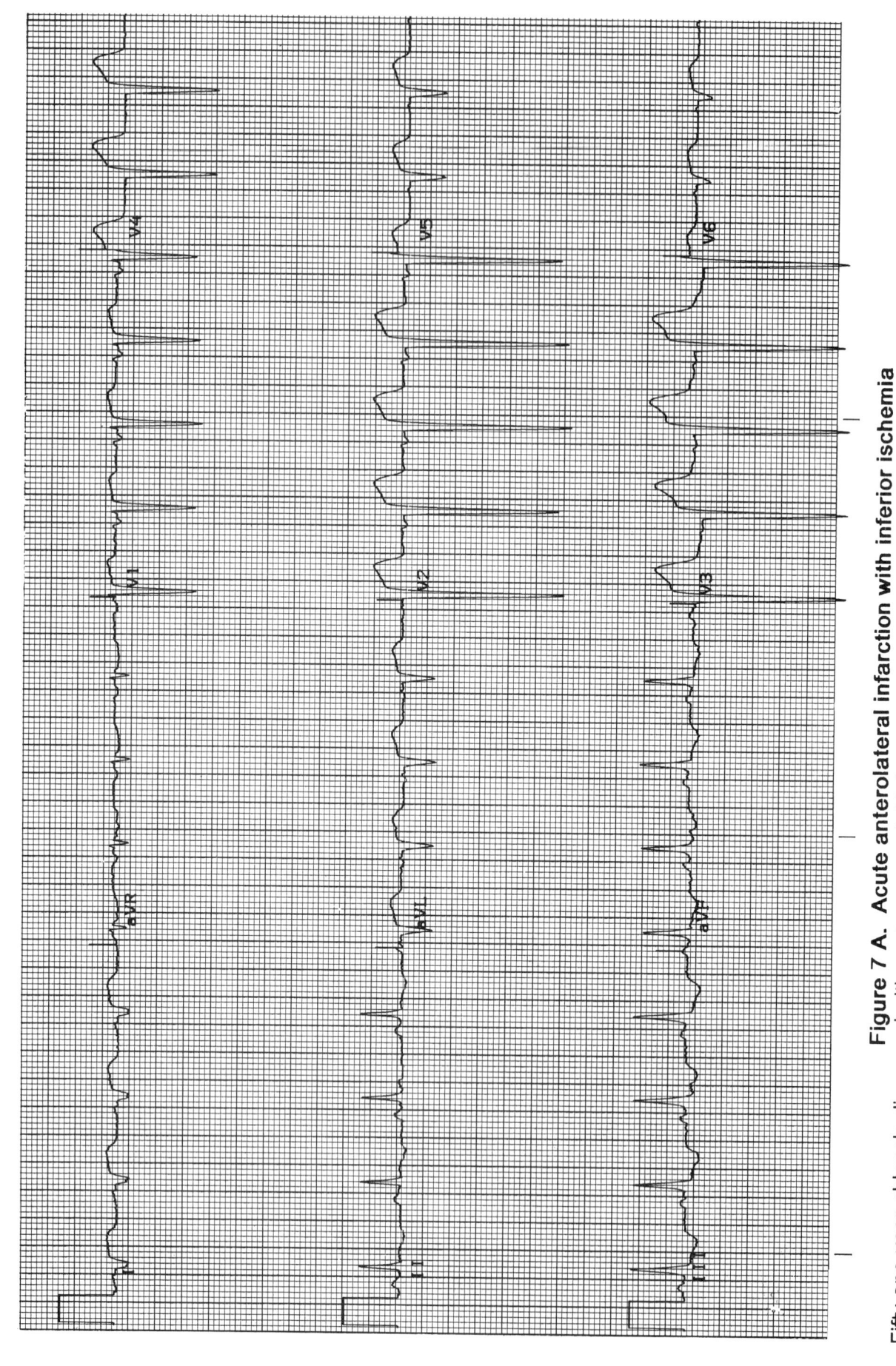

Fifty-one-year-old male diagnosed with acute myocardial infarction. Note the Q waves and elevated ST segments in leads V_2 through V_6, I, aVL. Also note the inverted T waves in II, III, aVF.

Chapter 7 — Myocardial Ischemia, Injury, and Infarction

In review:

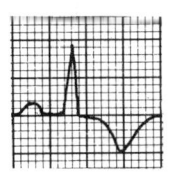

Myocardial ischemia causes inversion of the T waves over the affected area of the ventricle.

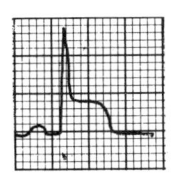

Myocardial injury causes elevation of the ST segments over the affected area of the ventricle.

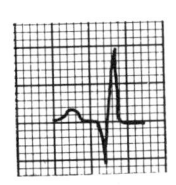

Myocardial infarction causes pathological Q waves over the affected area of the ventricle.

The age of infarction can be inferred from the 12 lead ECG as follows:

    Q waves only = OLD INFARCTION
    Q waves with elevated ST segments (with or without T wave inversion) = ACUTE INFARCTION
    Q waves with inverted T waves = AGE UNDETERMINED

Practice 12 lead ECG #1 on page 49 is an example of an anteroseptal myocardial infarction, age undetermined, with lateral ischemia.

QUESTION: What type of a hemiblock is present in practice 12 lead ECG #1?

ANSWER: LADH. The frontal plane axis is LAD quadrant -60°; there is a small q in I and a small r in II.

Practice 12 lead ECG #54 on page 160 is an example of an old anteroseptal myocardial infarction and an inferior infarction, age undetermined.

Figure 7 B on the following page is an example of an acute inferior myocardial infarction.

QUESTION: What ECG changes do you expect to see with an acute inferior myocardial infarction?

ANSWER: Pathological Q waves and elevated ST segments in the inferior leads II, III, aVF.

QUESTION: Do you need to see the ECG changes in all three leads?

ANSWER: No. However, you should see changes in at least two leads to be significant.

Examine Figure 7 B on the following page.

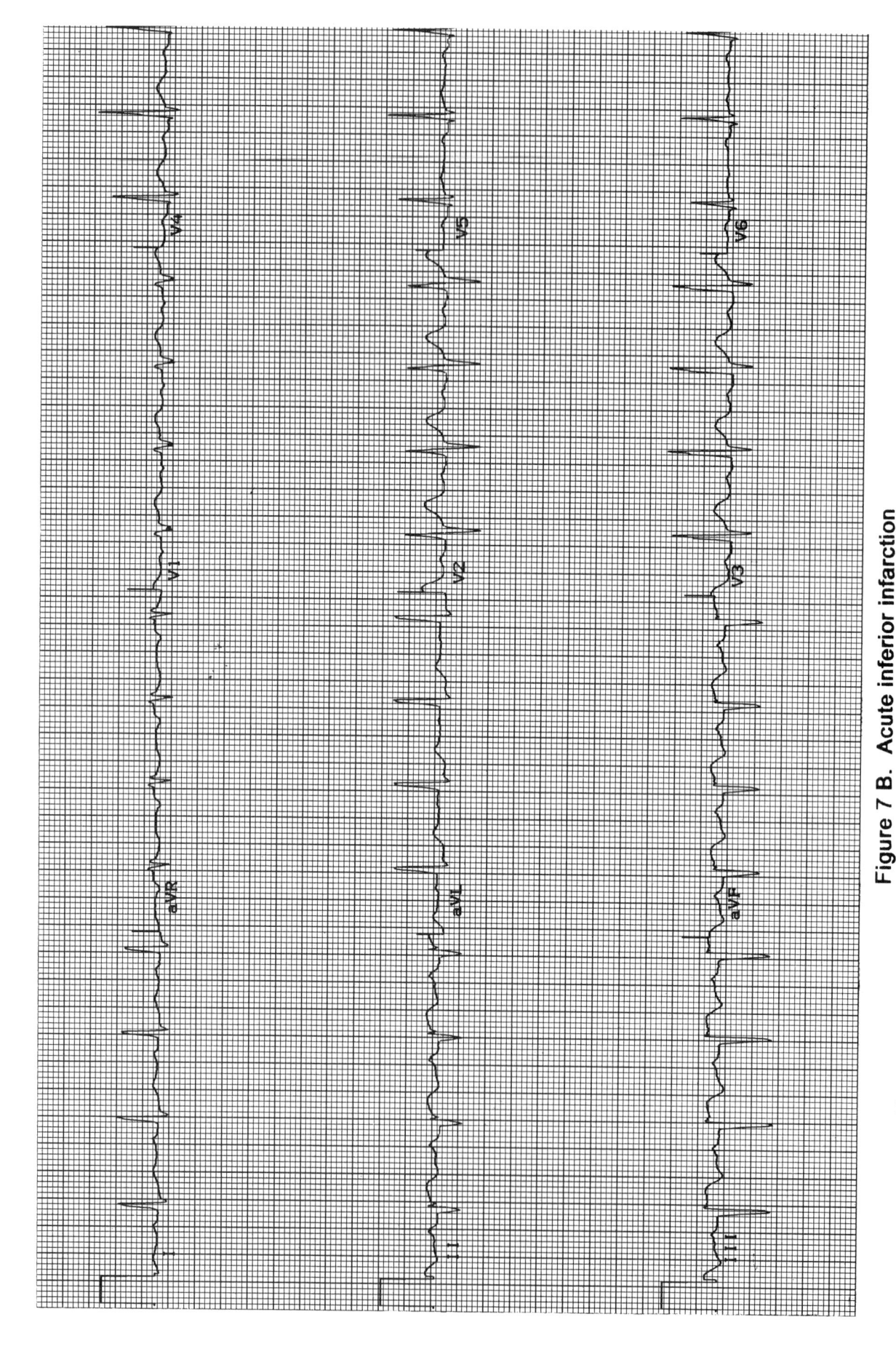

Figure 7 B. Acute inferior infarction
Note the pathological Q waves and elevated ST segments in the inferior leads II, III, aVF

Chapter 7 -- Myocardial Ischemia, Injury, and Infarction

RECIPROCAL CHANGES: ACUTE AND POSTERIOR

Unfortunately, the term *reciprocal* has two different meanings in 12 lead ECG interpretation and refers to two entirely different situations. This is very confusing to the beginner. In this text the terms have been modified to increase clarity:

1. Acute reciprocal changes
2. Posterior reciprocal changes

ACUTE RECIPROCAL CHANGES

During an acute infarction the anterior/lateral leads may show an inverse pattern to the inferior leads. For example, elevated ST segments in V_2 to V_6, I, aVL will often result in ST segment depression in the inferior leads II, III, aVF. Conversely, the elevated ST segments seen in II, III, aVF during an acute inferior infarction may show reciprocal ST segment depressions in one or more of the anterior/lateral leads V_2 to V_6, I, aVL. These inverse ECG patterns are called *acute reciprocal changes*.

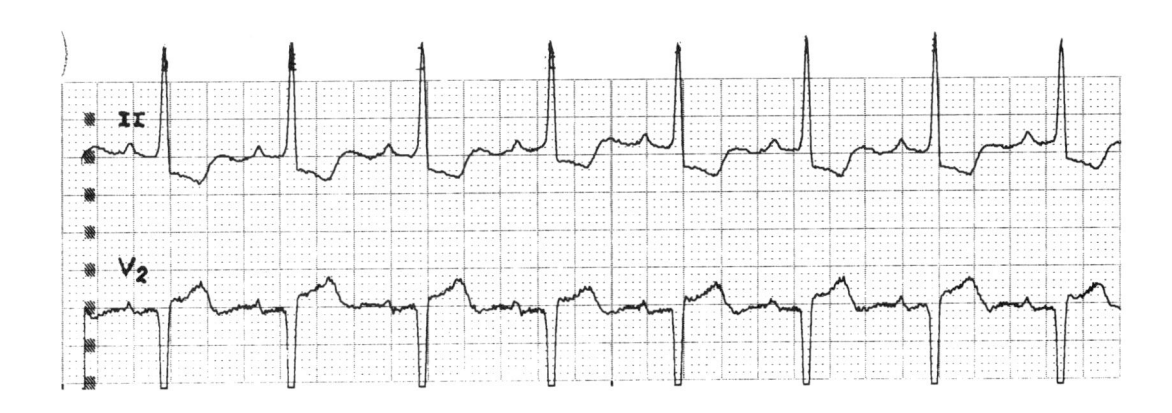

Note on the above strip the acute elevation of the ST segment in V_2 (bottom) and the acute reciprocal changes in lead II (top). The patient is having an acute infarction of the anterior wall seen in V_2 with acute reciprocal changes recorded in the inferior lead II.

Note the depressed ST segments in aVL in Figure 7 B on the previous page; these are acute reciprocal changes.

These acute reciprocal changes seen in the leads opposite the acute event are explained as electrical phenomena due to reciprocal electrical alterations. This phenomena is most often seen with extensive transmural myocardial infarction. The more extensive the infarction the more likely these changes will be present.

Figure 7 C on the following page is an example of an acute septal, anterolateral myocardial infarction with acute reciprocal changes recorded as depressed ST segments in the inferior leads.

Figure 7 C. Acute septal anterolateral infarction

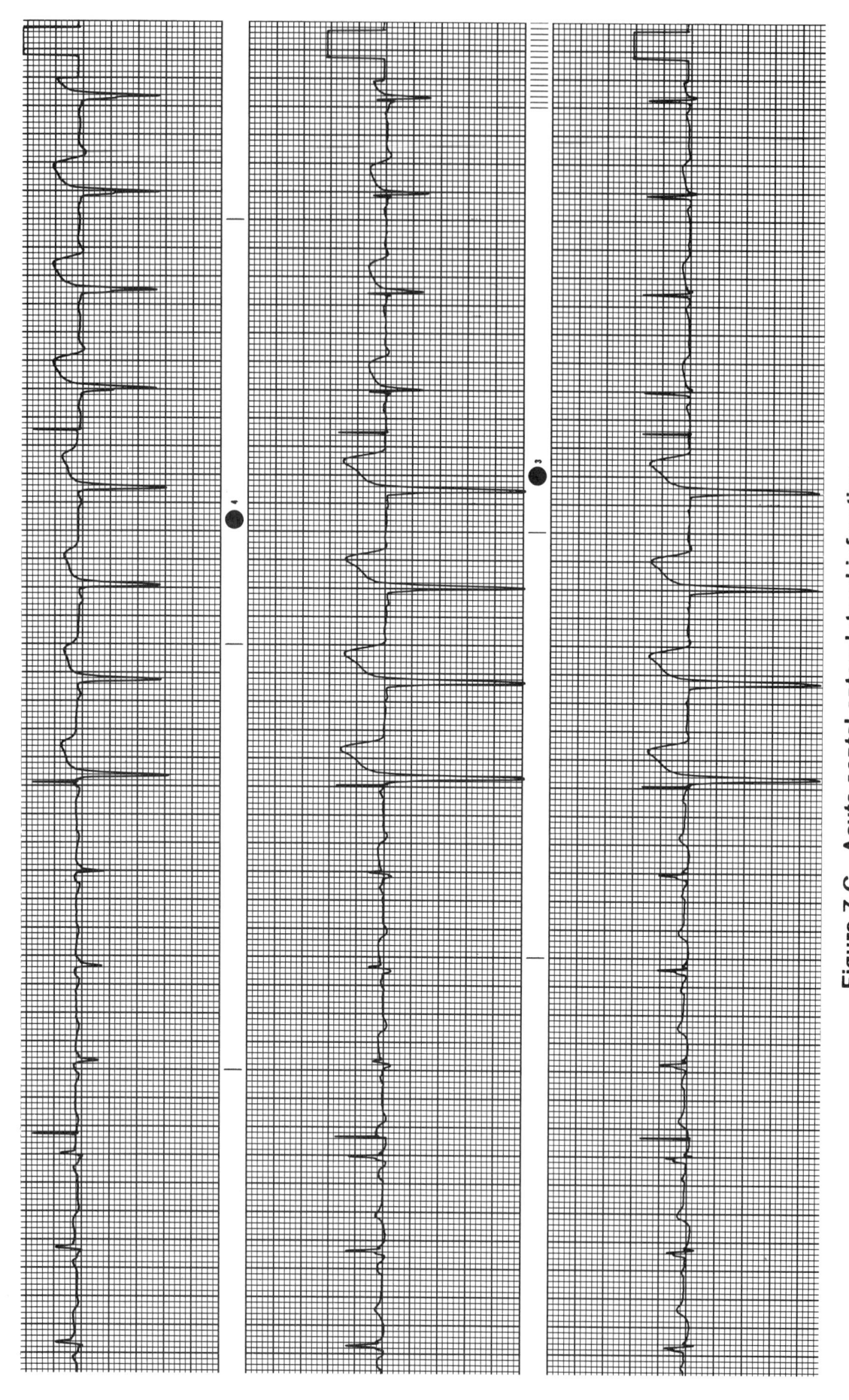

Note the elevated ST segments in V_1 through V_6 (acute injury) and the QS waves in V_1, V_2, V_3, V_4, aVL (infarction). Also note the depressed ST segments in II, III, aVF; these acute reciprocal changes (ST segment depression) in II, III, aVF are often seen during an acute myocardial infarction.

Chapter 7 — Myocardial Ischemia, Injury, and Infarction

POSTERIOR RECIPROCAL CHANGES

The term *reciprocal changes* is also used to denote the ECG changes that occur with posterior wall infarctions. This is an entirely different meaning of the word "reciprocal" than previously discussed.

Recall the location of V_1 and V_2 on the chest. These two leads usually see electrical forces moving away from them towards the intact posterior wall. The normal S waves in V_1 and V_2 result from the normal wave of ventricular depolarization moving towards the intact posterior (left) ventricle.

When the posterior wall is infarcted electrical forces no longer move towards it. The wave of depolarization will move away from the necrotic cells of the posterior wall towards the anterior surface. V_1 and V_2 will see these forces coming towards them and inscribe large R waves.

V_1 and V_2 normally have small r waves relative to their S wave. **Posterior infarctions will cause large R waves in V_1 and V_2.**

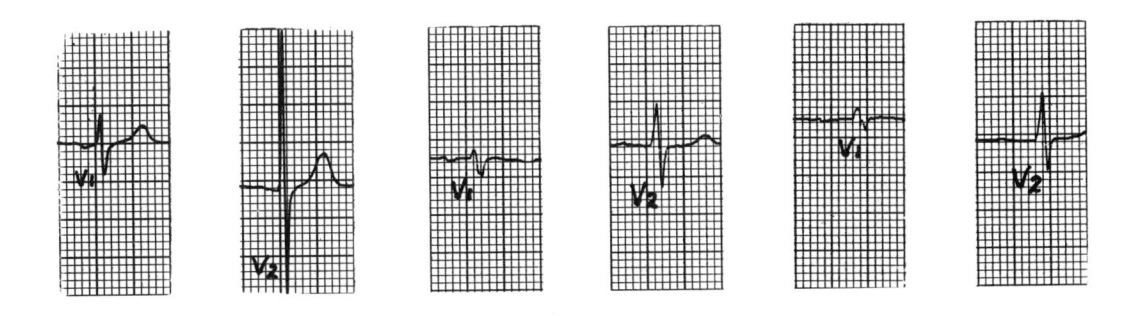

Posterior Myocardial Infarction V_1 and V_2

These large R waves in V_1 and V_2 are called *posterior reciprocal changes*; these reciprocal changes refer to the acute event in the posterior wall.

It is unfortunate that "reciprocal" is used with two entirely different meanings. But that is the state of the art. The terms acute reciprocal changes and posterior reciprocal changes are used herein for clarity.

Figure 7 D on the following page is an example of an inferior and posterior myocardial infarction.

Figure 7 D. Inferior and posterior myocardial infarction

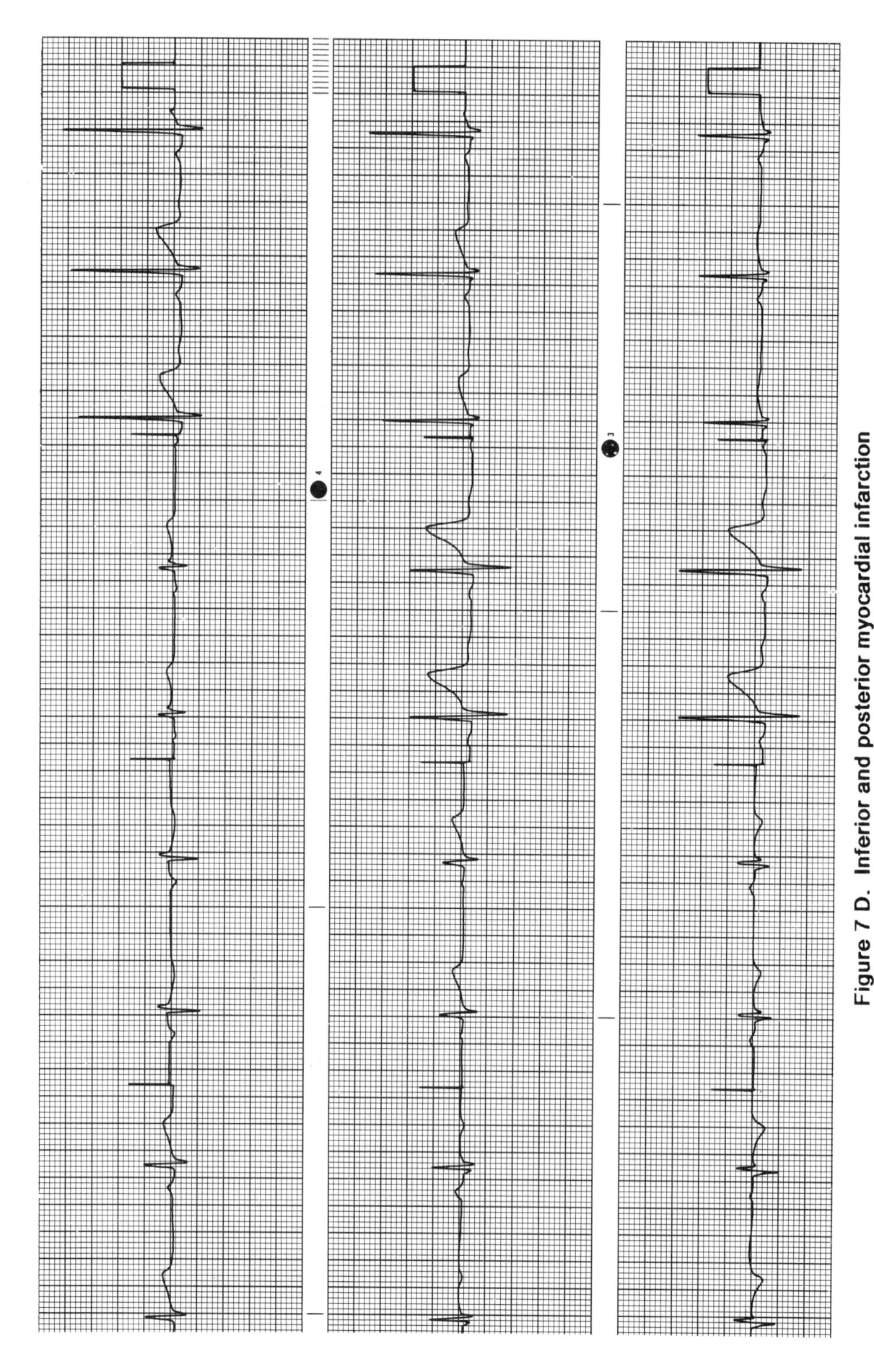

Note the pathological q waves in the inferior leads II, III, aVF, and the tall R waves in V_1, V_2. These tall R wave are reciprocal changes seen with posterior infarction.

Chapter 7 — Myocardial Ischemia, Injury, and Infarction

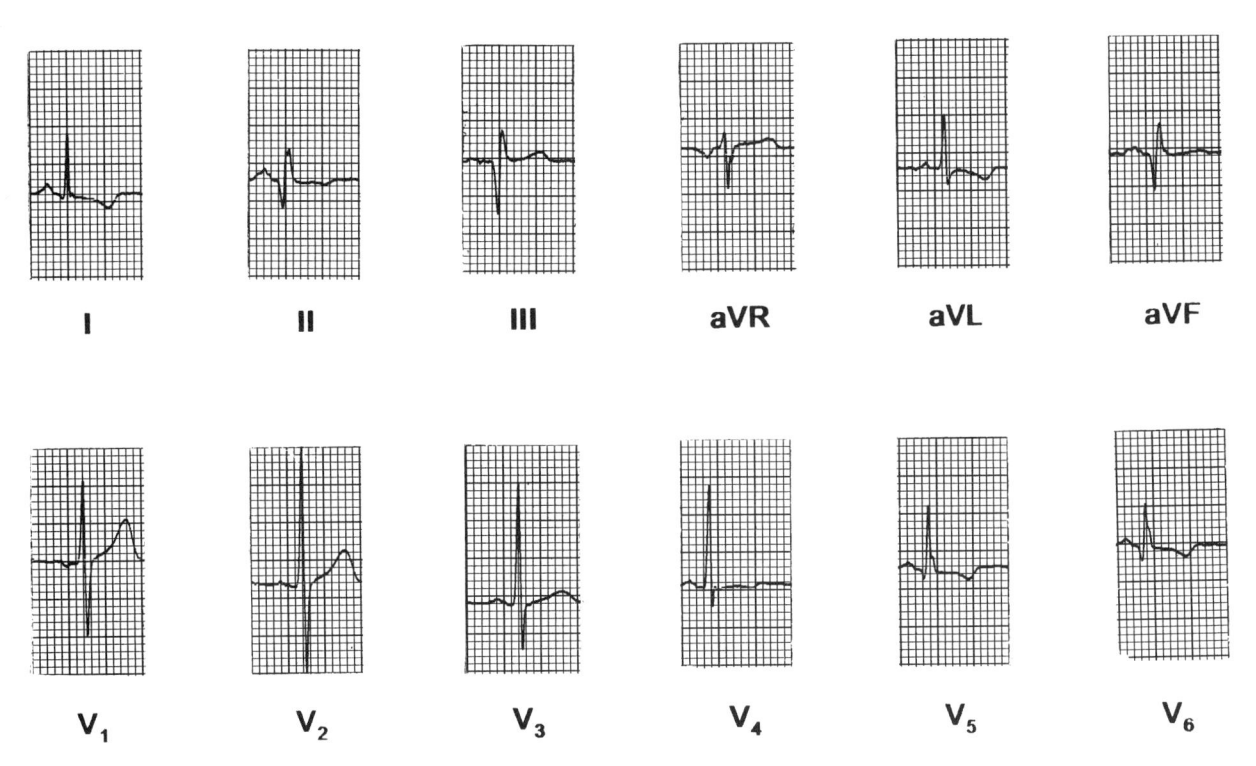

Figure 7 E. Inferoposterior myocardial infarction with lateral ischemia

In Figure 7 E note the tall R waves in V_1 and V_2 indicative of posterior infarction. There are also pathological Q waves in the inferior leads with inverted T waves in lead II: this is an inferoposterior infarction with lateral ischemia, age undetermined. Also note the inverted T waves in the lateral leads, I, aVL, V_5, V_6 indicative of lateral ischemia.

One way to assess for a posterior infarction is to turn the 12 lead upside down and backwards—hold it up to the light and look at V_1 and V_2. The following page is blank so you may try it. Turn the page upside down and backwards and you will see pathological q waves and inverted T waves in V_1 and V_2.

This is the Norman method of assessing posterior infarction.

Chapter 7 — **Myocardial Ischemia, Injury, and Infarction**

This page is blank so that you may see the posterior infarction using the Norman method. Turn this page upside down, hold it up to the light and you will be able to see the pathological q waves and inverted T waves in V_1 and V_2 in Figure 7 E on page 201.

Chapter 7 — Myocardial Ischemia, Injury, and Infarction

QUESTION: What other two conditions previously discussed cause tall R waves in V_1 and V_2?

ANSWER: Right ventricular hypertrophy and right bundle branch block.

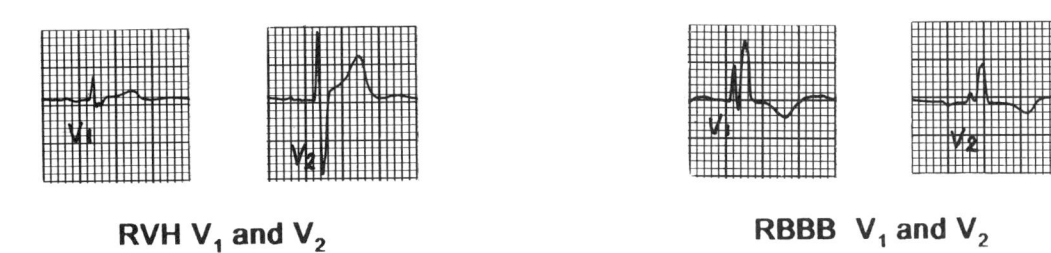

RVH V_1 and V_2   **RBBB V_1 and V_2**

Recall that the right coronary artery supplies the inferior and most of the posterior wall of the left ventricle. Whenever there is an inferior infarction you should be alert to the possibility of a posterior infarction.

Assessment of the R wave progression will alert you to the possibility of a posterior infarction because tall R waves in V_1 are abnormal. Tall R waves in the right precordial leads (V_1, V_2) alert you to look for conditions that cause tall R waves in these leads.

QUESTION: What three conditions have now been discussed that cause tall R waves in V_1 and V_2?

ANSWER:
1. Right ventricular hypertrophy
2. Right bundle branch block   cause tall R waves in V_1 and V_2
3. Posterior myocardial infarction

Chapter 7 — Myocardial Ischemia, Injury, and Infarction

SUBENDOCARDIAL INFARCTIONS

The ECG changes discussed have described *transmural* myocardial ischemia, injury, and infarction. Transmural means the entire thickness of the ventricular wall is affected.

Sometimes myocardial ischemia or infarction is limited to the inner layer of the heart. *Subendocardial infarction* means that only the inner half of the total thickness of the ventricular wall is involved.

ECG changes seen in acute subendocardial infarction are ST segment depression and T wave inversion in the leads facing the infarcted wall. The inversion of the T wave is often quite deep.

Figure 7 F below is an example of acute subendocardial infraction.

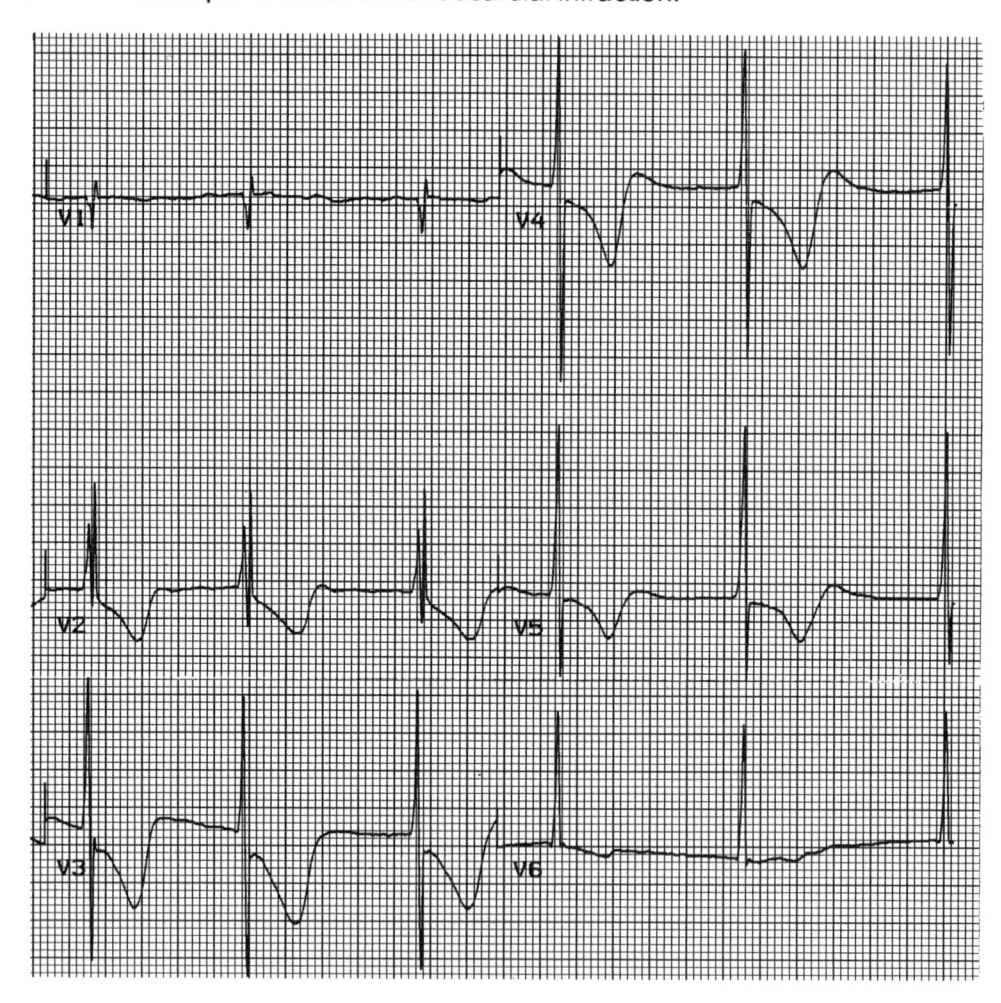

Figure 7 F. Anterolateral subendocardial infarction

Note the ST segment depression and T wave inversion V_2 through V_6.

Chapter 7 — Myocardial Ischemia, Injury, and Infarction

PRACTICE 12 LEAD ECGs #71-95

Assess the following practice 12 lead ECGs using these guidelines:

Basic rhythm:
Frontal plane axis:
R wave progression:
P wave:
Complex configuration and duration:
ST segment:
T wave:
Secondary ST-T changes:
VAT:
12 Lead ECG Interpretation:

Interpret practice 12 lead ECGs #71-80 as normal or abnormal and identify any areas of transmural myocardial ischemia, injury, infarction and any subendocardial infarctions. Answers begin on page 216.

Practice 12 lead ECGs #81-95 identify any chamber enlargements, intraventricular conduction defects, and/or areas of myocardial ischemia, injury, and/or infarction. Answers begin on page 234.

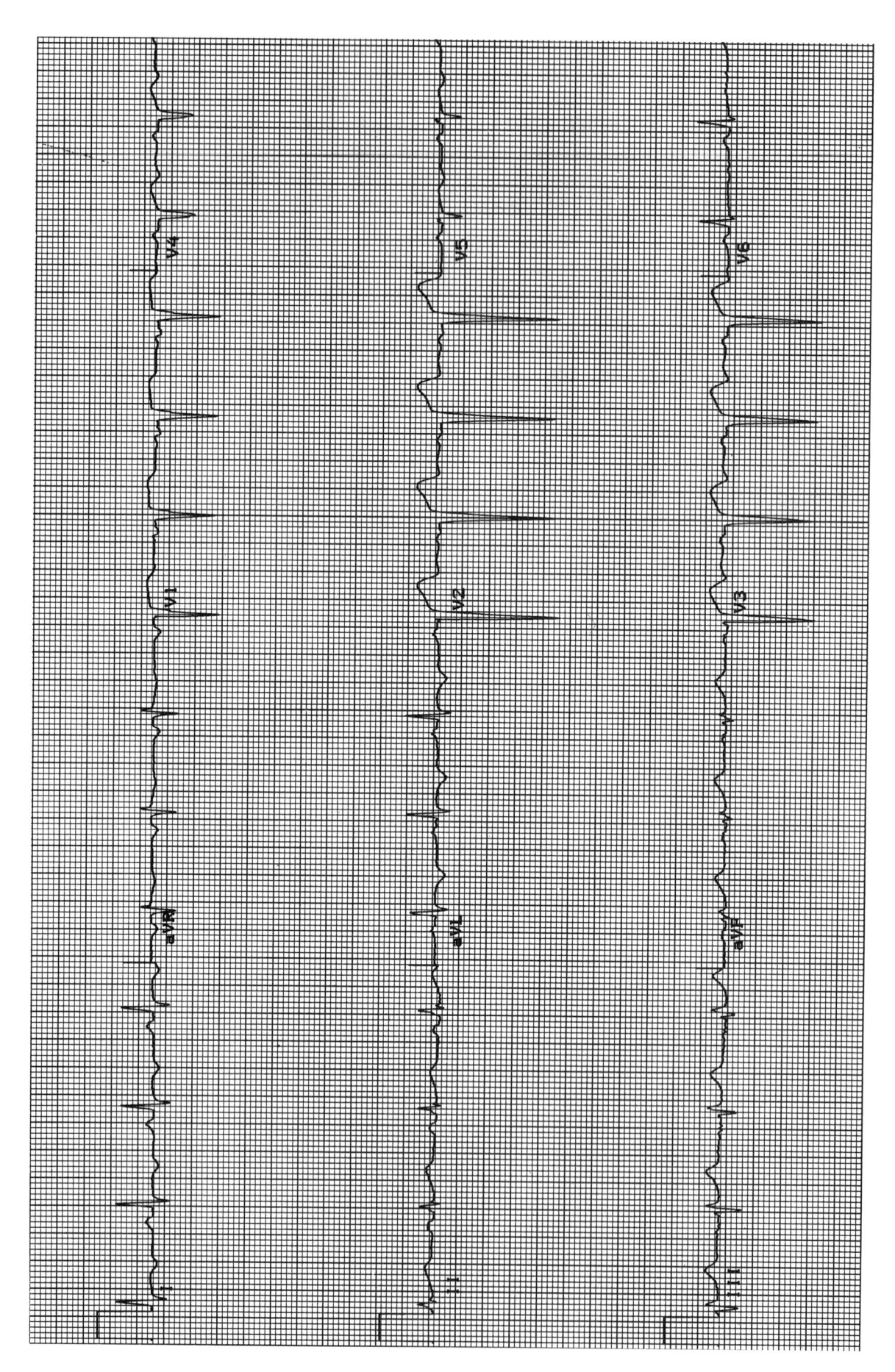

Practice 12 Lead ECG #71

Practice 12 Lead ECG #72

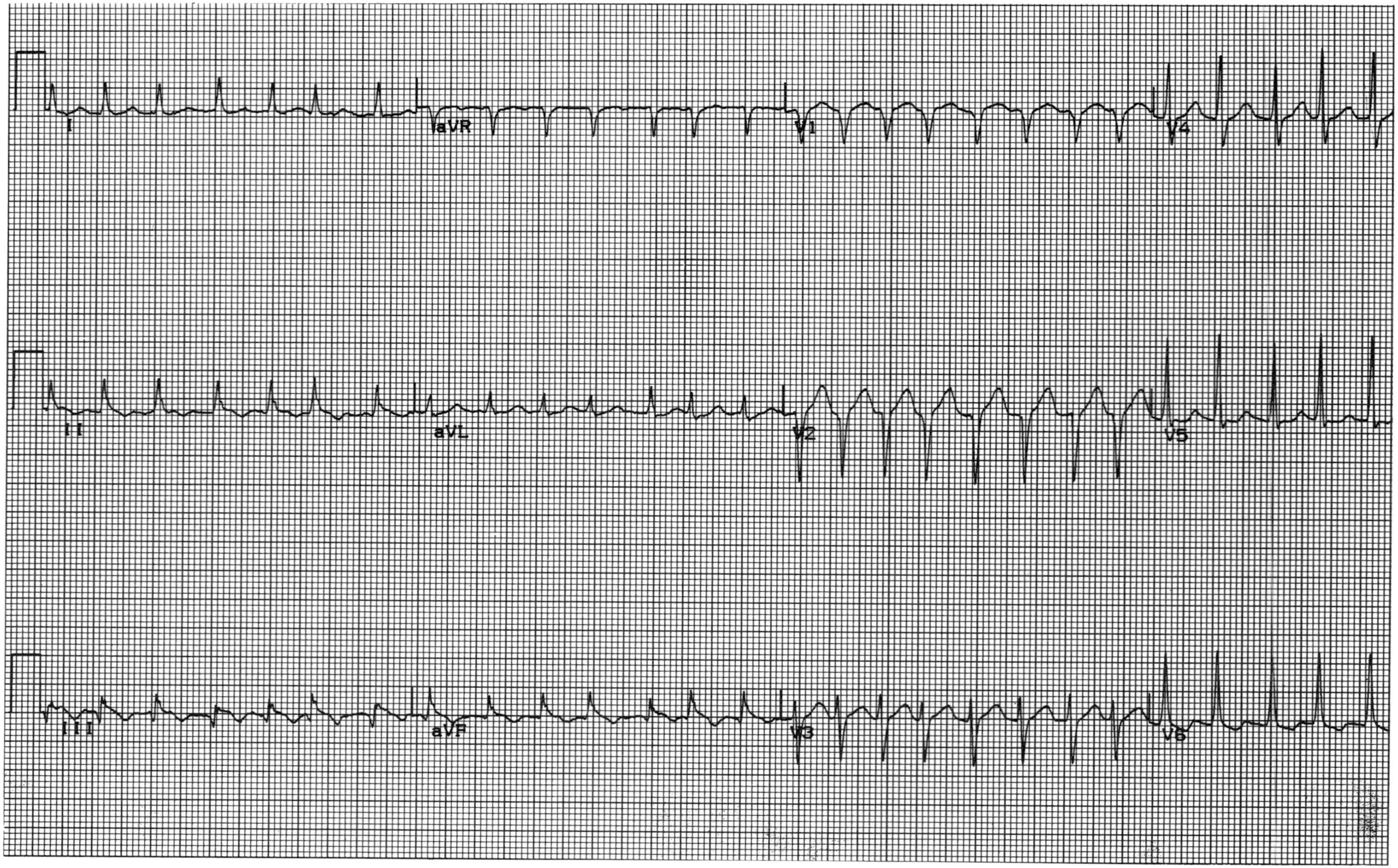

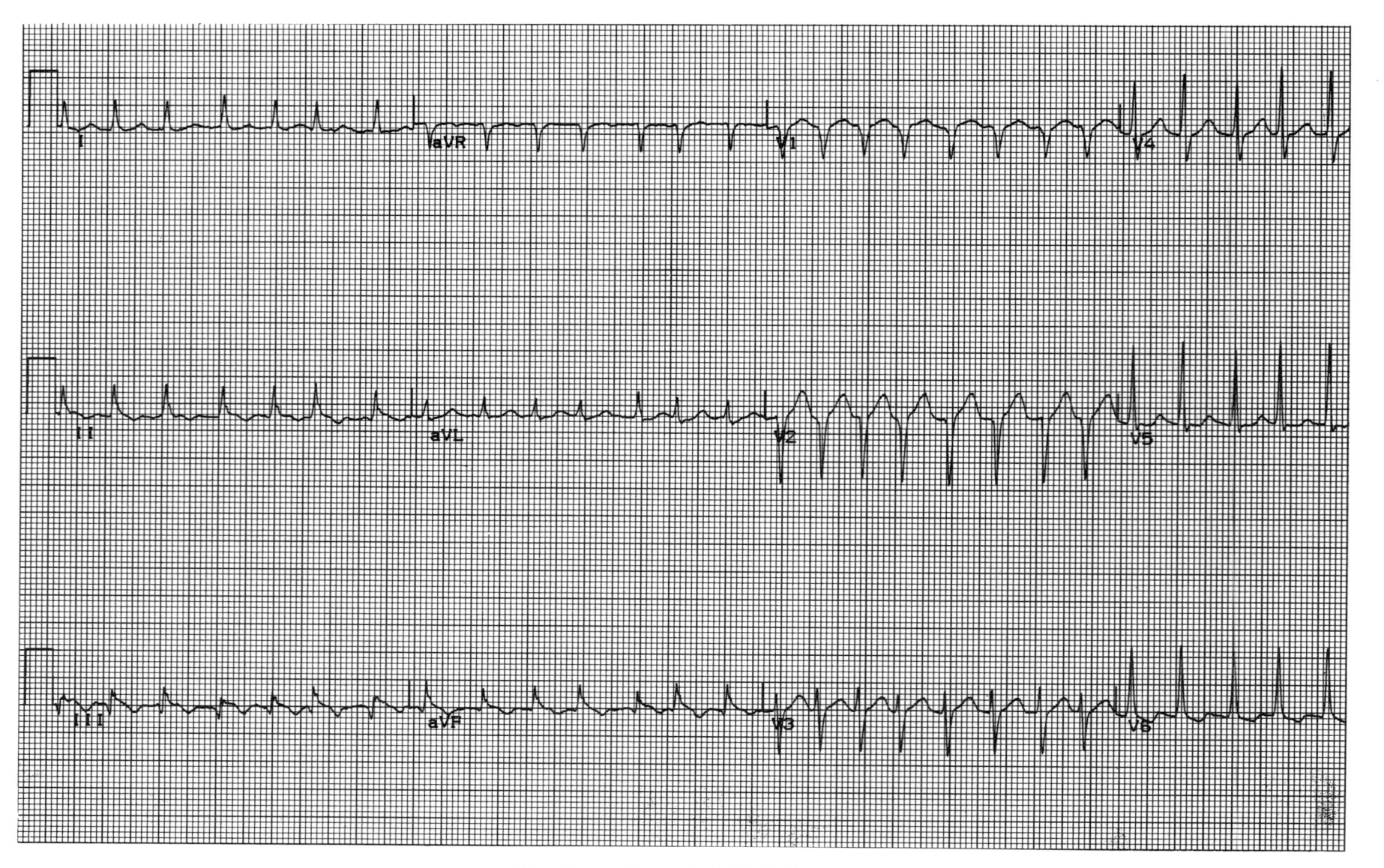

Practice 12 Lead ECG #73

Practice 12 Lead ECG #74

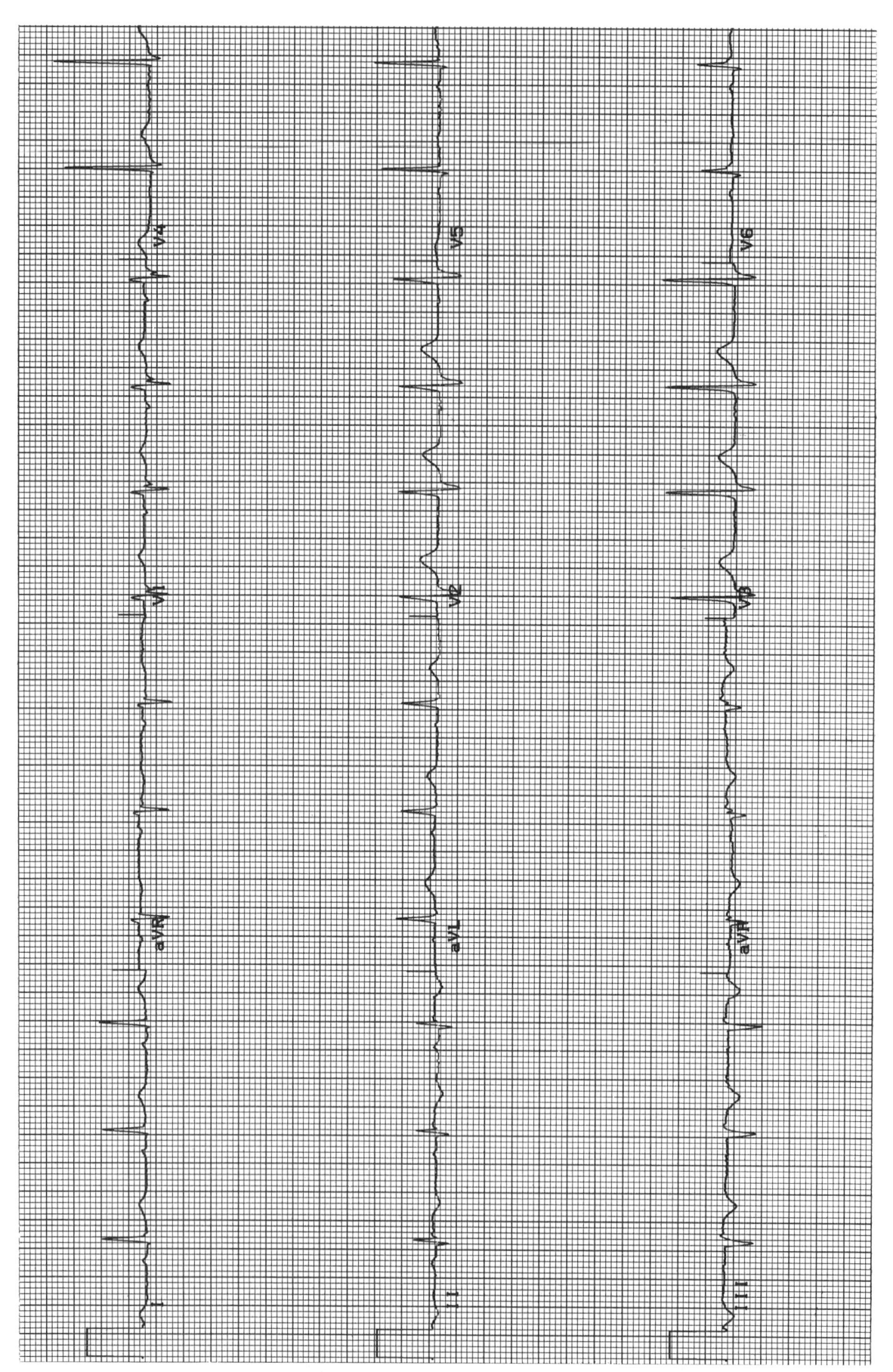

Practice 12 Lead ECG #75

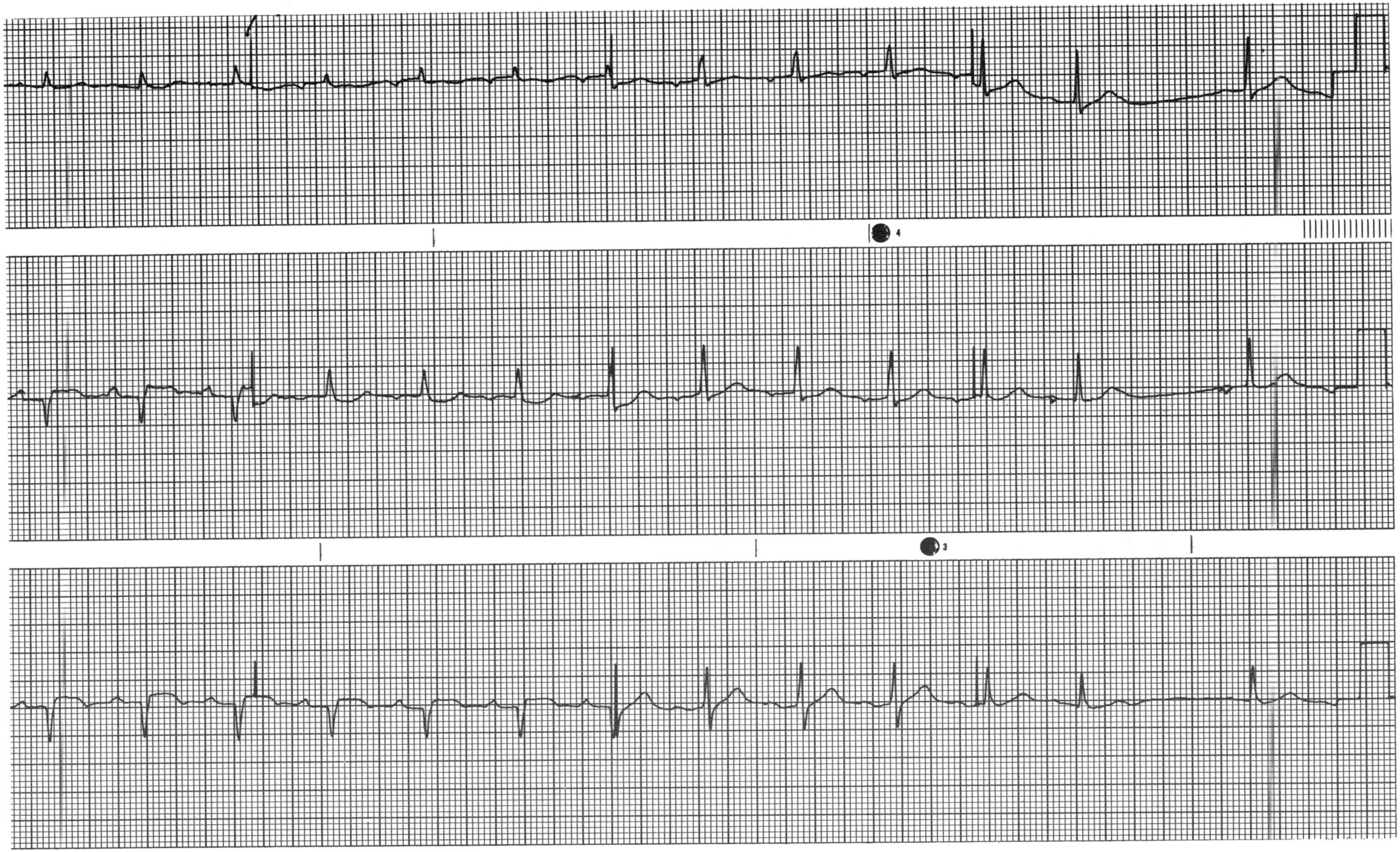

Practice 12 Lead ECG #76

Practice 12 Lead ECG #77

Practice 12 Lead ECG #78

Practice 12 Lead ECG #79

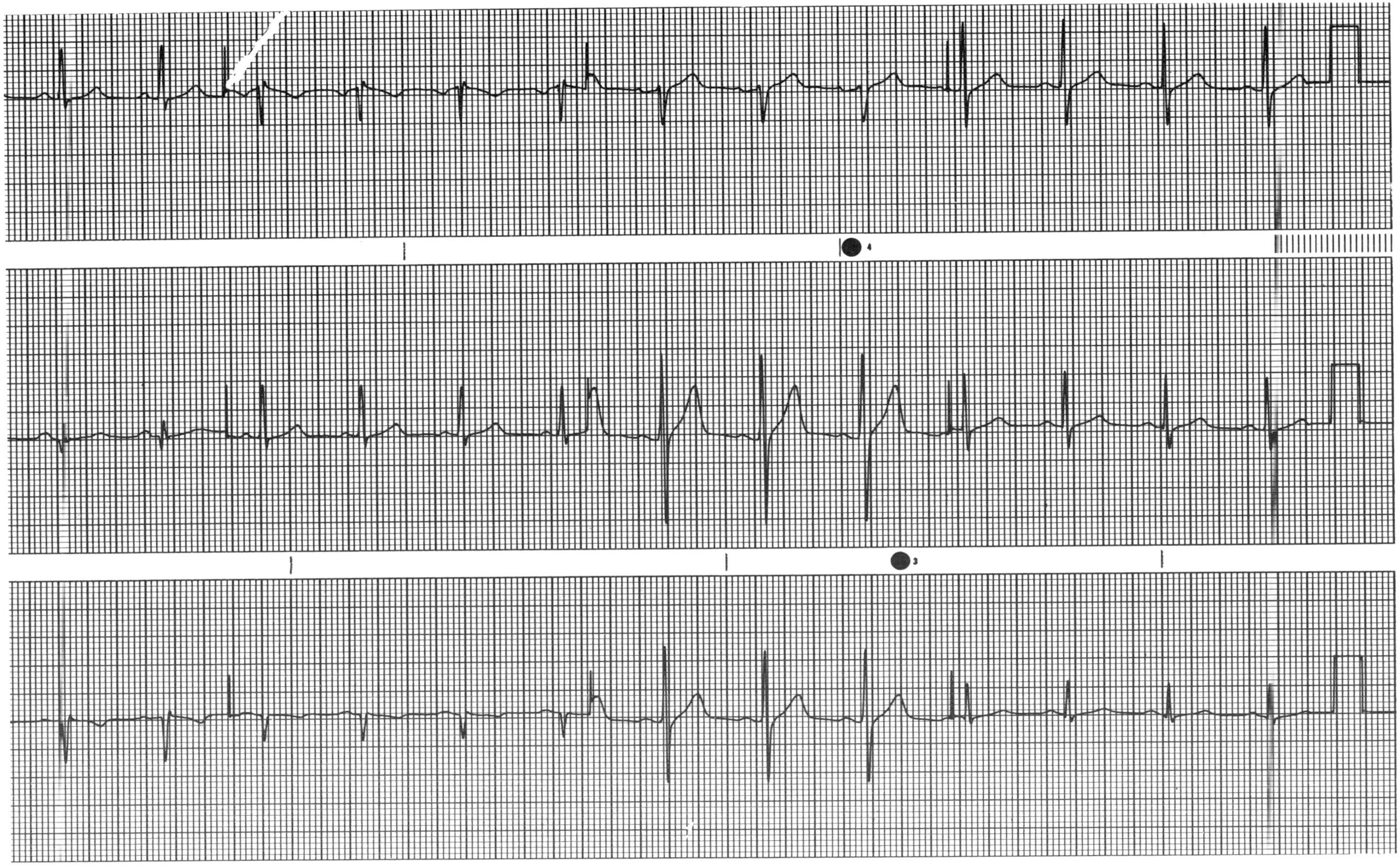

Practice 12 Lead ECG #80

Chapter 7 — Myocardial Ischemia, Injury, and Infarction

ANSWERS TO PRACTICE 12 LEAD ECGs #71-80

71. **Basic rhythm:** Normal sinus rhythm
    Frontal plane axis: Normal 0°
    R wave progression: Abnormal: No r wave in V_1, V_2, V_3, V_4; small r finally appears in V_5; transition occurs in V_6 — too late!
    Complex configuration: Abnormal: QS in V_1, V_2, V_3, V_4
    Complex duration: Normal
    P wave: Normal
    ST segment: Abnormal: Elevated in V_1, V_2, V_3
    T wave: Abnormal: Inverted in I, aVL; biphasic in V_4, V_5; flat in V_6
    12 Lead ECG Interpretation: Abnormal
    - Acute anteroseptal infarction with lateral ischemia

72. **Basic rhythm:** Normal sinus rhythm
    Frontal plane axis: Normal +60°
    R wave progression: Abnormal: QS in V_1 and V_2
    P wave: Normal
    Complex configuration: Abnormal: QS in V_1, V_2 as noted above
    Complex duration: Normal
    ST segment: Elevated in V_2
    T wave: Normal
    12 Lead ECG Interpretation: Abnormal
    - Septal infarction — the age of the infarction on the ECG is undetermined. Clinically, this is an acute situation in a 40-year-old male.

73. **Basic rhythm:** Atrial fibrillation with rapid ventricular response
    Frontal plane axis: Normal +30° (+40° corrected)
    R wave progression: Abnormal: No r in V_1 or V_2; r in V_3 with transition in V_4 and normal R waves in V_5 and V_6
    Complex configuration: Abnormal: QS pattern in V_1 and V_2
    Complex duration: Normal: 0.08 second
    P wave: No identifiable P waves
    ST segment: Depressed in V_6
    T wave: Abnormal: Inverted in II, III, aVF
    12 Lead ECG Interpretation: Abnormal
    - Atrial fibrillation with rapid ventricular response
    - Septal infarction, age undetermined with inferior ischemia

Chapter 7 — Myocardial Ischemia, Injury, and Infarction

74. **Basic rhythm:** Sinus tachycardia
    Frontal plane axis: Normal 0°
    R wave progression: Normal
    Complex configuration: Abnormal: Pathological q waves in II, III, aVF. One might question if the q wave in lead II is pathological or not. The amplitude of the q in leads III and aVF leave no doubt that these are pathological q waves.
    Complex duration: Normal
    P wave: Normal
    ST segment: Normal
    T wave: Abnormal: Inverted in II, III, aVF, V_3, V_4, V_5, V_6
    12 Lead ECG Interpretation: Abnormal
    - Sinus tachycardia
    - Inferior infarction, age undetermined with lateral ischemia
    The clinical presentation is an acute myocardial infarction of a 60-year-old female with chest pain and shortness of breath

75. **Basic rhythm:** Normal sinus rhythm
    Frontal plane axis: LAD quadrant -30° (-15° corrected)
    R wave progression: Normal
    Complex configuration: Pathological q/Q waves in II, III, aVF
    Complex duration: Normal: 0.08 seconds
    P wave: Normal
    ST segment: Normal
    T wave: Abnormal: Inverted in II, III, aVF
    12 Lead ECG Interpretation: Abnormal
    - Inferior infarction, age undetermined
    - The abnormal left axis deviation can be accounted for by the inferior infarction

76. **Basic rhythm:** Sinus arrhythmia
    Frontal plane axis: LAD quadrant: -60° (-70° corrected)
    R wave progression: Abnormal with tall R waves in V_1, V_2
    Complex configuration: Abnormal as noted above plus pathological Q waves in II, III, aVF
    Complex duration: Normal
    P wave: Normal
    ST segment: Abnormal: Depressed in V_2; elevated in II, III, aVF
    T wave: Abnormal: Inverted in III, aVF
    12 Lead ECG Interpretation: Abnormal
    - Marked sinus arrhythmia
    - Acute inferoposterior infarction

    Recall that tall R waves in V_1, V_2 are reciprocal changes seen with posterior infarctions. If you were to turn this tracing upside down and backwards, there would be pathological Q waves and inverted T waves in V_1 and V_2.

Chapter 7 — Myocardial Ischemia, Injury, and Infarction

77. **Basic rhythm:** Normal sinus rhythm
    Frontal plane axis: Normal +60°
    R wave progression: Abnormal with loss of anterior forces in V_2, V_3, V_4
    Complex configuration: Abnormal: QS in V_2, V_3
    Complex duration: Normal
    P wave: Normal
    ST segment: Abnormal: Elevated in I, aVL, V_2, V_3, V_4, V_5, V_6; depressed in III, aVF
    T wave: Normal
    12 Lead ECG Interpretation: Abnormal
    - Acute anterior myocardial infarction with lateral injury
    Notice the acute reciprocal ST depressions in the inferior leads III and aVF

78. **Basic rhythm:** Normal sinus rhythm
    Frontal plane axis: LAD quadrant -30° (-45° corrected)
    R wave progression: Abnormal with loss of anterior forces
    Complex configuration: Abnormal: QS in V_2, V_3, V_4; rS in V_5
    Complex duration: Normal
    P wave: Normal
    ST segment: Abnormal: Elevated in V_2, V_3, V_4 (minimally); depressed in II
    T wave: Abnormal: Inverted I, II, aVL, aVF, V_5, V_6
    12 Lead ECG Interpretation: Abnormal
    - Anterior myocardial infarction, age undetermined with lateral and inferior ischemia
    - Abnormal left axis deviation is probably due to the area of infarction

79. **Basic rhythm:** Sinus rhythm
    Frontal plane axis: Normal 0° (+15° corrected)
    R wave progression: Abnormal: QS in V_1, V_2, rsR' in V_3
    Complex configuration: Abnormal as noted above
    Complex duration: Normal: 0.08 seconds
    P wave: Normal
    ST segment: Abnormal: Depressed in I, II, aVL, V_4, V_5, V_6; elevated in V_1, V_2
    T wave: Abnormal: Inverted in I, II, III, aVL, aVF, V_3, V_4, V_5, V_6
    12 Lead ECG Interpretation: Abnormal
    - Acute septal infarction
    - Inferior, anterior, and lateral subendocardial infarction

80. **Basic rhythm:** Normal sinus rhythm
    Frontal plane axis: LAD quadrant -30°
    R wave progression: Normal
    Complex configuration: Abnormal with pathological q/Q waves in II, III, aVF
    Complex duration: Normal: 0.08 seconds
    P wave: Normal
    ST segment: Normal
    T wave: Abnormal: Inverted in III, aVF
    12 Lead ECG Interpretation: Abnormal
    - Inferior infarction, age undetermined

Practice 12 lead ECGs #81-95 follow, with answers beginning on page 234.

Practice 12 Lead ECG #81

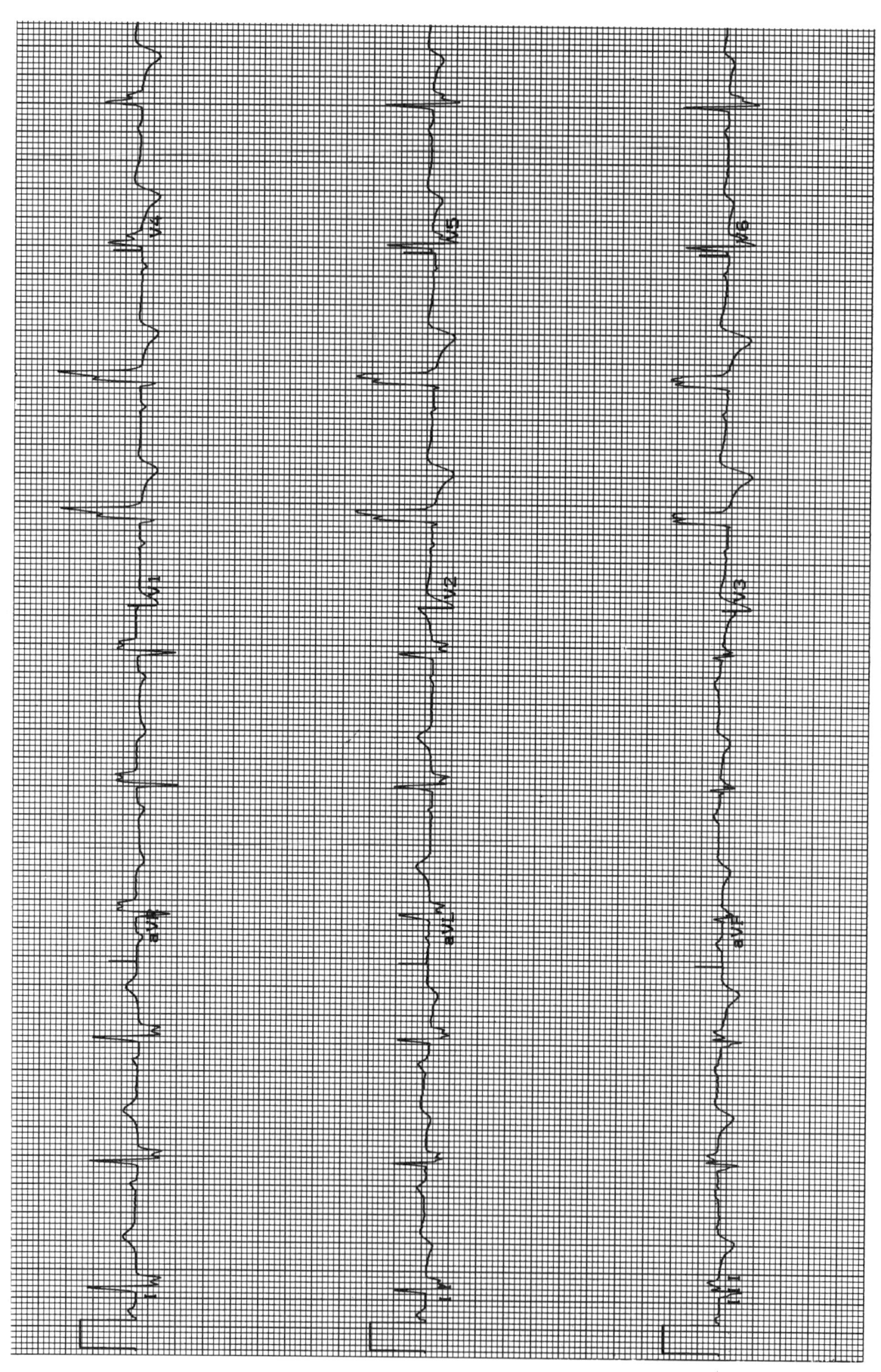

Practice 12 Lead ECG #82

Practice 12 Lead ECG #83

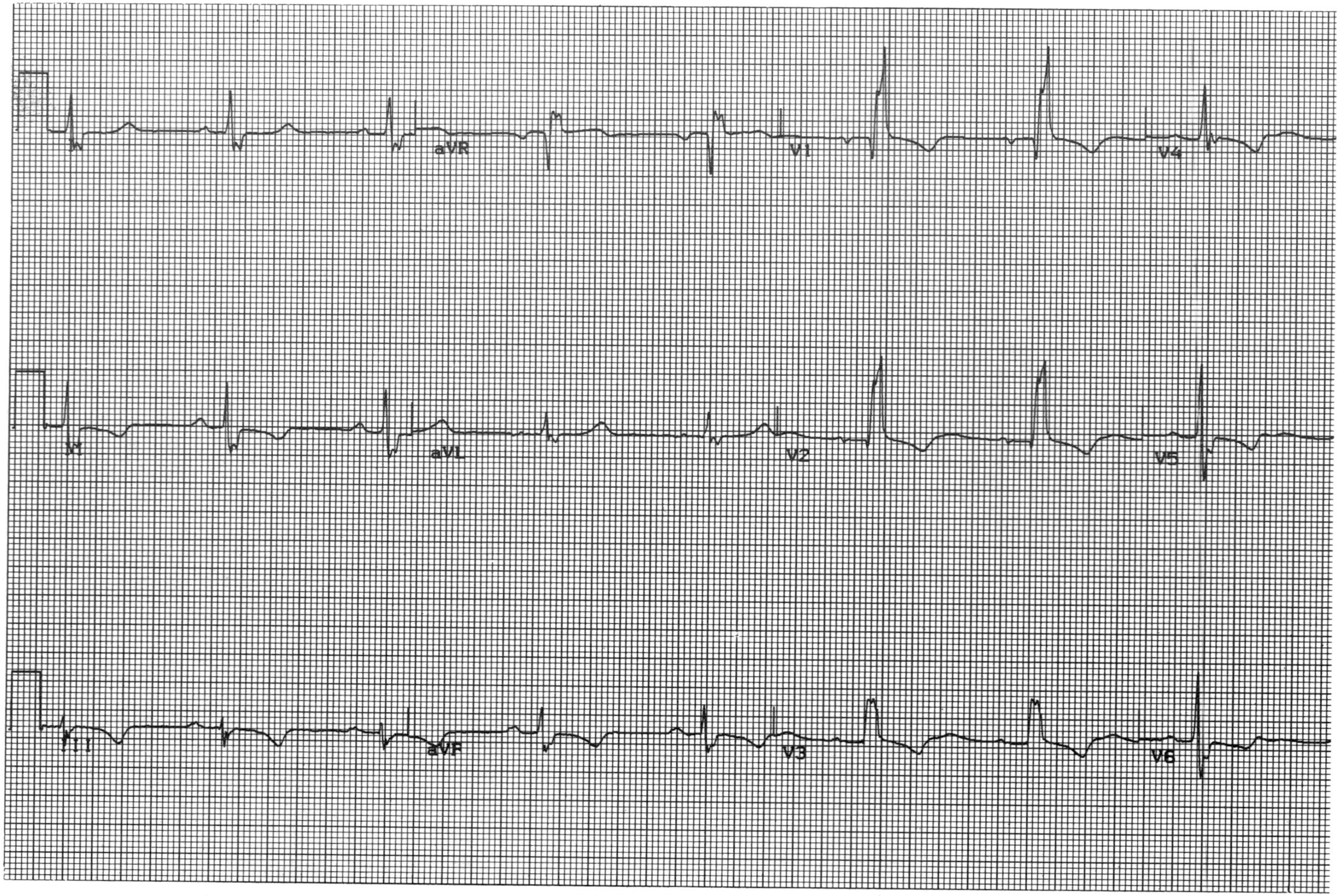

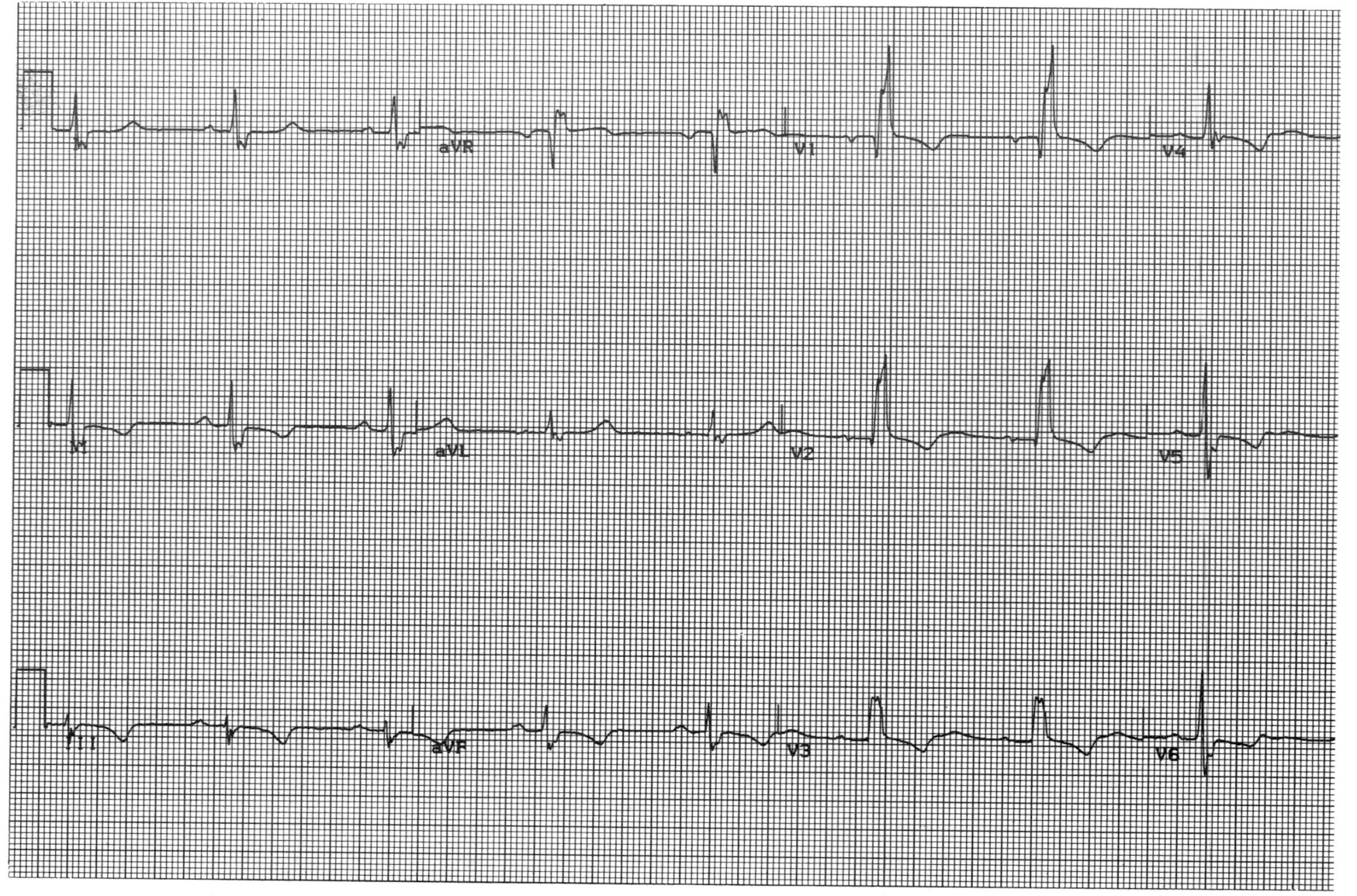

Practice 12 Lead ECG #84

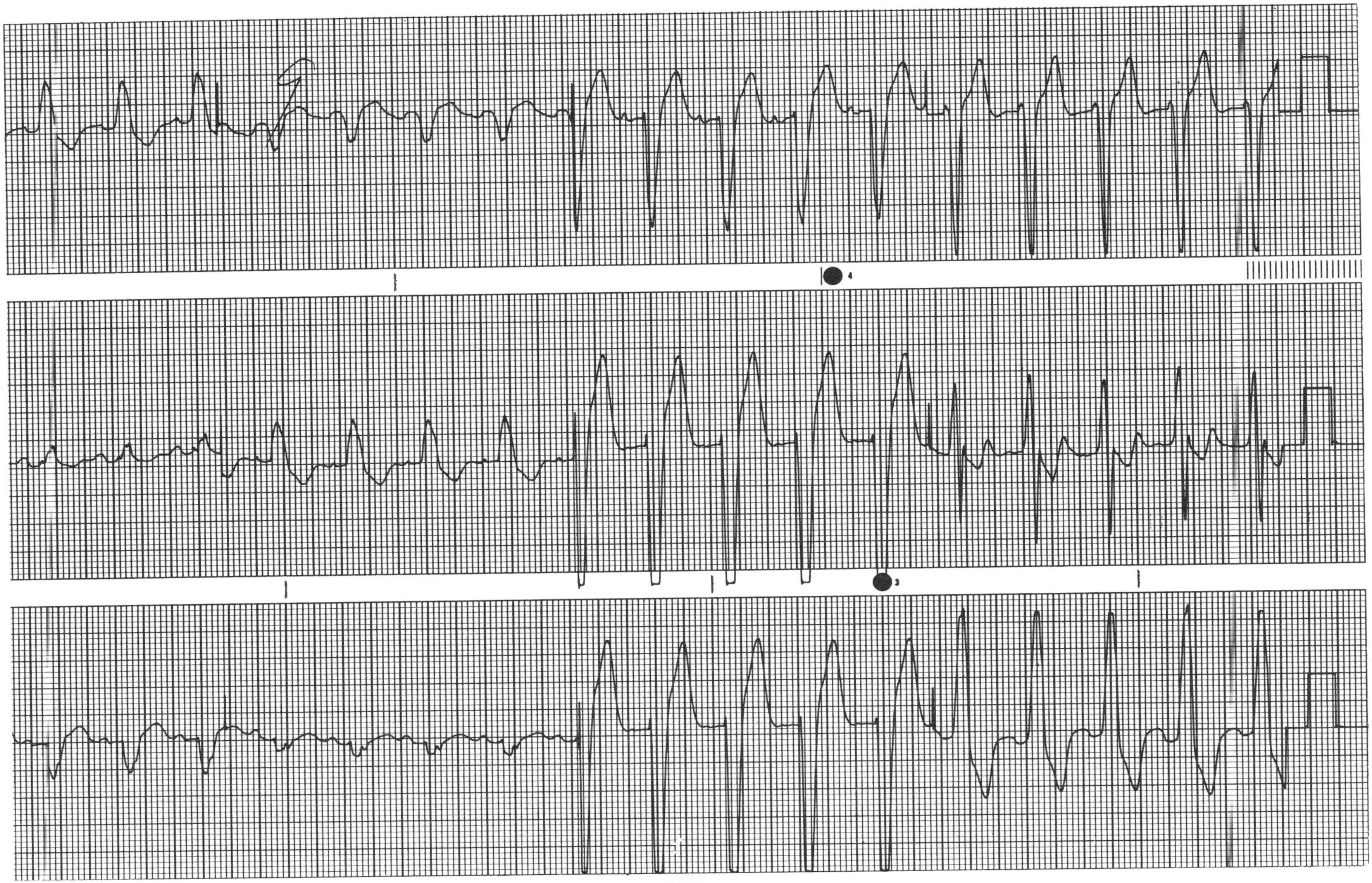

Practice 12 Lead ECG #85

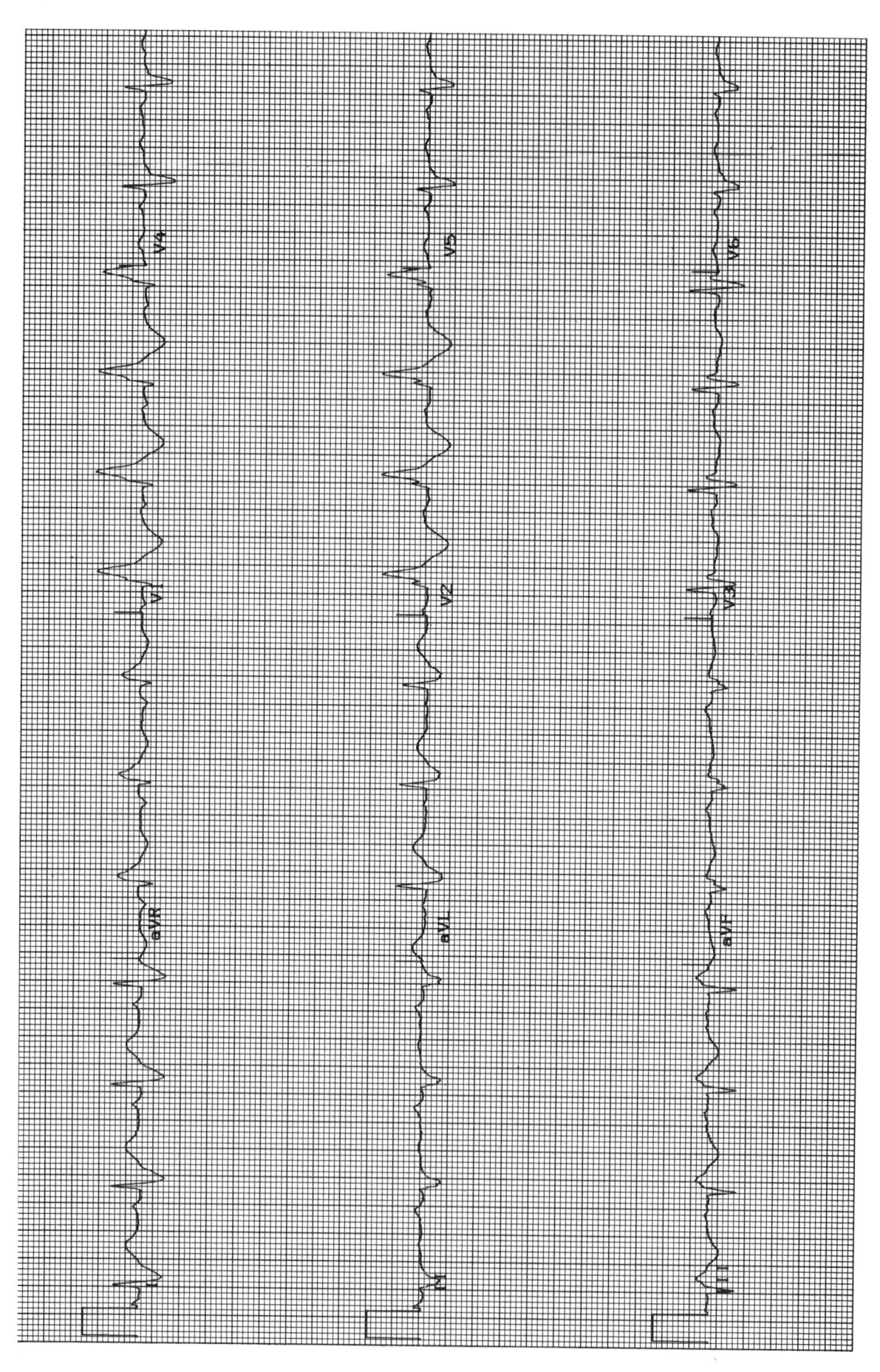

Practice 12 Lead ECG #86

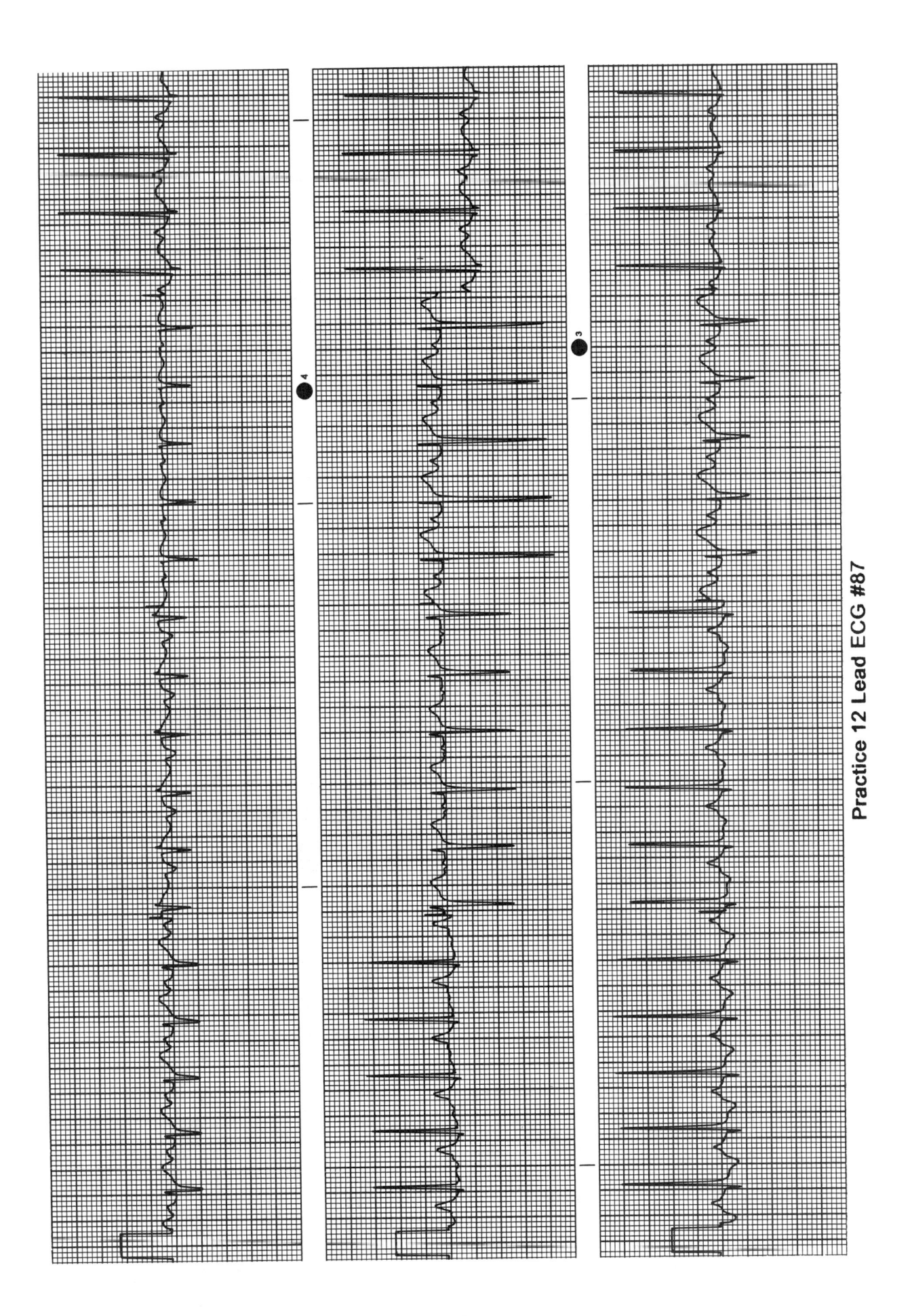

Practice 12 Lead ECG #87

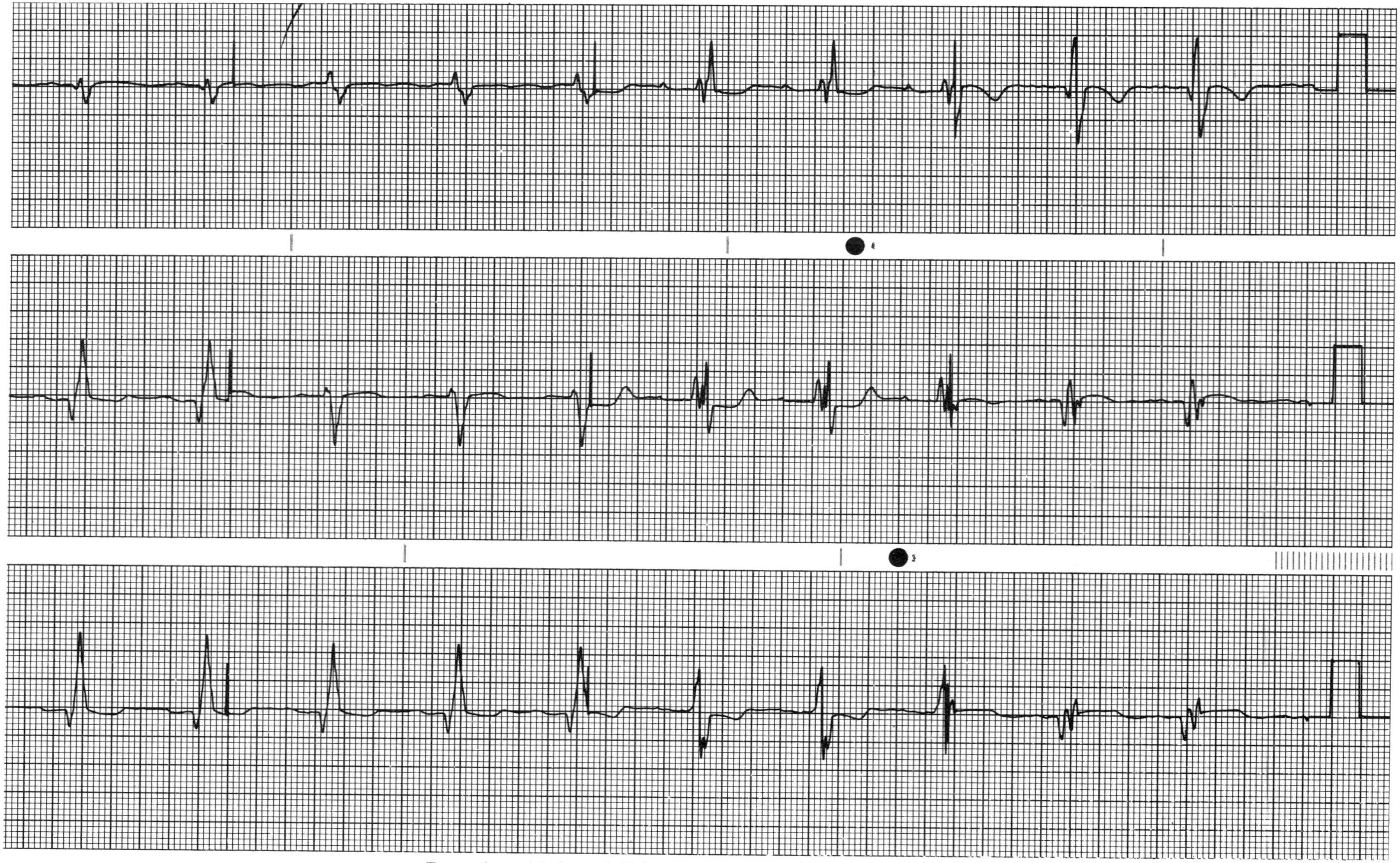

Practice 12 Lead ECG #88

Practice 12 Lead ECG #89

Practice 12 Lead ECG #90

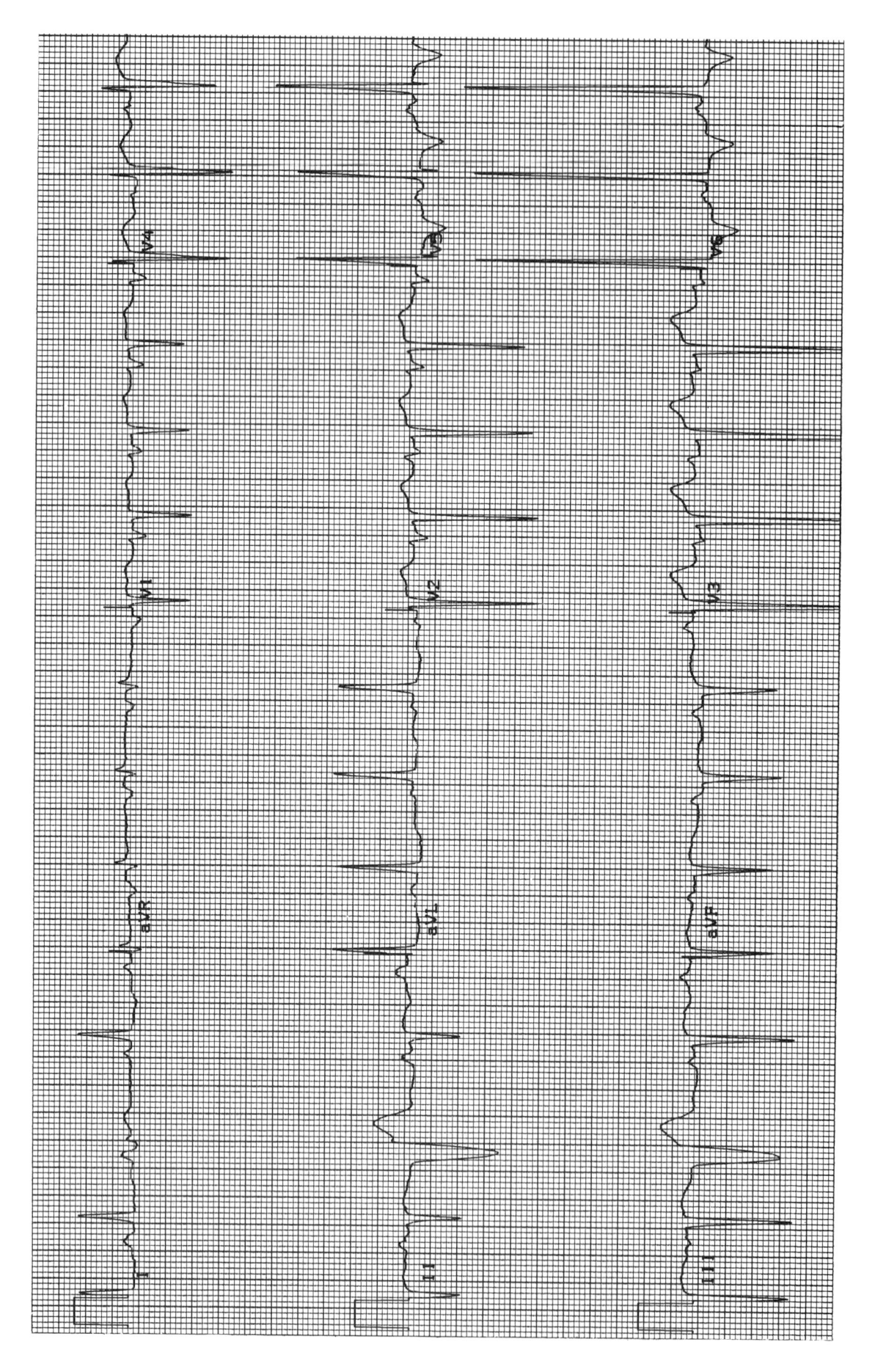

Practice 12 Lead ECG #91

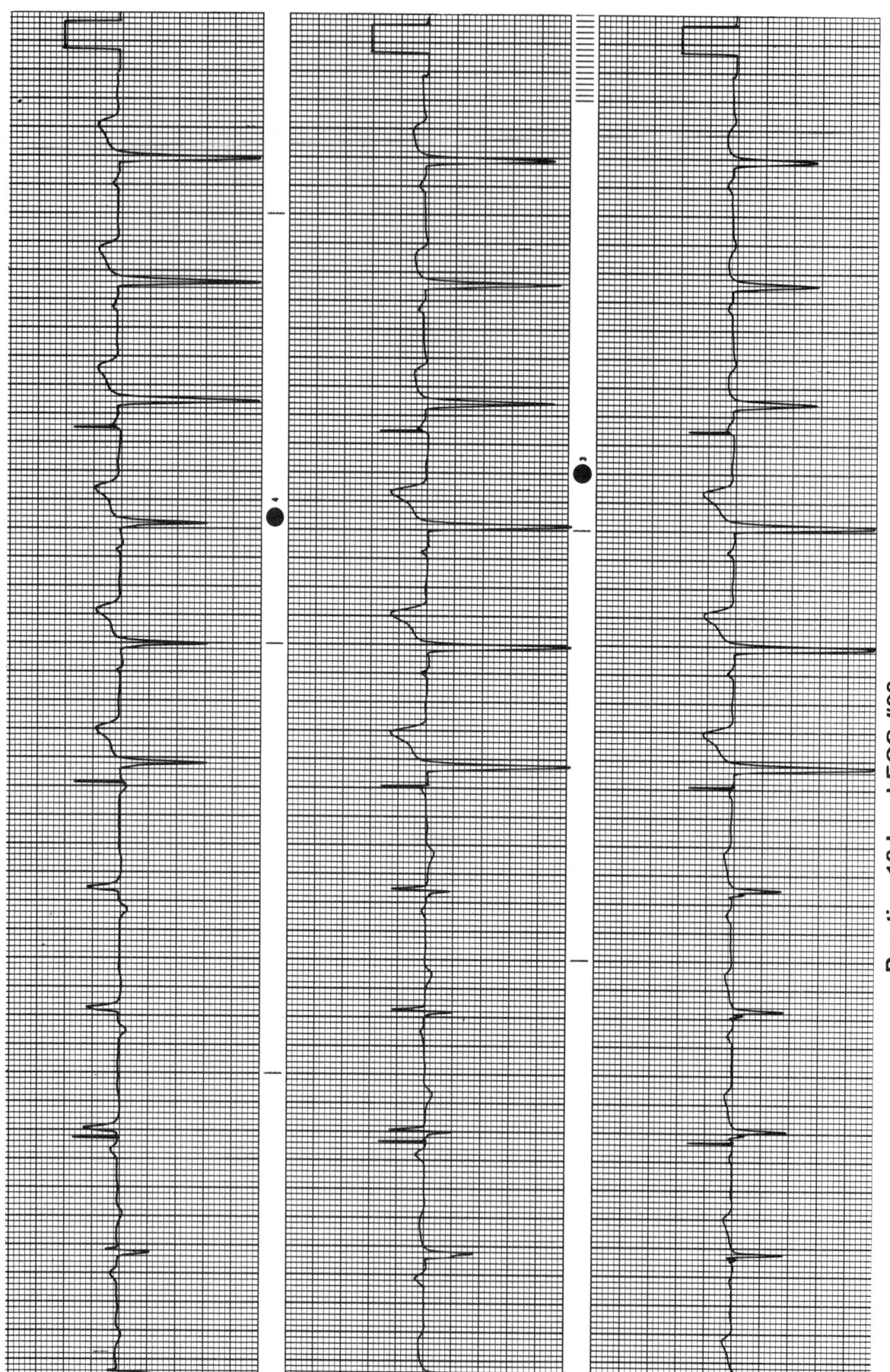

Practice 12 Lead ECG #92

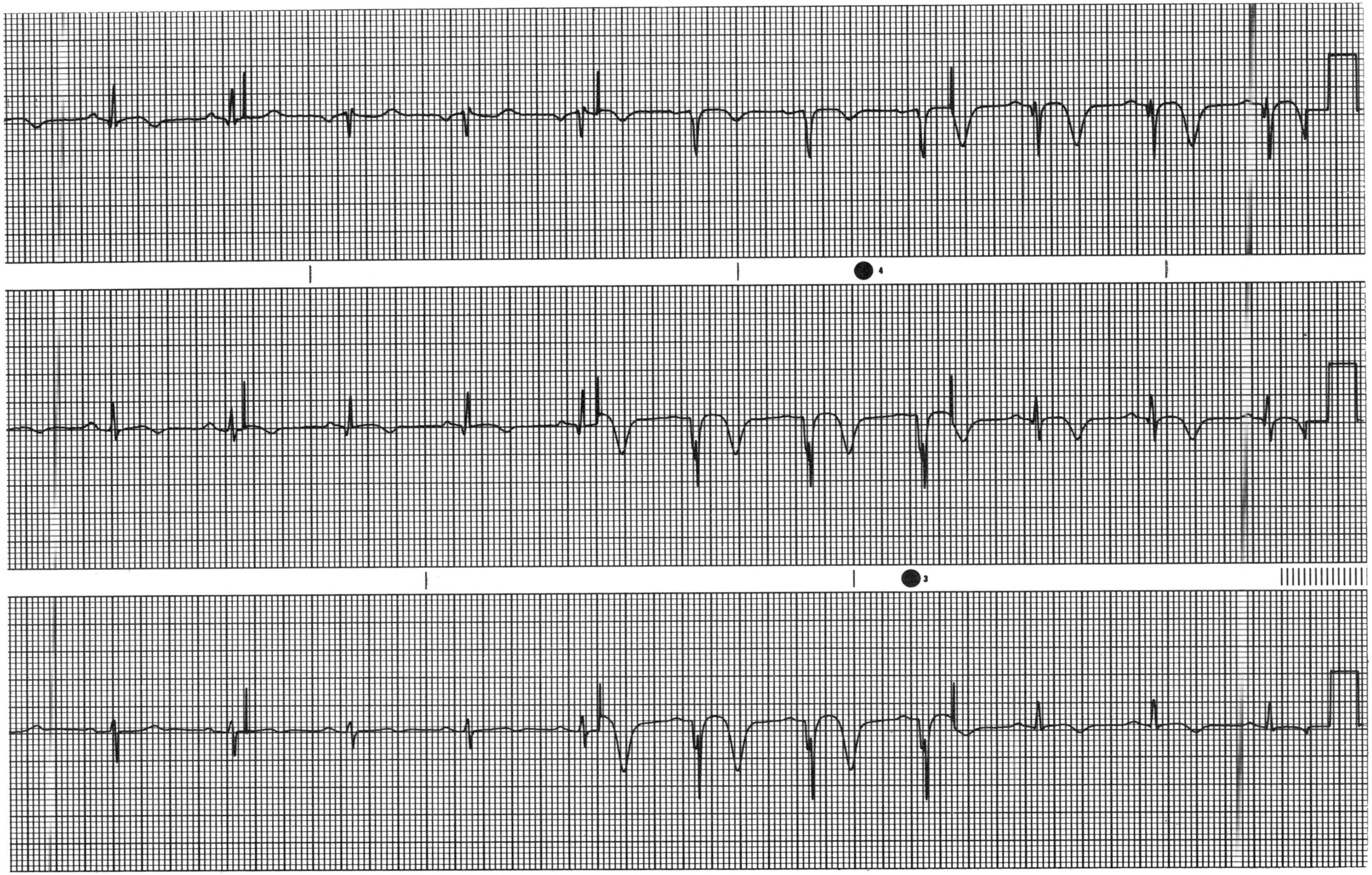

Practice 12 Lead ECG #93

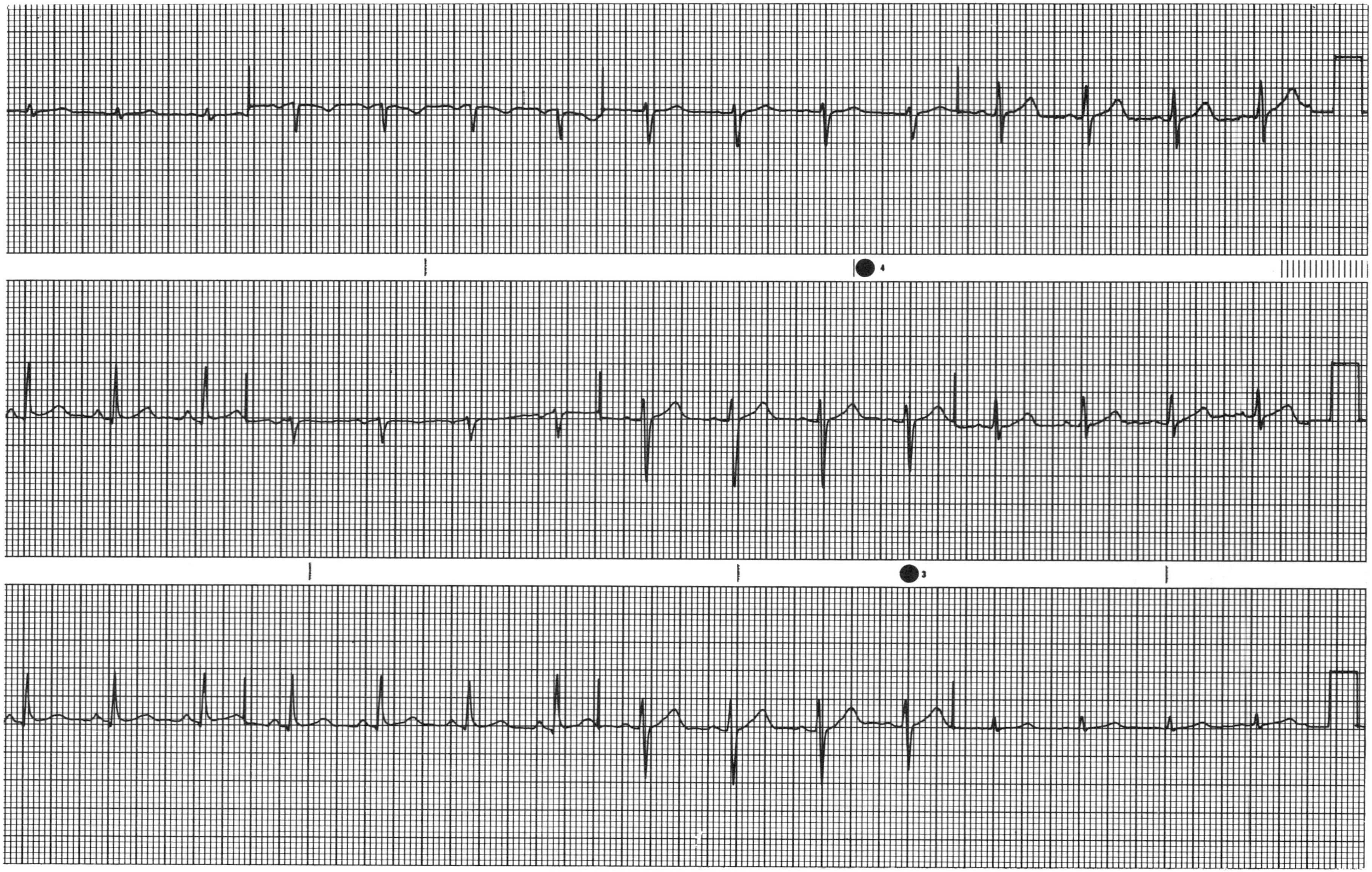

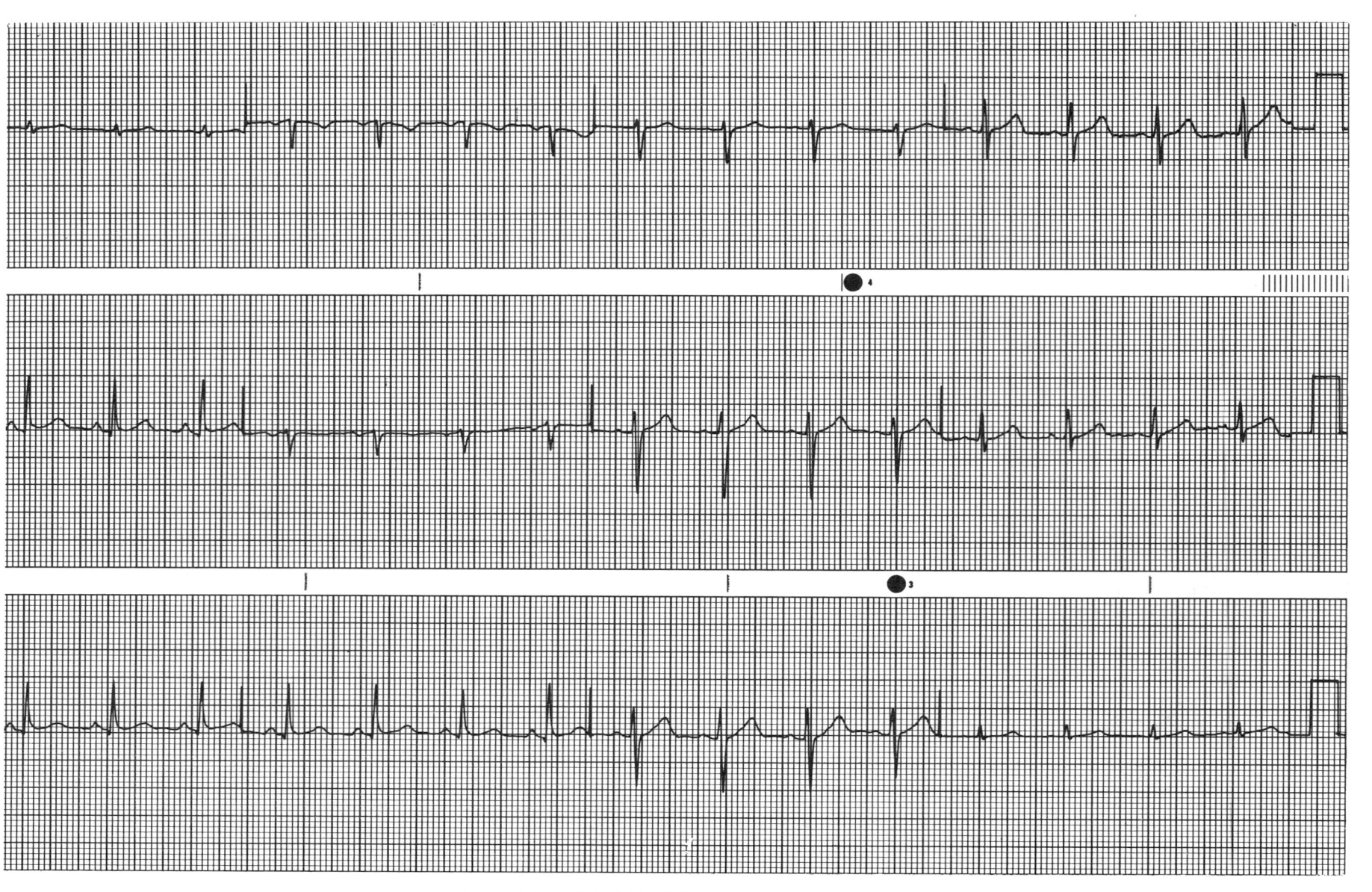

Practice 12 Lead ECG #94

Practice 12 Lead ECG #95

Chapter 7 — Myocardial Ischemia, Injury, and Infarction

ANSWERS TO PRACTICE 12 LEAD ECGs #81-95

81. **Basic rhythm:** Normal sinus rhythm
    Frontal plane axis: Normal +90°
    R wave progression: Normal
    Complex configuration: Normal
    Complex duration: Normal
    P wave: Normal
    ST segment: Normal
    T wave: Normal
    12 Lead ECG Interpretation: Normal

82. **Basic rhythm:** Normal sinus rhythm
    Frontal plane axis: Normal 0°
    R wave progression: Abnormal: qRR' in V_1, V_2; RR' in V_3; R'r in V_4; Rss' in V_5, V_6 (The s waves are deep and slurred for these leads)
    Complex configuration: Abnormal as noted above and Rss' in I, II; q r r' in III
    Complex duration: Abnormal: 0.14 seconds
    P wave: Normal
    Secondary ST-T changes: V_1, V_2
    T wave: Abnormal: Inverted in II, III, aVF, V_3, V_4, V_5, V_6
    12 Lead ECG Interpretation: Abnormal
       - Right bundle branch block
       - Septal infarction, aged undetermined with inferolateral ischemia

83. **Basic rhythm:** Normal sinus rhythm
    Frontal plane axis: Normal +90°
    R wave progression: Abnormal: Loss of anterior forces in V_2; QS in V_3, V_4; qr in V_5; qR in V_6
    Complex configuration: Abnormal as noted above
    Complex duration: Normal
    P wave: Abnormal: Wide and notched in II, III and aVF; abnormal P terminal in V_1
    ST segment: Normal
    T wave: Abnormal: Inverted in I, aVL, V_5, V_6
    12 Lead ECG Interpretation: Abnormal
        - P mitrale
        - Anterolateral infarction, age undetermined

84. **Basic rhythm:** Sinus bradycardia
    Frontal plane axis: Normal 0° (+10° corrected)
    R wave progression: Abnormal: qRR' in V_1, V_2
    Complex configuration: Abnormal as noted above and R'/S' in many leads
    Complex duration: Abnormal: 0.14 seconds
    P wave: Normal
    Secondary ST-T changes: V_1, V_2
    T wave: Inverted in III, AVF, V_3, V_4
    12 Lead ECG Interpretation: Abnormal
        - Sinus bradycardia
        - Right bundle branch block
        - Septal infarction, age undetermined with anterior and inferior ischemia

Chapter 7 — Myocardial Ischemia, Injury, and Infarction

85. **Basic rhythm:** Sinus tachycardia
    Frontal plane axis: Normal 0° (LAD quadrant -10° corrected)
    R wave progression: Abnormal: rS in V_1; rS with no progression of r wave in V_2, V_3, V_4
    Complex configuration: Abnormal as noted above and RR' in other leads
    Complex duration: Abnormal: 0.14 seconds
    P wave: Normal
    Secondary ST-T changes: I, aVL, V_5, V_6
    ST segment: Abnormal: Elevated in V_1, V_2, V_3, V_4
    12 Lead ECG Interpretation: Abnormal
    - Sinus tachycardia
    - Left bundle branch block

86. **Basic rhythm:** Normal sinus rhythm
    Frontal plane axis: LAD quadrant -90° (-80° corrected)
    R wave progression: Abnormal: qRR' in V_1; rR' in V_2; RSr' in V_3; rs in V_4, V_5, V_6
    Complex configuration: As noted above with QS or qs in II, III, aVF
    Complex duration: Abnormal: 0.16 seconds
    P wave: Normal
    Secondary ST-T changes: V_1, V_2
    T wave: Abnormal: Inverted in III, aVF
    12 Lead ECG Interpretation: Abnormal
    - Right bundle branch block
    - Inferior and septal infarction, age undetermined

87. **Basic rhythm:** Sinus tachycardia
    Frontal plane axis: Normal +90° (RAD quadrant +100° corrected)
    R wave progression: Normal: Transition in V_4 is a normal variant
    Complex configuration: Normal
    Complex duration: Normal: 0.08 seconds
    P wave: Abnormal: Tall and peaked in II and aVF; peaked in III
    ST segment: Normal
    T wave: Abnormal: Inverted in II, III, aVF
    12 Lead ECG Interpretation: Abnormal
    - Sinus tachycardia
    - P pulmonale
    - Consider inferior ischemia

Chapter 7 — Myocardial Ischemia, Injury, and Infarction

88. **Basic rhythm:** Normal sinus rhythm with first degree AV heart block (PRi = 0.24 seconds)
    Frontal plane axis: Normal +90° (RAD quadrant +100° corrected)
    R wave progression: Abnormal: rsR' in V_1, V_2; transition occurs in V_3 but the normal tall R waves of V_4, V_5, V_6 are replaced with qRS in V_4 and pathological q waves in V_5 and V_6.
    Complex configuration: Abnormal as noted above and pathological q waves in II, III, aVF; R' in many leads.
    Complex duration: Abnormal: 0.14 seconds
    P wave: Normal
    Secondary ST-T changes: V_1, V_2
    T wave: Abnormal: Flat in II, III, aVF; inverted in V_3, V_4, V_5, V_6
    12 Lead ECG Interpretation: Abnormal
    - First degree AV heart block
    - Right bundle branch block
    - Inferior and lateral myocardial infarction, age undetermined, with anterior ischemia

89. **Basic rhythm:** Sinus arrhythmia
    Frontal plane axis: Normal 0° (LAD quadrant -10° corrected)
    R wave progression: Abnormal: Normal r wave in V_1 does not increase in V_2, V_3, V_4 = loss of anterior forces; transition abnormally occurs in V_5
    Complex configuration: Abnormal as noted above and RR' in aVL; r r'S in aVF; loss of physiological q waves in I, aVL, V_5, V_6
    Complex duration: Abnormal: 0.12 seconds
    P wave: Normal
    Secondary ST-T changes: V_5, V_6, I, aVL
    12 Lead ECG Interpretation: Abnormal
    - Sinus arrhythmia
    - Left bundle branch block

90. **Basic rhythm:** Normal sinus rhythm with occasional PVCs
    Frontal plane axis: LAD quadrant -60°
    R wave progression: Abnormal: loss of anterior forces
    Complex configuration: Abnormal as noted above and QS in II, III, aVF; S > 25 mm in V_3; R > 25 mm in V_6
    Complex duration: Normal: 0.10 seconds
    P wave: Abnormal: Wide and notched in II; abnormal P terminal in V_1
    Secondary ST-T: I, aVL, V_5, V_6
    12 Lead ECG Interpretation: Abnormal
    - PVCs
    - Inferior infarction, age undetermined
    - P mitrale
    - Left ventricular hypertrophy
    Estes score for this patient:

Voltage criteria	3
Secondary ST-T changes (not on digitalis)	3
Complex interval greater than 0.09 seconds	1
Abnormal P terminal in V_1	3
TOTAL	10

Chapter 7 — Myocardial Ischemia, Injury, and Infarction

91. **Basic rhythm:** Normal sinus rhythm
    Frontal plane axis: Normal: 0° (LAD quadrant -5° corrected)
    R wave progression: Abnormal: Large R in V_1. Recall that large R waves in V_1 may indicate RVH, RBBB, or posterior infarction.
    Complex configuration: Abnormal: Q waves in II, III, aVF
    Complex duration: Normal: 0.08 seconds
    P wave: Normal: II, III, aVF have artifact
    ST segment: Normal
    T wave: Abnormal: Inverted in I, II, aVL, aVF, V_5, V_6
    12 Lead ECG Interpretation: Abnormal
    - Inferoposterior infarction with lateral ischemia, age undetermined

92. **Basic rhythm:** Normal sinus rhythm
    Frontal plane axis: No man's land quadrant -120°
    R wave progression: Abnormal: No r wave in any precordial lead
    Complex configuration: Abnormal: QS in V_1 through V_6; Qr in I, aVL; Q in II, aVF
    P wave: Normal
    ST segment: Abnormal: Elevated in V_1, V_2, V_3, V_4
    T wave: Abnormal: Inverted in I, aVL, V_5, V_6
    12 Lead ECG Interpretation: Abnormal
    - Acute anteroseptal infarction
    - Lateral infarction, age undetermined

93. **Basic rhythm:** Normal sinus rhythm
    Frontal plane axis: Normal 0°
    R wave progression: Abnormal: QS in V_1, V_2, V_3, V_4; transition in V_5
    Complex configuration: Abnormal as noted above
    P wave: Normal
    ST segment: Normal
    T wave: Abnormal: Inverted in I, II, aVL, aVF, V_1 through V_6
    12 Lead ECG Interpretation: Abnormal
    - Anteroseptal infarction, age undetermined, with inferior and lateral ischemia

94. **Basic rhythm:** Normal sinus rhythm
    Frontal plane axis: Normal +90°
    R wave progression: Normal
    Complex configuration: Normal: Transition in V_4 – a normal variant
    Complex duration: Normal: 0.08 seconds
    P wave: Normal
    ST segment: Normal
    T wave: Normal
    12 Lead ECG Interpretation: Normal

Chapter 7 — Myocardial Ischemia, Injury, and Infarction

95. **Basic rhythm:** Normal sinus rhythm
    Frontal plane axis: Normal 0°
    R wave progression: Abnormal: R wave in V_1 has more amplitude than the S wave in V_1
    Complex configuration: Abnormal as noted above and pathological Q waves in II, III, aVF
    P wave: Normal
    ST segment: Normal
    T wave: Abnormal: Inverted in I, II, aVL, aVF, V_5, V_6
    12 Lead ECG Interpretation: Abnormal
    - Inferoposterior infarction with lateral ischemia, age undetermined

CHAPTER 8
SUPRAVENTRICULAR ABERRANCY VERSUS VENTRICULAR ECTOPY

THE SCOPE OF THE PROBLEM

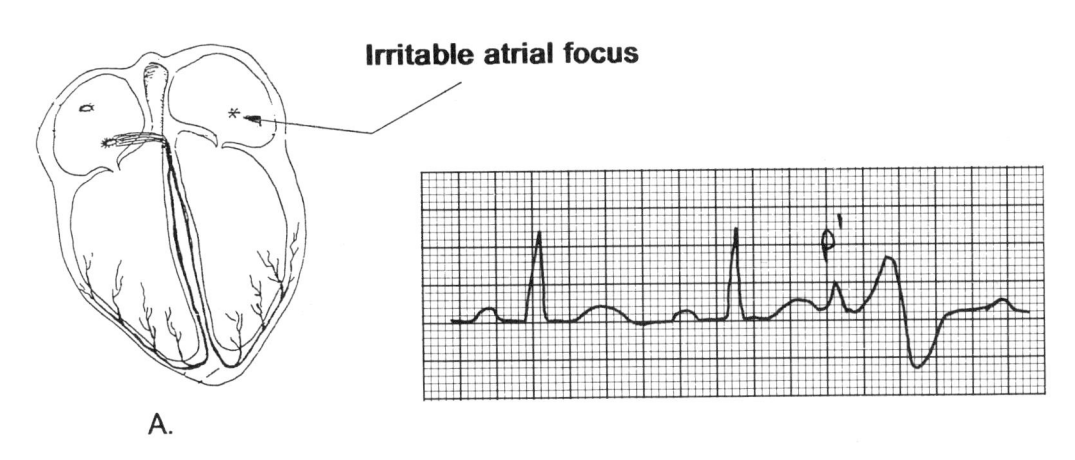

A.

In picture A above, a PAC interrupts the normal sinus rhythm while the right ventricle is still in its refractory period; the left ventricle has recovered from the previous sinus beat and accepts conduction of the PAC. The left ventricle depolarizes, and in the meantime the right ventricle recovers and is depolarized abnormally via the Purkinje fibers. This abnormal depolarization of one of the ventricles results in abnormal repolarization with the ST-T going in the opposite direction to the main part of the complex as depicted in the ECG above.

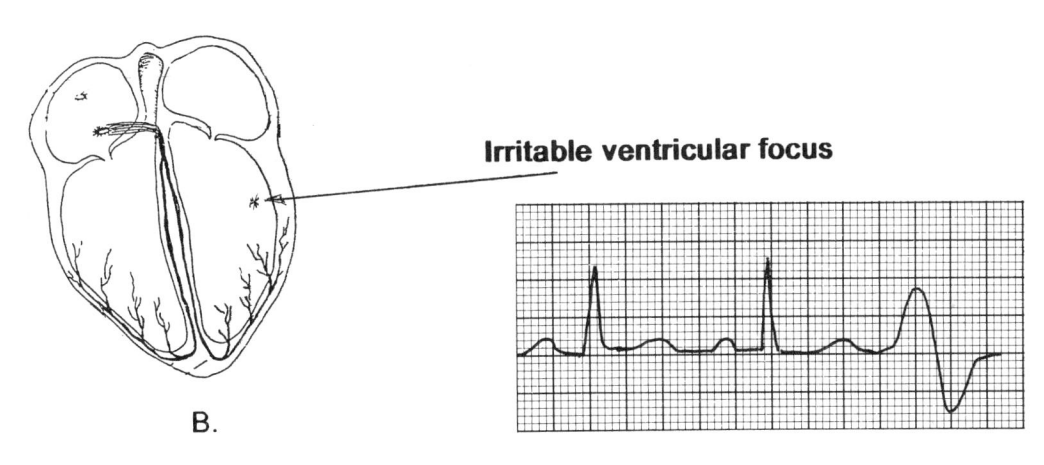

B.

In picture B above, a PVC interrupts the normal sinus rhythm. The PVC depolarizes the ventricles abnormally. This abnormal depolarization results in abnormal repolarization with the ST-T going in the opposite direction to the main part of the complex.

The scope of the problem is that the PAC that conducted aberrantly in picture A looks very much like the PVC in picture B.

Chapter 8 — Supraventricular Aberrancy Versus Ventricular Ectopy

Furthermore, the irritable ectopic in the atria that caused the PAC may develop into PAT with aberrant conduction to the ventricles:

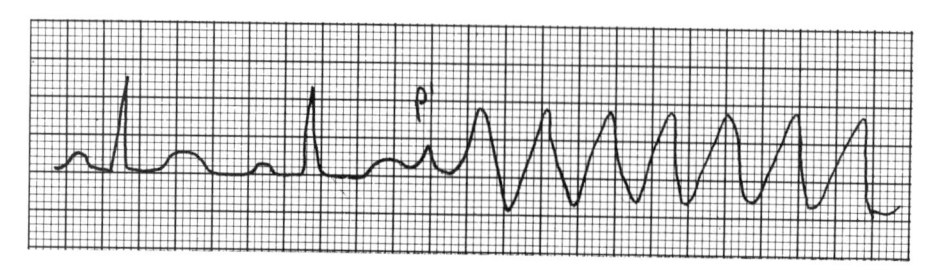

Paroxysmal Atrial Tachycardia with Aberrant Conduction

... and the PVC may also take over as pacemaker resulting in ventricular tachycardia:

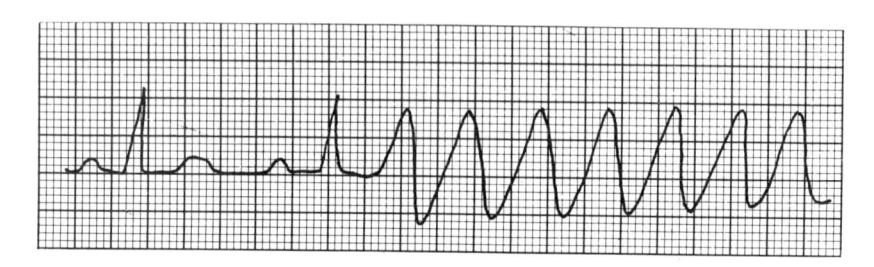

Ventricular Tachycardia

Again, the problem is that PAT with aberrant conduction looks like ventricular tachycardia on the ECG. The supraventricular tachycardia mimics ventricular tachycardia and vice versa.

Supraventricular aberrancy is a temporary form of abnormal intraventricular conduction of a supraventricular impulse. Supraventricular aberrancy results from an unequal refractory period of the bundle branches. As described in picture A, a supraventricular impulse arrived when one of the bundle branches was able to conduct and the other bundle branch was still in its refractory period. The abnormal PAC was inscribed due to the aberrant pathway through the ventricles.

The right bundle branch has a longer refractory period than the left bundle branch and is more likely to be responsible for aberrant ventricular conduction, i.e., supraventricular aberrancy.

Supraventricular aberrancy may occur with a single premature beat such as a PAC or a PJC or with arrhythmias such as sinus tachycardia, atrial tachycardia, uncontrolled atrial fibrillation, atrial flutter, and junctional tachycardia.

Ventricular ectopy refers to the ectopic site's origin in the ventricles such as PVCs or ventricular tachycardia.

Researchers have attempted to develop decisive criteria to make an accurate ECG diagnosis of supraventricular aberrancy versus ventricular ectopy. They have been unsuccessful. One must make a reasonable interpretation based on available ECG clues. Some ECG clues favor supraventricular aberrancy while others favor ventricular ectopy as follows.

Chapter 8 — Supraventricular Aberrancy Versus Ventricular Ectopy

ECG CHARACTERISTICS OF SUPRAVENTRICULAR ABERRANCY

1. **Ashman's Phenomena:** The refractory period of the ventricular conduction system is affected by the preceding cycle length. When there is a long R to R cycle the refractory period will be long. When there is a short R to R cycle the refractory period will be short.

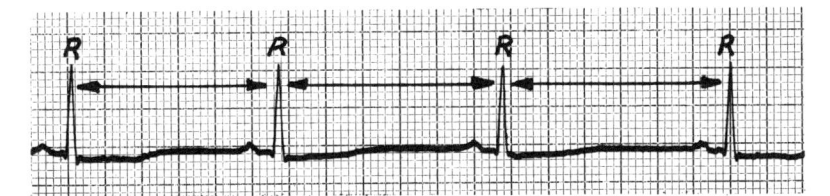

   In the strip above, the ventricles have "set themselves up" for another long refractory period. Therefore, if the next beat is early it may arrive during the ventricular refractory period. If both bundle branches are in their absolute refractory period the impulse would just not conduct. However, if one of the bundle branches has recovered but one is still refractory, the impulse will be conducted to the ventricles aberrantly.

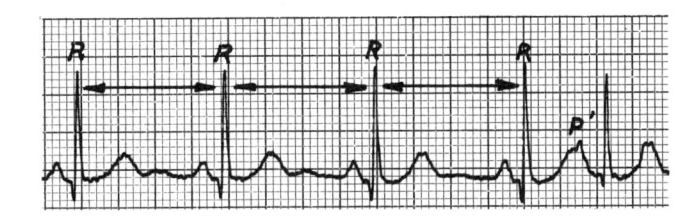

   Supraventricular aberrancy is favored when a premature impulse follows a long R to R cycle length. This is *Ashman's phenomena*.

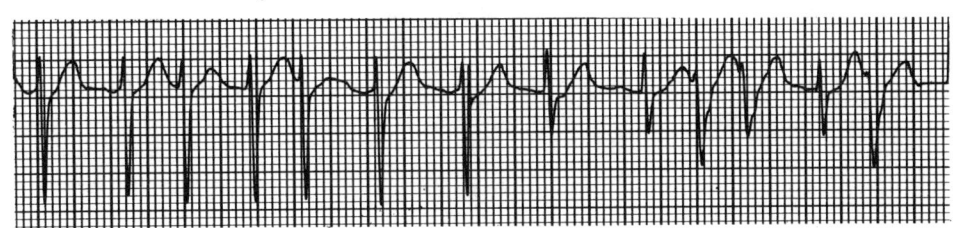

   Ashman's Phenomena

   NOTE: the first premature beat that conducts aberrantly (10th beat) ends a short cycle preceded by a long cycle. Ashman's phenomena is also called the *long-short ventricular cycle*.

2. **Triphasic pattern in V_1 (rsR'):** Aberrantly conducted supraventricular complexes often have right bundle branch block ECG morphology because the right bundle branch has a longer refractory period than the left. The triphasic rabbit ear pattern in V_1 favors supraventricular aberrancy.

Chapter 8 — Supraventricular Aberrancy Versus Ventricular Ectopy

3. **Complex duration less than 0.14 seconds.** Supraventricular complexes with aberrancy conduct normally via one of the bundle branches. The aberrant complex is wide because of abnormal conduction through <u>one</u> ventricle. Although the overall conduction is delayed, it is <u>usually</u> completed in less than 0.14 seconds.

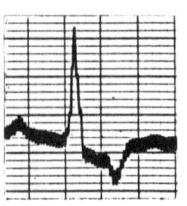

4. **Initial vector similar to that of the normally conducted beats.** One of the bundle branches has recovered from the previous stimulus so the premature complex will likely begin conduction the same way the normal complex began conduction. If the initial vector of the normal beat is positive, i.e., an R wave, and the initial vector of the aberrant beat is also positive — this favors supraventricular aberrancy.

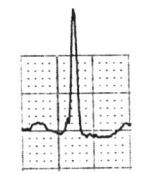

   Normal Beat 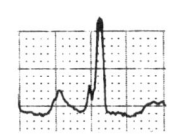   **Aberrantly Conducted Beat**

   NOTE: The initial vector is the same in the normal beat as in the aberrantly conducted beat. The same initial vector favors supraventricular aberrancy.

   Supraventricular aberrancy is favored if the initial vector of the normal beat is negative and the initial vector of the aberrant beat is also negative.

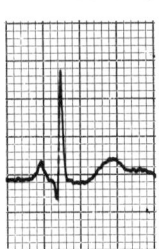

   Normal Beat 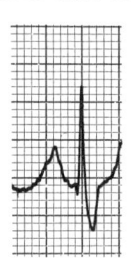   **Aberrantly Conducted Beat**

   NOTE: The initial vector of the normal beat and the aberrantly conducted beat are both negative, i.e., q waves. The same or similar initial vector favors supraventricular aberrancy.

5. **Premature P' (P prime).** The P' of the aberrantly conducted beat is often hidden in the T wave. That's the reason it conducts abnormally — it falls in the refractory period of the previous beat.

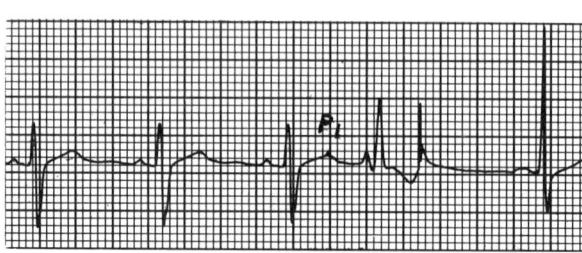

Chapter 8 — Supraventricular Aberrancy Versus Ventricular Ectopy

6. **Noncompensatory pause.** PACs usually have a noncompensatory pause. To measure for a compensatory or a noncompensatory pause, measure the distance between three sinus beats, 1-2-3, on the strip below:

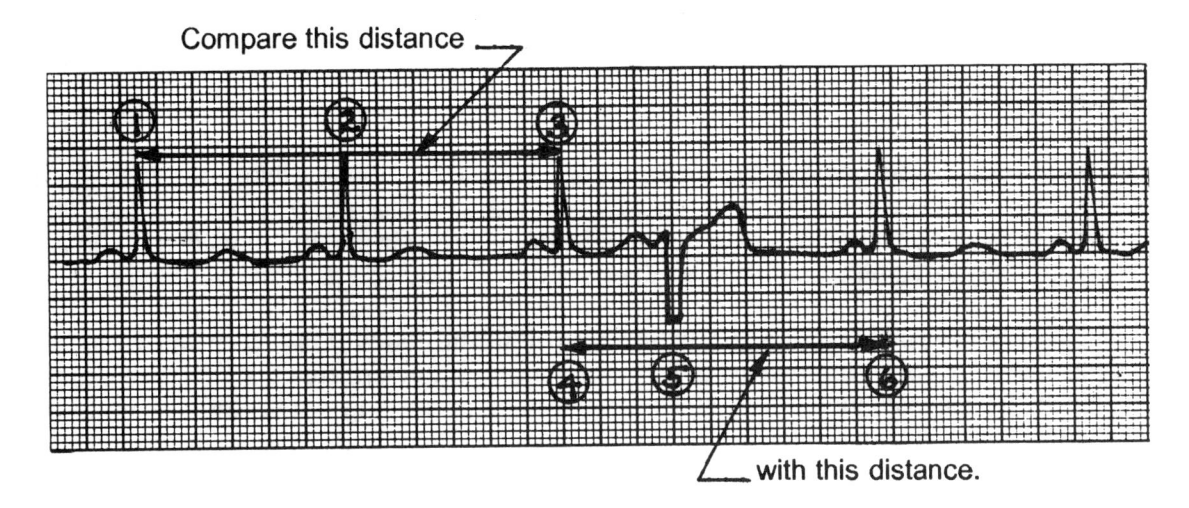

Noncompensatory pause

... then compare that distance between three beats, one of which includes the premature beat (4-5-6). In the above example the distance between 1-2-3 (three sinus beats) is not the same as the distance between 4-5-6 (sinus, premature, sinus beats). When the distance is NOT the same it is a NONCOMPENSATORY PAUSE. PACs usually have a noncompensatory pause.

When the distance is the same it is called a COMPENSATORY PAUSE. PVCs usually have a compensatory pause:

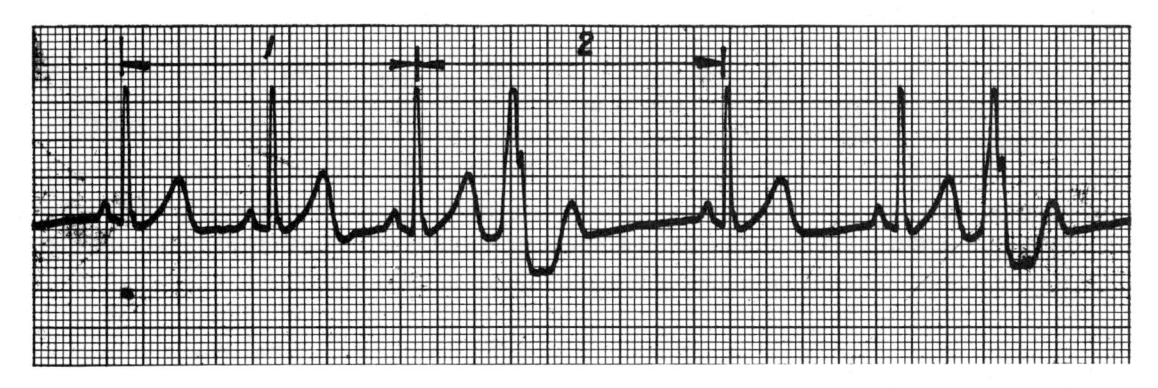

Compensatory pause

In the above strip the distance between the first three sinus beats (1) is the same as the distance between (2) three beats, one of which includes the PVC: this is a compensatory pause.

Chapter 8 — Supraventricular Aberrancy Versus Ventricular Ectopy

QUESTION: The presence of a noncompensatory pause favors supraventricular aberrancy over ventricular ectopy.

A. True
B. False

ANSWER. A. True

7. **Ventricular rate greater than 170 BPM.** Recall the inherent firing rate of the ventricles is 15 to 40 times per minute. Irritable foci in the atria fire at much faster rates. The atrial rate in atrial fibrillation is 350 to 600 times per minute. One of the functions of the AV node is to delay rapid atrial impulses so they are not conducted 1:1 to the ventricles.

8. **Carotid sinus massage or other vagal maneuvers may terminate or slow a supraventricular tachycardia.** These vagal maneuvers exert a negative dromotropic effect at the AV node. Therefore, arrhythmias originating above the AV node may be slowed by these maneuvers but arrhythmias originating below the AV node would not be affected.

In summary, the above ECG characteristics favor supraventricular aberrancy over ventricular ectopy but they are not absolutes.

The long-short ventricular cycle, Ashman's phenomena, may occur with ventricular ectopics.

The right bundle branch block ECG morphology in V_1 is expected with supraventricular aberrancy due to the longer refractory period of the right bundle branch. However, left bundle branch block morphology is also seen with supraventricular aberrancy and right bundle branch block morphology is seen with ventricular ectopics.

Aberrantly conducted beats usually have a rate greater than 170 BPM and a complex duration less than 0.14 seconds but neither of these are proof positive of supraventricular aberrancy.

The presence of a P^I preceding an aberrant complex does not completely rule out a ventricular ectopic. A PAC may occur and inscribe the P^I, but there is nothing to prevent a PVC from firing immediately after the premature atrial ectopic.

On the other hand, if you are trying to distinguish a PAC with aberrancy from a PVC and there is a

(1) P^I and
(2) a noncompensatory pause,

. . . odds are very much in favor of the PAC with aberrancy.

Chapter 8 — Supraventricular Aberrancy Versus Ventricular Ectopy

ECG CHARACTERISTICS OF VENTRICULAR ECTOPY

Generally speaking, the opposite of the ECG characteristics of supraventricular aberrancy just described are the ECG characteristics of ventricular ectopy.

1. **Absence of P'.** P' are often difficult to see because they are hidden in the T wave; be sure they are absent. Also, remember that the absence of a P' will occur with some junctional arrhythmias.

2. **Compensatory pause.** PVCs usually have a compensatory pause. To measure for a compensatory pause, measure the distance between three sinus beats (1-2-3 on the strip below).

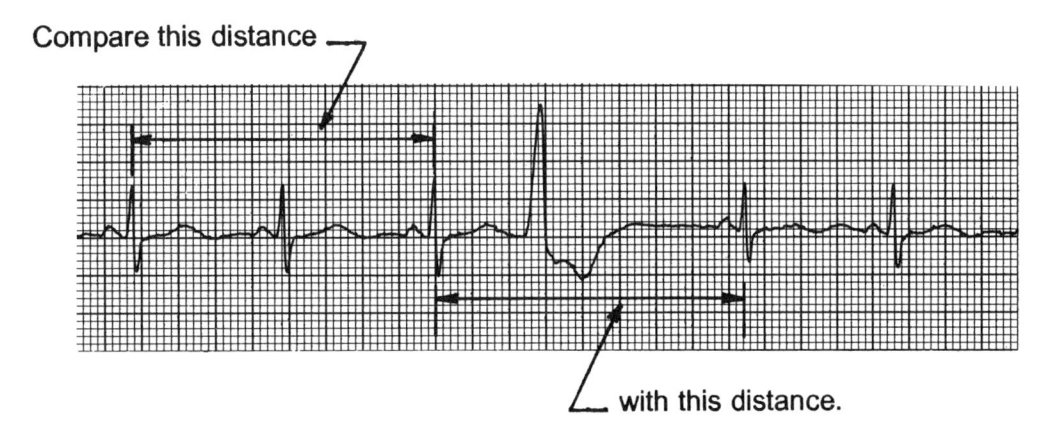

Compare this distance with this distance.

QUESTION: In the above strip a compensatory pause is present.

ANSWER: True. When the distance is the same it is a compensatory pause. PVCs usually have a compensatory pause as the sinus rhythm is not disturbed by the ventricular ectopic beat.

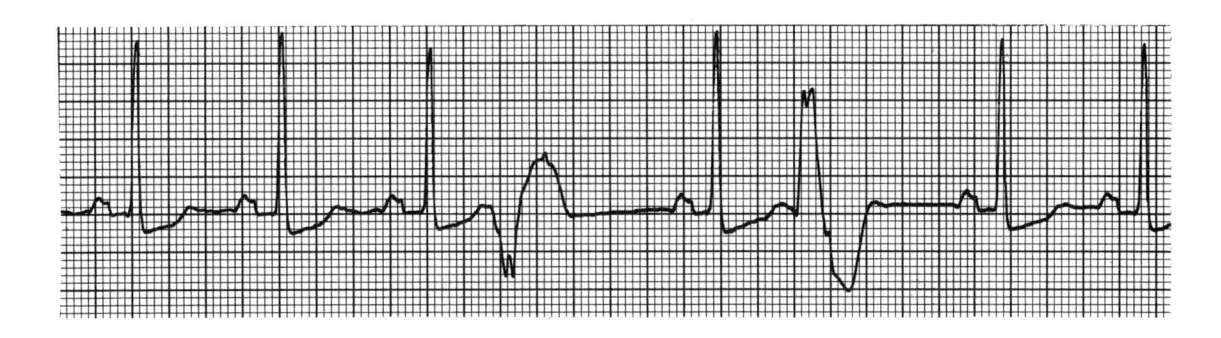

PVCs with compensatory pause

3. **Axis deviation**

   a. Left axis deviation or no man's land quadrant favors right ventricular ectopy.
   b. Right axis deviation favors left ventricular ectopy.

Chapter 8 -- Supraventricular Aberrancy versus Ventricular Ectopy

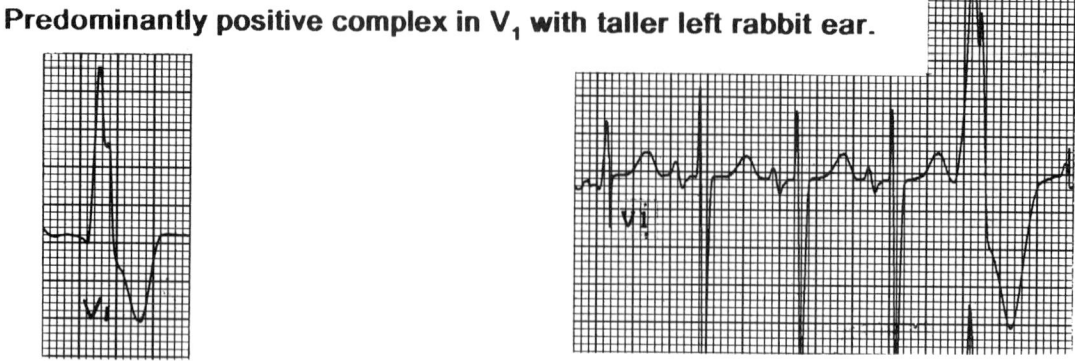

4. **Predominantly positive complex in V_1 with taller left rabbit ear.**

   In the two strips above, the left (first) rabbit ear of the PVC is taller than the second rabbit ear. When this morphology occurs in V_1, odds are very high in favor of ventricular ectopy.

5. **QS or rS in V_6** favors left ventricular ectopy.

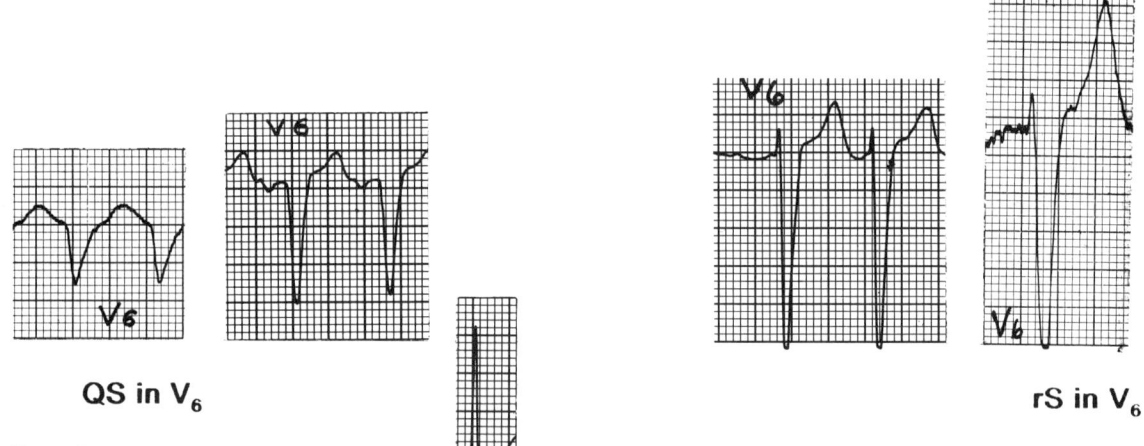

   QS in V_6 rS in V_6

   Recall the normal complex in V_6 is   . With left ventricular ectopy the impulse begins on the left and moves away from the positive electrode of V_6 resulting in a primarily negative complex, i.e., QS or rS.

   With left ventricular ectopy the impulse begins on the left and moves away from the positive electrode of V_6 resulting in a primarily negative complex.

6. **Fat initial r wave greater than 0.03 seconds in V_1** favors right ventricular ectopy.

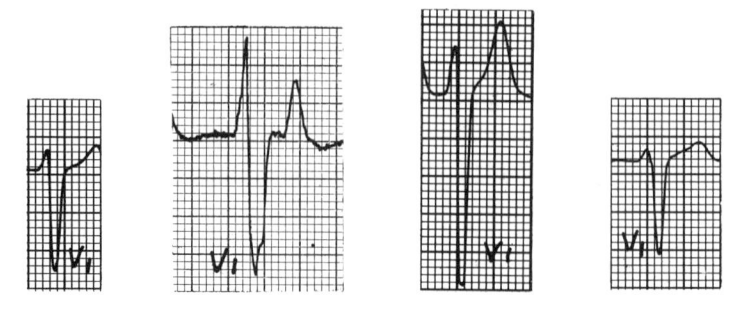

   Fat initial R in V_1 greater than 0.03 seconds in duration

Chapter 8 — Supraventricular Aberrancy versus Ventricular Ectopy

7. **Complex duration greater than 0.14 seconds.**

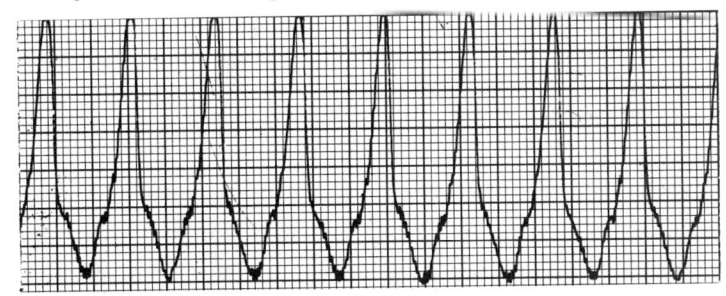

8. **Ventricular rate between 130 and 170 BPM.**

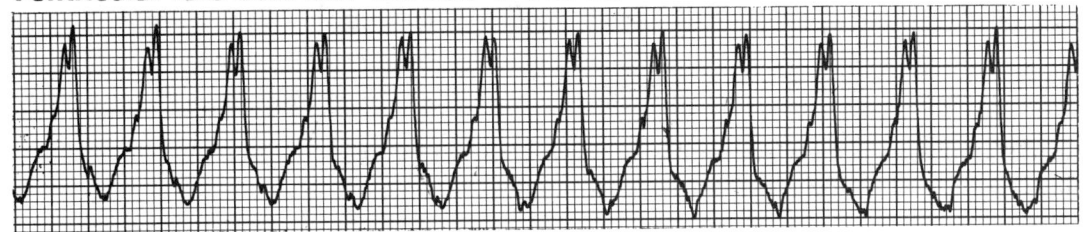

   Recall the inherent firing rate of the ventricles is 15 to 40 times per minute.

9. **Concordant pattern:** presence of all positive or all negative complexes across the precordium V_1 through V_6. Concordant pattern only occurs in three situations: (1) Wolfe-Parkinson-White syndrome, (2) ventricular tachycardia, and (3) septal-anterolateral infarction.

   Refer to practice 12 lead ECG #92 on page 230 for an example of a negative concordant pattern.

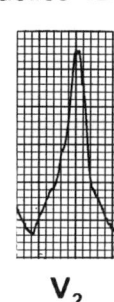

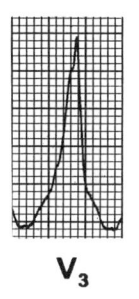

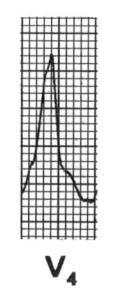

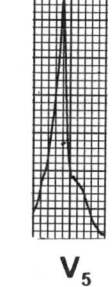

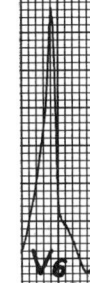

   V_1 V_2 V_3 V_4 V_5 V_6

   Concordant pattern with all positive complexes

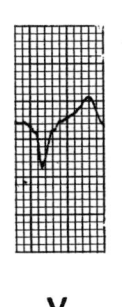

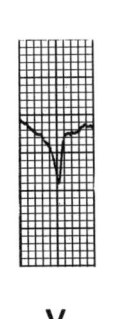

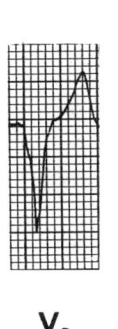

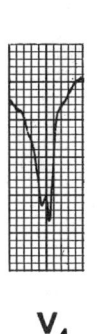

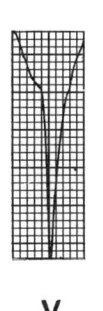

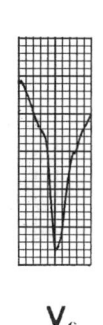

   V_1 V_2 V_3 V_4 V_5 V_6

   Concordant pattern with all negative complexes

Chapter 8 — Supraventricular Aberrancy versus Ventricular Ectopy

10. **Fusion beats** are also known as Dressler beats and summation beats.

    When a supraventricular and a ventricular pacemaker spread through the heart at the same time, they meet and merge together. A fusion beat is the result of this merging. On the ECG, the complex has some characteristics from each of the sources of its origin.

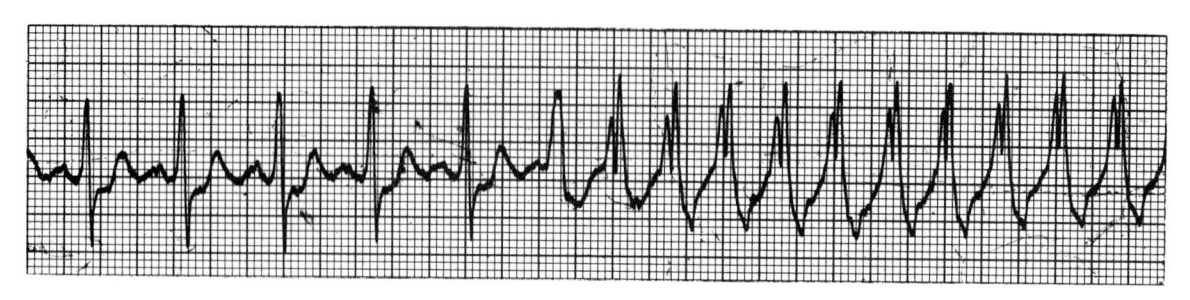

    In the above strip the sixth beat is a fusion beat. It looks a little like the sinus beats which proceed it and a little like the ventricular beats that follow it.

11. **Monophasic or biphasic pattern in V_1** favors ventricular ectopy.

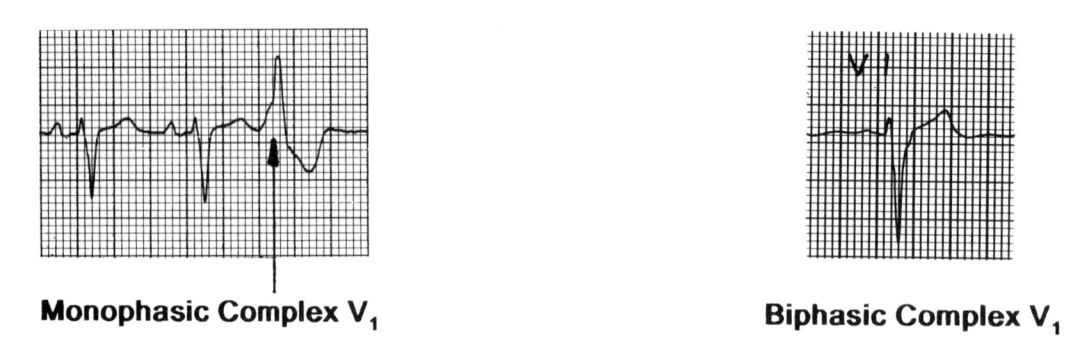

    Monophasic Complex V_1   **Biphasic Complex V_1**

    Recall that a triphasic complex in V_1 favors supraventricular aberrancy.

12. **AV dissociation.** Evidence of two separate pacemakers for the atria and the ventricles favors ventricular ectopy.

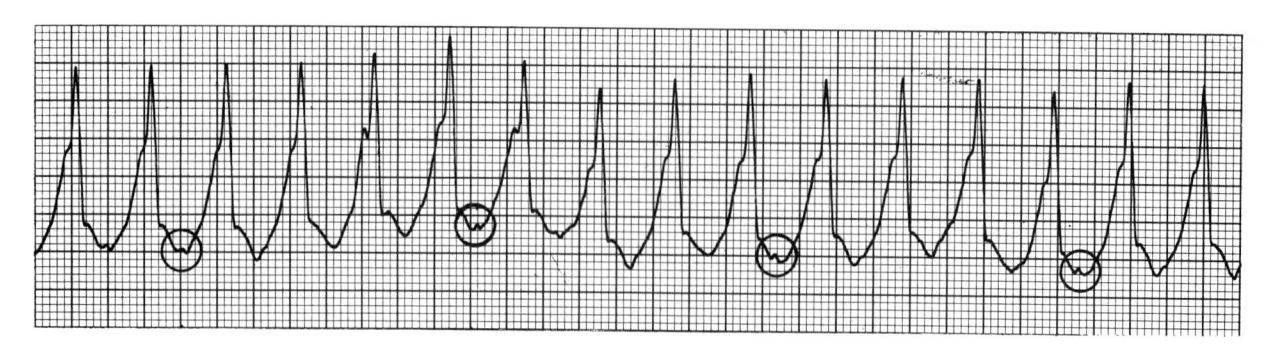

    AV Dissociation

    Note the P waves (circled) beating independently of the ventricular pacemaker.

Chapter 8 — Supraventricular Aberrancy Versus Ventricular Ectopy

SUMMARY

Recent electrophysiological studies with endocardial mapping techniques are casting doubt on the accuracy of interpreting supraventricular aberrancy versus ventricular ectopy with the body surface ECG alone.

Knowledge of this topic will at least give rise to a search for the origin of the aberrantly conducted arrhythmias and decrease the *lidocaine reflex* and the inappropriate use of other medications.

SUPRAVENTRICULAR ABERRANCY	VENTRICULAR ECTOPY
Ashman's phenomena	Fusion beats
Triphasic complex V_1	Biphasic or predominantly positive complex in V_1 with taller left rabbit ear
Initial vector the same or similar	Opposite initial vector
P prime (P')	Absence of P prime
Noncompensatory pause	Compensatory pause
Ventricular rate 170 or greater	Ventricular rate less than 170
Slowed or terminated by vagal maneuvers	Unaffected by vagal maneuvers
Complex duration less than 0.14 seconds	Complex duration $\geq$ 0.14 seconds
	QS or rS in V_6
	Fat initial r greater than 0.03 seconds in V_1
	Concordant pattern
	Evidence of AV dissociation
	Left, right, or no man's land axis deviation

Chapter 8 -- Supraventricular Aberrancy versus Ventricular Ectopy

PRACTICE STRIPS

On the following strips identify clues for supraventricular aberrancy and ventricular ectopy, then interpret the strip. Answers begin on page 257.

SUPRAVENTRICULAR ABERRANCY versus VENTRICULAR ECTOPY
PRACTICE STRIPS #1-20

1.

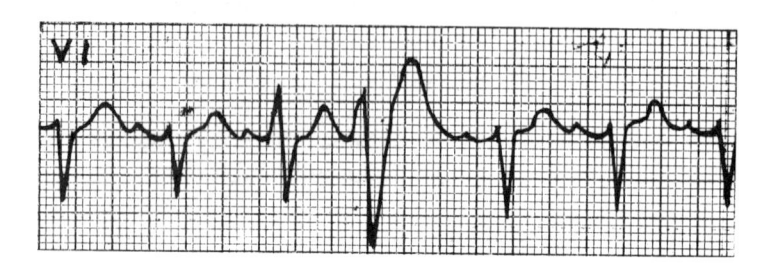

2.

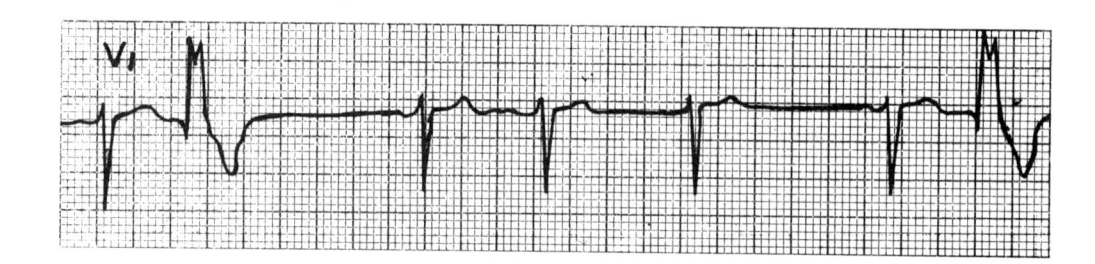

3.

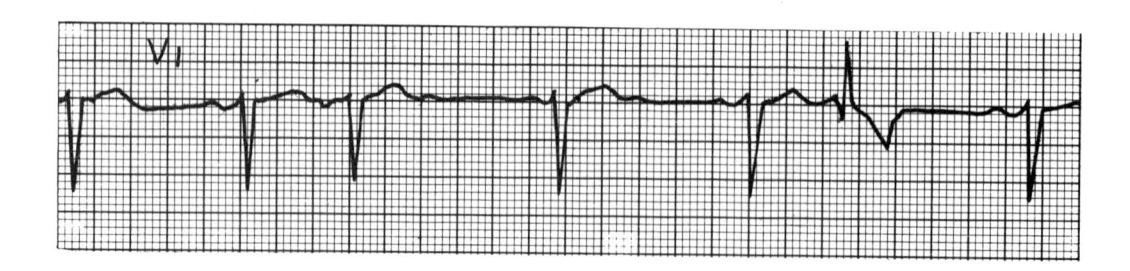

Chapter 8 — Supraventricular Aberrancy versus Ventricular Ectopy

4.

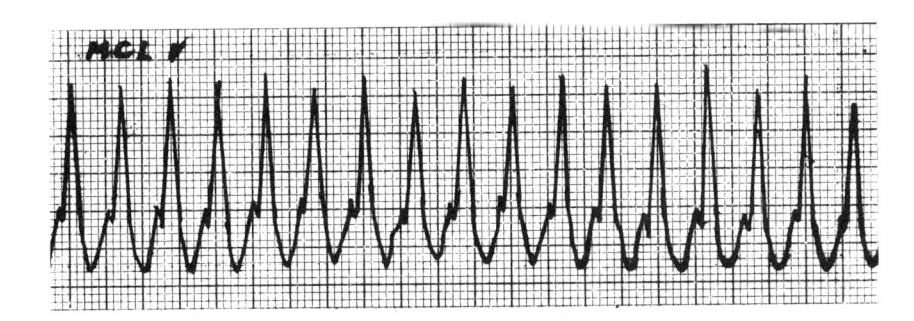

5.

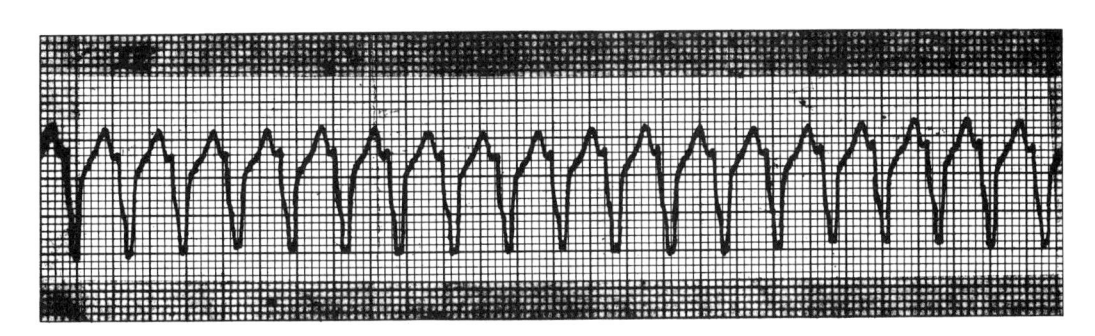

6.

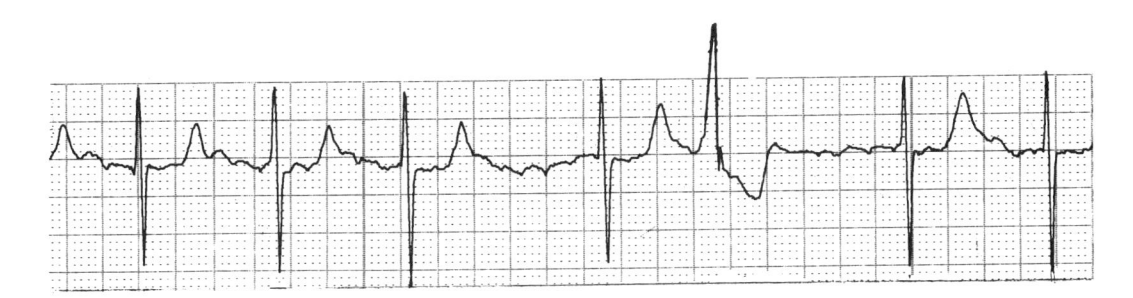

7.

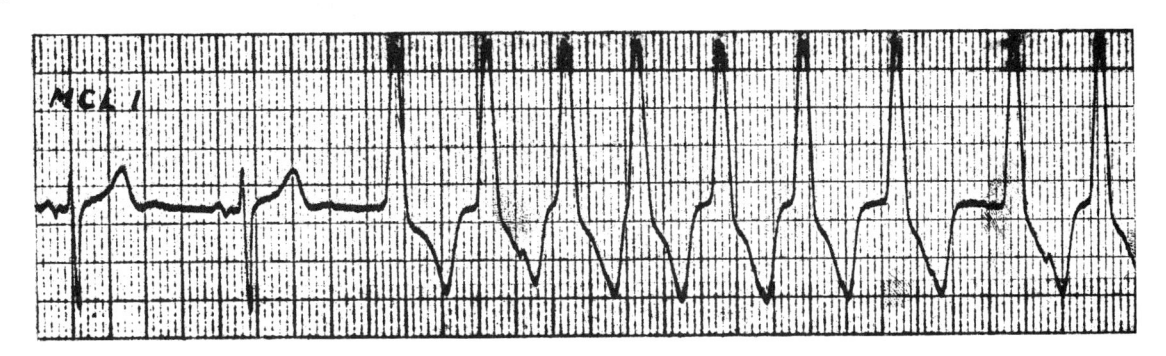

Chapter 8 -- Supraventricular Aberrancy versus Ventricular Ectopy

8.

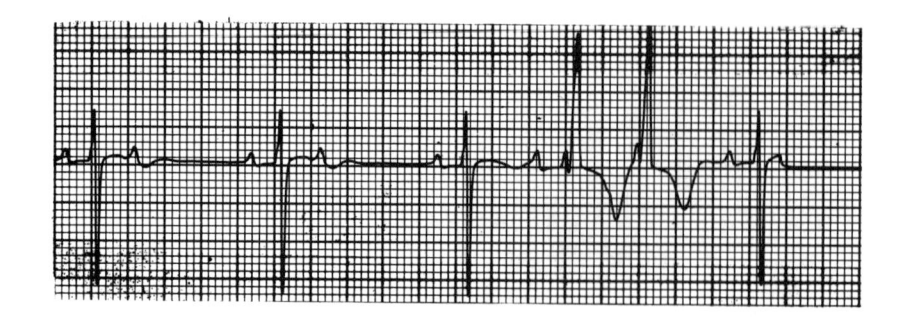

9.

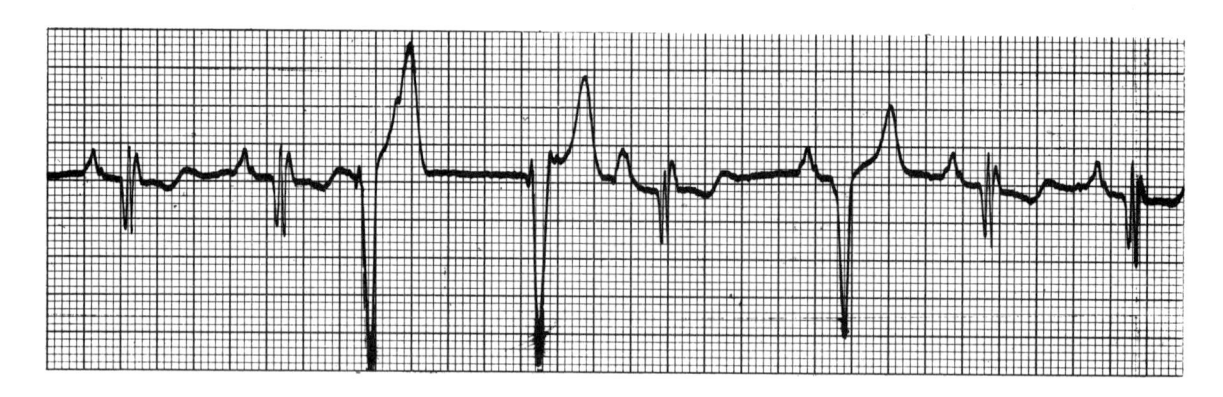

10.

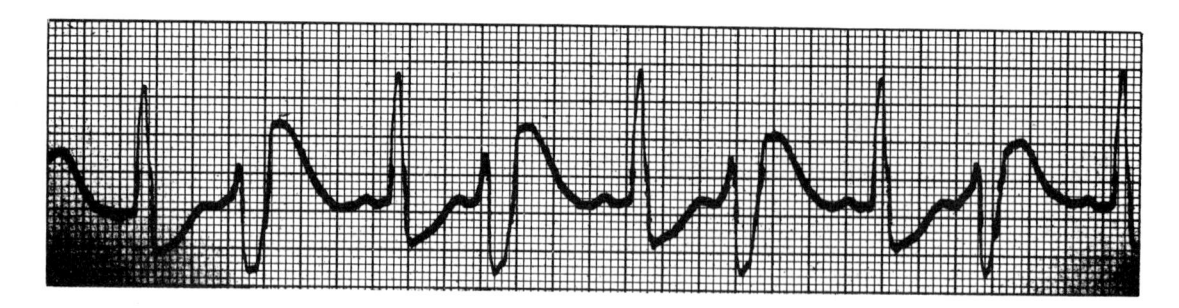

#11

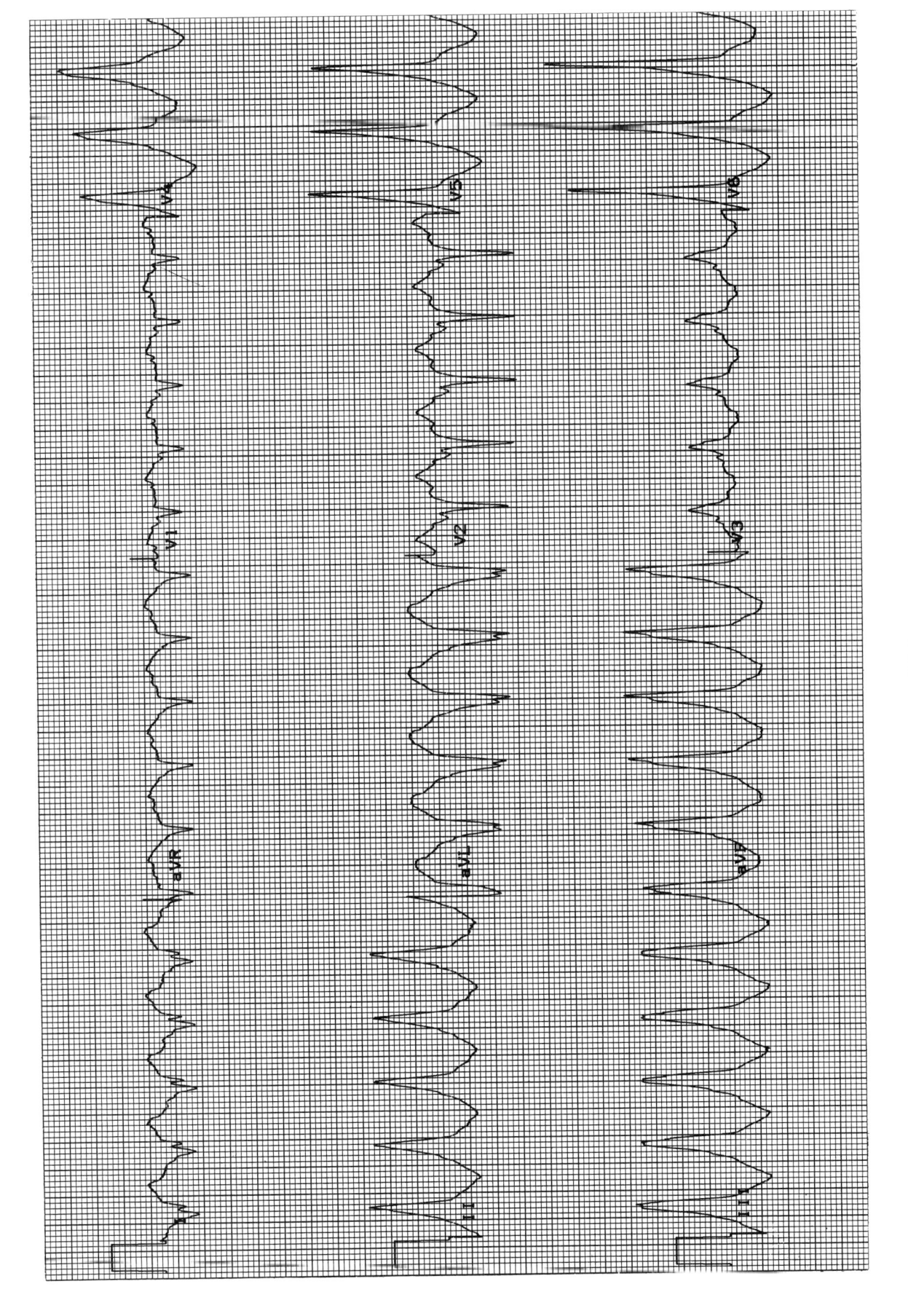

Chapter 8 -- Supraventricular Aberrancy versus Ventricular Ectopy

12.

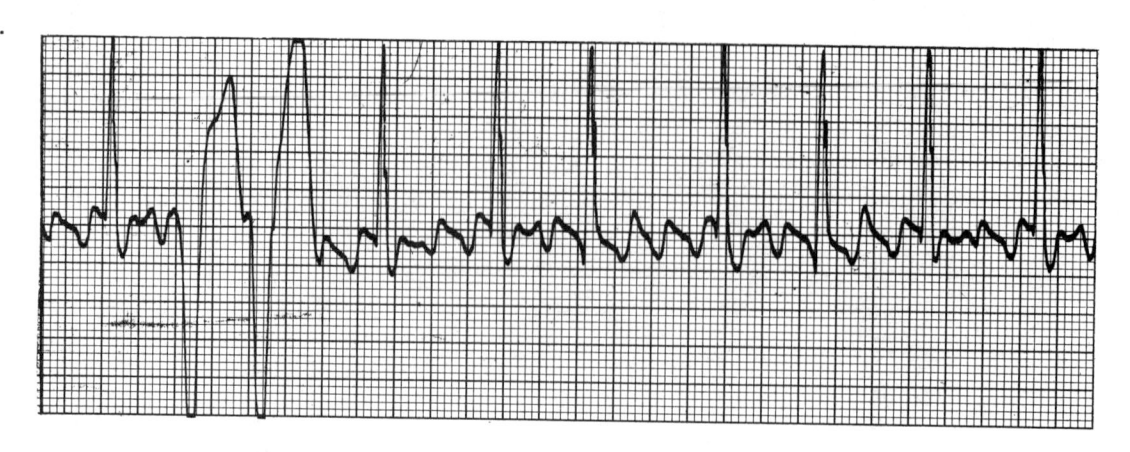

13.

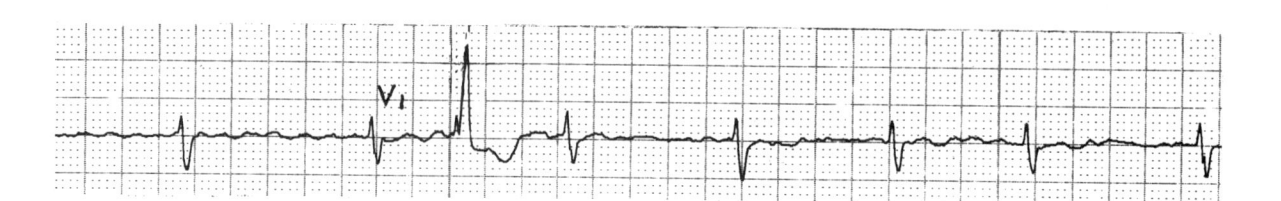

14.

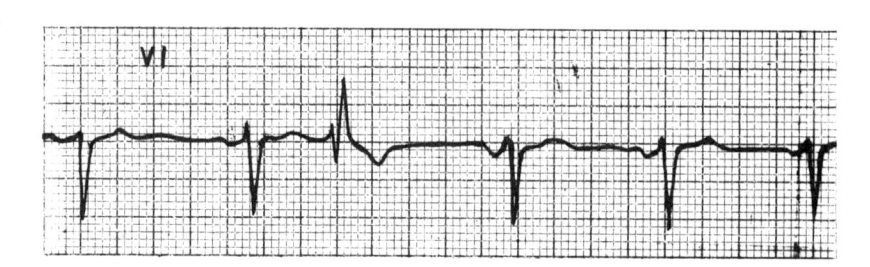

15.

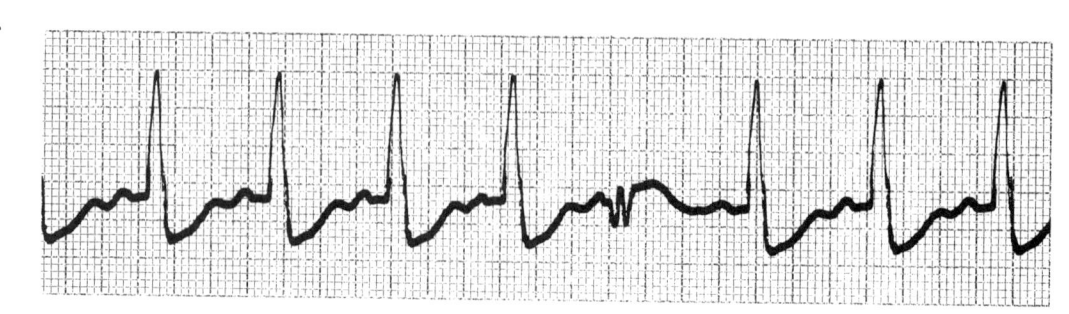

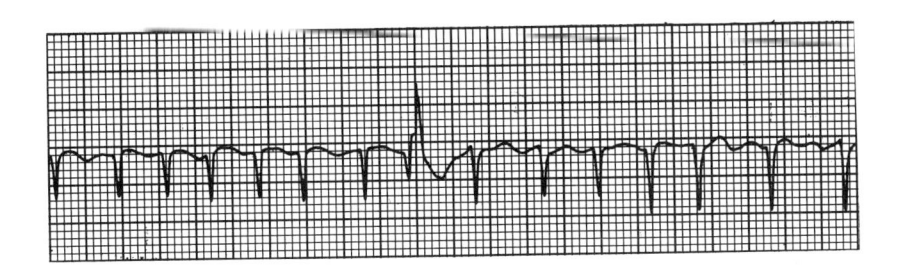

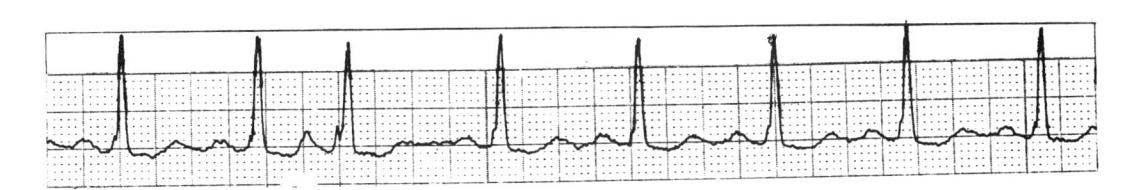

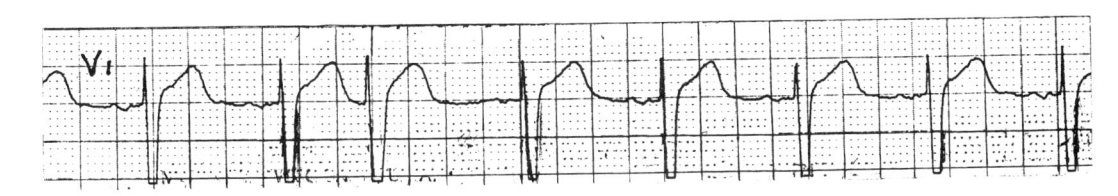

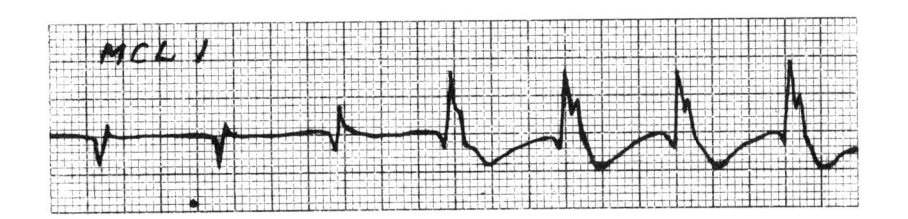

Chapter 8 -- Supraventricular Aberrancy versus Ventricular Ectopy

16.

17.

18.

19.

255

Chapter 8 -- Supraventricular Aberrancy versus Ventricular Ectopy

20.

Chapter 8 — Supraventricular Aberrancy Versus Ventricular Ectopy

ANSWERS ABERRANCY VERSUS ECTOPY PRACTICE STRIPS #1-20

1. Sinus tachycardia with one PVC (4th) and one fusion beat (3rd)

    Ventricular ectopy clues:

    - Fat initial r in V_1 greater than 0.3 seconds
    - Fusion beat (3rd)
    - Compensatory pause
    - Complex duration of PVC greater than 0.14 seconds

2. Atrial fibrillation, controlled with two PVCs (3rd and 8th beats)

    Ventricular ectopy clues:

    - Taller left rabbit ears in V_1
    - Initial vector is opposite:

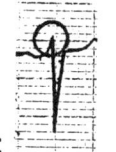

        The normal sinus beat is: initial vector (∧)

        The aberrantly conducted beat is: initial vector (∨)

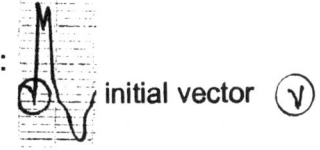

    - Complex duration greater than 0.14 seconds

3. Normal sinus rhythm with two PACs (3rd and 6th beat)

    Supraventricular aberrancy clues for 6th beat:

    - Initial vector is the same
    - Complex duration of aberrantly conducted beats is less than 0.14 seconds
    - rsR' in V_1
    - Ashman's phenomena: Note the long R to R cycle which precedes the aberrantly conducted beat.

4. Atrial tachycardia with aberrant conduction

    Supraventricular aberrancy clues:

    - Ventricular rate 210 BPM
    - rsR' in MCL_1 (MCL_1 is similar to V_1)

Chapter 8 — Supraventricular Aberrancy Versus Ventricular Ectopy

5. PAT with aberrancy:

    Supraventricular aberrancy clues:

    - Ventricular rate 210 BPM
    - Duration of complex is less than 0.14 seconds

6. Atrial fibrillation, controlled with one aberrantly conducted beat (5th).

    Supraventricular aberrancy clues:

    - Ashman's phenomena
    - Complex duration of aberrantly conducted beat is less than 0.14 second
    - rR' in V_1 (first rabbit ear is shorter than the second one)
    - Initial vector is similar

7. Normal sinus rhythm with ventricular tachycardia.

    Ventricular ectopy clues:

    - Ventricular rate less than 170
    - Taller left rabbit ear in V_1
    - Evidence of AV dissociation (the P wave is seen in the ST segment)
    - Complex duration of aberrantly conducted beats is 0.14 seconds

8. Sinus bradycardia with two aberrantly conducted PACs (4th and 5th beats)

    Supraventricular aberrancy clues:

    - Ashman's phenomenon
    - Presence of P'
    - Complex duration of aberrantly conducted beats is less than 0.14 seconds
    - Initial vector similar
    - rsR' pattern in V_1

9. NSR with IVCD, first degree AV heart block, possible biatrial enlargement, 2 PVCs (3rd and 4th beats), and one fusion beat (6th).

    Ventricular ectopy clues:

    - Fusion beat
    - PVCs have initial vector opposite that of the sinus beats
    - Complex duration of PVCs is 0.14 seconds

Chapter 8 — Supraventricular Aberrancy Versus Ventricular Ectopy

10. Ventricular bigeminy

    Ventricular ectopy clues:

    - Fusion beat (note the hybrid configuration of the next to the last beat)
    - Fat initial r wave
    - PVC complex duration is 0.18 seconds

11. Ventricular tachycardia

    Ventricular ectopy clues:

    - Right axis deviation
    - Complex duration 0.20 seconds
    - No P'

12. Atrial flutter with variable conduction and sequential PVCs

    Ventricular ectopy clues:

    - Initial vector of PVCs is opposite that of the normally conducted beats
    - Duration of PVCs is 0.14 seconds
    - Rate of PVCs is 150 BPM
    - No P'

13. Atrial fibrillation with one aberrantly conducted beat (3rd)

    Supraventricular aberrancy clues:

    - Ashman's phenomena
    - rR' in V_1
    - Complex duration < 0.14 seconds

14. Sinus arrhythmias with one PAC (3rd beat)

    Supraventricular aberrancy clues:

    - Initial vector the same
    - Complex duration less than 0.14 seconds
    - P' present
    - Noncompensatory pause
    - rsR' pattern in V_1
    - Ashman's phenomena

Chapter 8 – Supraventricular Aberrancy Versus Ventricular Ectopy

15. Normal sinus rhythm with one PVC (5th beat)

    Ventricular ectopy clues:

    - Compensatory pause
    - Initial vector of PVC opposite that of the sinus beats
    - PRI preceding the aberrant beat is only 0.08 seconds

16. Uncontrolled atrial fibrillation with one PAC with aberrancy (8th beat)

    Supraventricular aberrancy clues:

    - Ashman's phenomena
    - Complex duration less than 0.14 seconds
    - Initial vector is similar

17. Normal sinus rhythm with one aberrant PAC (3rd beat) lead II

    Supraventricular aberrancy clues:

    - P'
    - Noncompensatory pause
    - Initial vector is similar
    - Complex duration of PAC is less than 0.14 seconds
    - Ashman's phenomena (long-short cycle)

18. Normal sinus rhythm with one aberrant PAC (3rd beat). This is a simultaneous recording in V_1 of #17 above. Notice how the P' is hidden in the T wave of the preceding beat in this lead.

19. Normal sinus rhythm with fusion beat and ventricular tachycardia

    Ventricular ectopy clues:

    - Fusion beat (3rd beat)
    - Taller left rabbit ear in MCL_1 (V_1)
    - Complex duration 0.16 seconds

20. Normal sinus rhythm with frequent PVCs

    Ventricular ectopy clues:

    - Taller left "rabbit ear" in V_1
    - PVC has rS pattern in V_6
    - PVCs have compensatory pause
    - Complex duration of PVCs is 0.16 seconds

CHAPTER 9
EFFECTS OF DRUGS AND ELECTROLYTES ON THE ECG

Many medications and electrolyte disturbances cause changes on the ECG and may indicate therapeutic and/or toxic effects. All areas of the ECG may be altered due to therapeutic and toxic effects of medications and changes in serum electrolytes. It is difficult to assess the 12 lead ECG for these changes without a clinical picture of the patient reflecting medications and laboratory values of electrolytes and drug levels.

CHANGES IN WAVES, INTERVALS, AND SEGMENTS

Common ECG changes due to medications and electrolytes include but are not limited to the following:

P wave: Increases or decreases in amplitude and becomes flat, inverted, and notched.

PR interval: Increases.

Complex: Increases or decreases in amplitude and increases in width.

ST segment: Depression and elevation.

T wave: Increases and decreases in amplitude; becomes flat, biphasic, notched, and inverted.

ST-T wave changes: The ST-T wave changes are primary changes. Some medications and abnormal serum electrolytes affect the action potential of the cardiac cell causing these ST segment and/or T wave changes.

U wave: Increases in amplitude. Prominent U waves can easily be mistaken for T waves and a QU interval may be misinterpreted as a prolonged QT interval.

QT interval: Shortens or prolongs in duration indicating repolarization abnormalities.

Except for the QT interval, the normal values for the above have previously been discussed.

QT INTERVAL

The normal QT interval is rate dependent. There is an inverse relationship between the QT interval and the heart rate.

QUESTION: As the heart rate increases the QT interval decreases.

A. True
B. False

ANSWER: A. True. The QT interval decreases as the heart rate increases.

Chapter 9 — Effects of Drugs and Electrolytes on the ECG

There are many charts and formulas used to calculate the normal QT interval. One rule of thumb is that the QT interval should be no more than half the R to R interval. This was previously discussed on page 15.

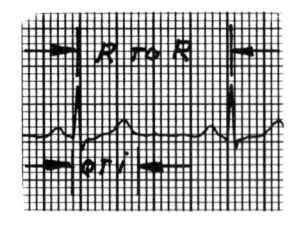

Normal QTi 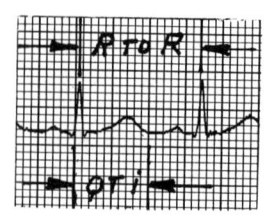   **Prolonged QTi**

This rule is a guideline for identifying the presence of a prolonged QT interval.

QTc is the QT interval corrected for heart rate. The upper limit of the QTc is 0.41 seconds for women and 0.39 seconds for men. Minor deviations from these normal limits are usually not significant.

Another general guideline to assess the QTc is a formula stated by Te-Chuan Chou, M.D.:

NORMAL QTI AT HEART RATE OF 70 IS 0.33 TO 0.40 SECONDS.

QTI CHANGES 0.02 SECONDS FOR EVERY CHANGE OF 10 BPM.

Example: Heart rate is 80 (has changed 10 BPM from 70). The QTI changes 0.02 seconds from the normal range of 0.33 to 0.40 seconds given for rate of 70 BPM.

QUESTION: In this example, will you add the 0.02 seconds or subtract it?

A. Add it
B. Subtract it

ANSWER: B. Subtract it. The heart rate has increased, so the QTI will decrease.

```
              0.33   to   0.40
             -0.02       -0.02
80 BPM: QTc = 0.31   to   0.38 seconds
```

This formula can be used as a general rule of thumb for heart rates between 45 and 115 BPM.

Chapter 9 — Effects of Drugs and Electrolytes on the ECG

The QT interval can be abnormally PROLONGED by certain drugs such as quinidine, procainamide, and disopyramide, and electrolyte disturbances such as hypokalemia or hypocalcemia. In hypothermia, the repolarization of the heart muscle cells are prolonged and the QT interval is prolonged. Myocardial ischemia, infarction, and subarachnoid hemorrhage may also prolong the QT interval. A prolonged QT interval may predispose to potentially lethal ventricular arrhythmias and death.

The QT interval may be SHORTENED by medications such as digitalis and abnormal serum electrolytes such as hypercalcemia and hyperkalemia.

EFFECTS OF DIGITALIS ON THE ECG

The earliest ECG changes with the administration of digitalis are usually a decrease in the amplitude of the T wave, shortening of the QT interval, and sagging of the ST segment. The T wave may become biphasic with an initial negative part followed by a positive terminal part. These changes are more commonly seen in leads with tall R waves. In leads with primarily negative complexes (aVR, V_1), the ST segment may be slightly elevated and rounded upward - a coving effect.

DIGITALIS EFFECT

Note the classical sagging "scooped" appearance of the ST segments in this patient with a digitalis level of 1.8.

The classical ST segments seen with digitalis administration is also described as a backward checkmark:

✓ A regular checkmark

\/ A backward checkmark

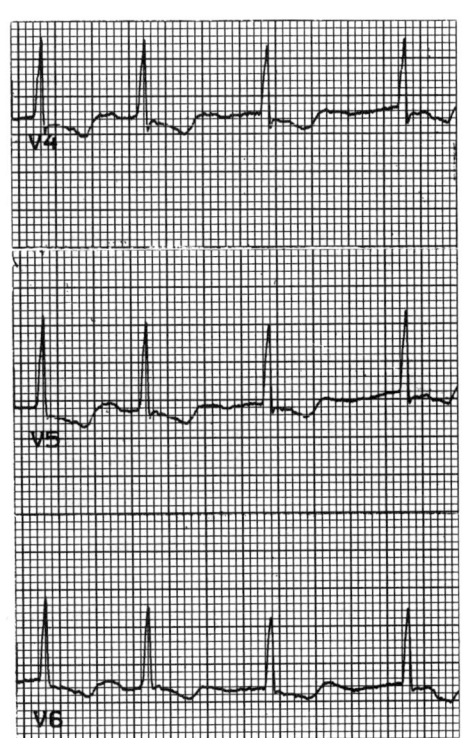

The amplitude of the U wave may increase with the administration of digitalis. This is usually best seen in V_2, V_3, and V_4.

Other nonspecific ST-T wave changes may occur with digitalis administration.

Any arrhythmia and all degrees of AV heart block can be caused by digitalis intoxication.

Chapter 9 -- Effects of Drugs and Electrolytes on the ECG

Digitalis is most often administered as digoxin.

The therapeutic serum level of digoxin is 0.5 to 2.0 ng/ml.

There is a narrow margin between the therapeutic and toxic levels.

ECG changes associated with digitalis are not significantly correlated with the degree of digitalization and may be absent in obvious cases of intoxication.

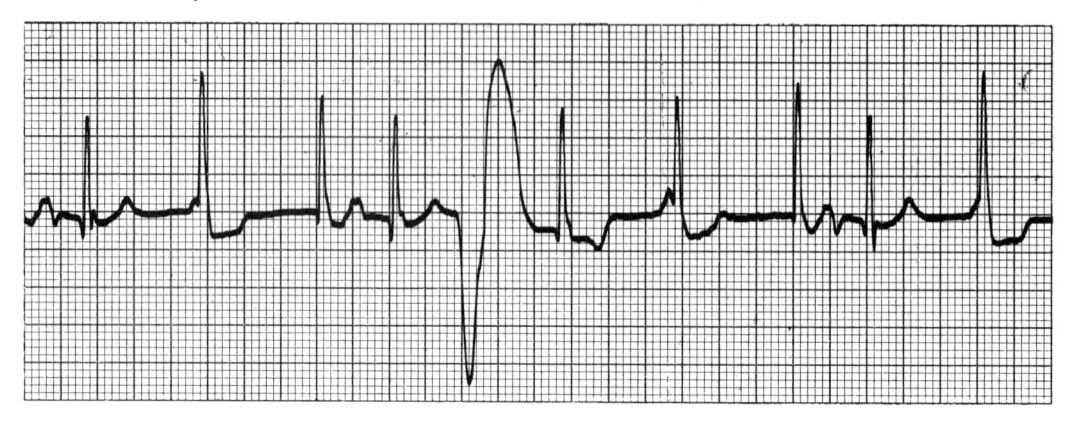

Figure 9 A

The digoxin level in the above patient is 4.0 ng/ml. Note the depressed ST-T segment, chaotic rhythm, and the ventricular irritability manifested by frequent PVCs.

In summary, the effects of digitalis on the ECG include:

1. ST segment depression.

2. Depressed amplitude of the T wave. The T wave may become biphasic or inverted.

3. Shortening of the QT interval.

4. Increase of the amplitude of the U wave.

5. Any arrhythmia, including AV heart blocks, may be caused by digitalis intoxication.

Chapter 9 — Effects of Drugs and Electrolytes on the ECG

QUINIDINE EFFECTS ON THE ECG: THERAPEUTIC AND TOXIC

The therapeutic level of quinidine is 2.3 to 5 ug/ml. Therapeutic effects on the ECG include a decrease in the amplitude of the T wave, increased duration and/or T wave inversion. The U wave may become prominent and it may be difficult to tell a U wave from a T wave. ST segment depression and prolongation of the QT interval occur as well as notching and widening of the P wave.

The ST segment and T and U wave changes due to quinidine administration imitate those seen in hypokalemia. It is difficult to assess a 12 lead ECG for drug and electrolyte changes without the clinical picture of the patient reflecting medications, and laboratory values of electrolytes and drug levels.

Toxic effects of quinidine include widening of the complex, various degrees of AV heart block, marked sinus bradycardia and/or sinus arrest, and ventricular arrhythmias with syncope and sudden death. More than 25 percent increase in the duration of the complex above the pre-treatment complex is considered a sign of toxicity; the physician must be notified and the medication discontinued.

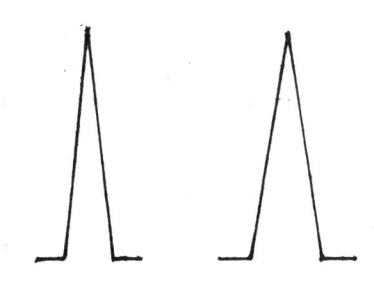

The duration of the complex has increased from 0.06 seconds to 0.09 seconds, a 50% increase after quinidine administration = toxicity.

An increase in the PR interval occurs when the serum concentration reaches a very high level, usually above 10 ug/liter. AV heart block, sinus bradycardia, sinus arrhythmia, sinus arrest, and ventricular ectopic beats, including ventricular tachycardia, are all considered ECG signs of quinidine toxicity.

In summary, the effects of quinidine on the ECG include:

THERAPEUTIC EFFECTS

1. **Decrease in the amplitude of the T wave or T wave inversion.**

2. **Depression of the ST segment.**

3. **Increase in the amplitude of the U wave.**

4. **Prolongation of the QT interval.**

5. **Widening and notching of the P wave.**

Chapter 9 — Effects of Drugs and Electrolytes on the ECG

TOXIC EFFECTS

1. Increase in the width of the complex more than 25 percent of the pretreatment complex.

2. AV heart block.

3. Ventricular arrhythmias.

4. Marked sinus bradycardia, sinus arrhythmia, and sinus arrest due to decrease in the automaticity of the sinus node.

OTHER MEDICATIONS

Other medications such as procainamide, disopyramide phosphate (Norpace), the phenothiazines, and tricyclic antidepressants have ECG effects similar to quinidine.

EFFECTS OF ELECTROLYTES ON THE ECG

The ECG is regarded to be a fairly accurate reflection of a patient's electrolyte status, especially potassium and calcium. Serum electrolyte determinations, however, are the most effective method of assessing electrolyte balance.

HYPERKALEMIA

The normal serum potassium is 3.5 to 5.0 mEq/L. Hyperkalemia affects both depolarization (P, QRS) and repolarization (ST segment and T wave).

Narrowing and peaking of the T wave is the first ECG change with hyperkalemia; the T wave assumes a characteristic tented shape and its amplitude may increase. These T wave changes are usually best seen in the precordial leads.

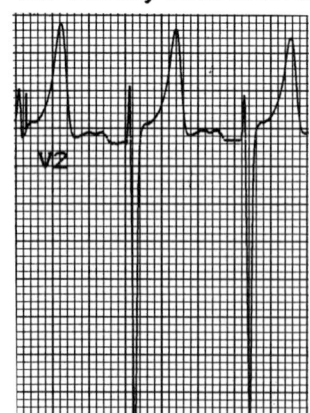

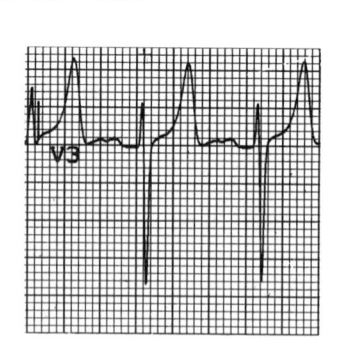

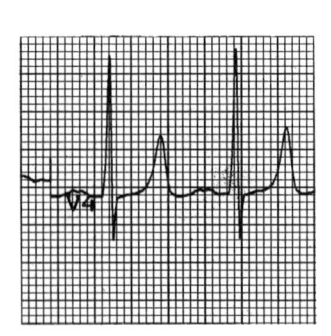

T Wave Changes with Hyperkalemia

The P waves become smaller and may disappear entirely with further potassium elevation. Advanced hyperkalemia causes a delay in the intraventricular conduction and the complex widens. As the potassium continues to rise, the width of the complex further increases and the ST segment elevates. Advanced hyperkalemia will inscribe a large sine wave pattern on the ECG, a terminal event if not reversed.

Chapter 9 -- Effects of Drugs and Electrolytes on the ECG

Other cardiac arrhythmias associated with hyperkalemia include AV heart blocks: first, second, third degree. Junctional arrhythmias will be diagnosed when the P wave disappears. Death in hyperkalemic patients is most commonly caused by ventricular tachycardia, ventricular fibrillation, and asystole.

The succession of the ECG changes seen with hyperkalemia is pictorially presented:

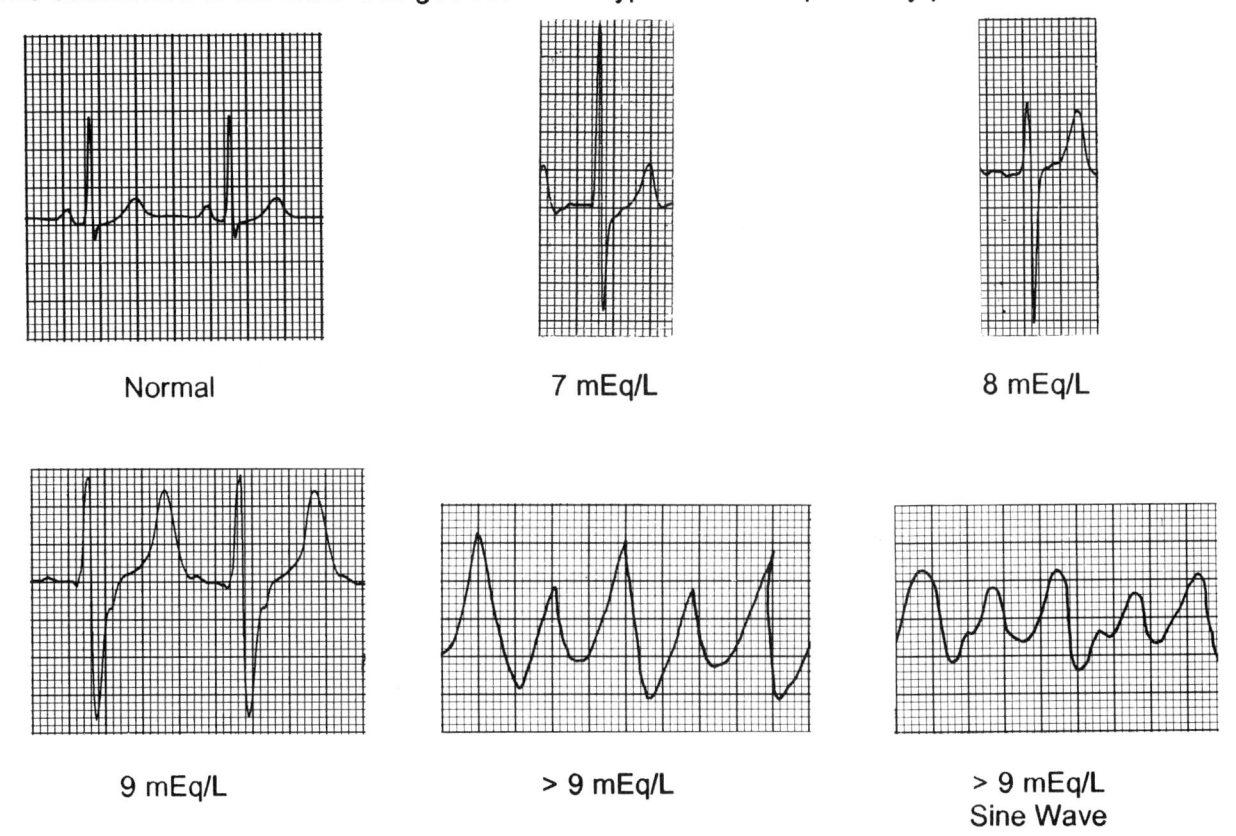

Normal   7 mEq/L   8 mEq/L

9 mEq/L   > 9 mEq/L   > 9 mEq/L
Sine Wave

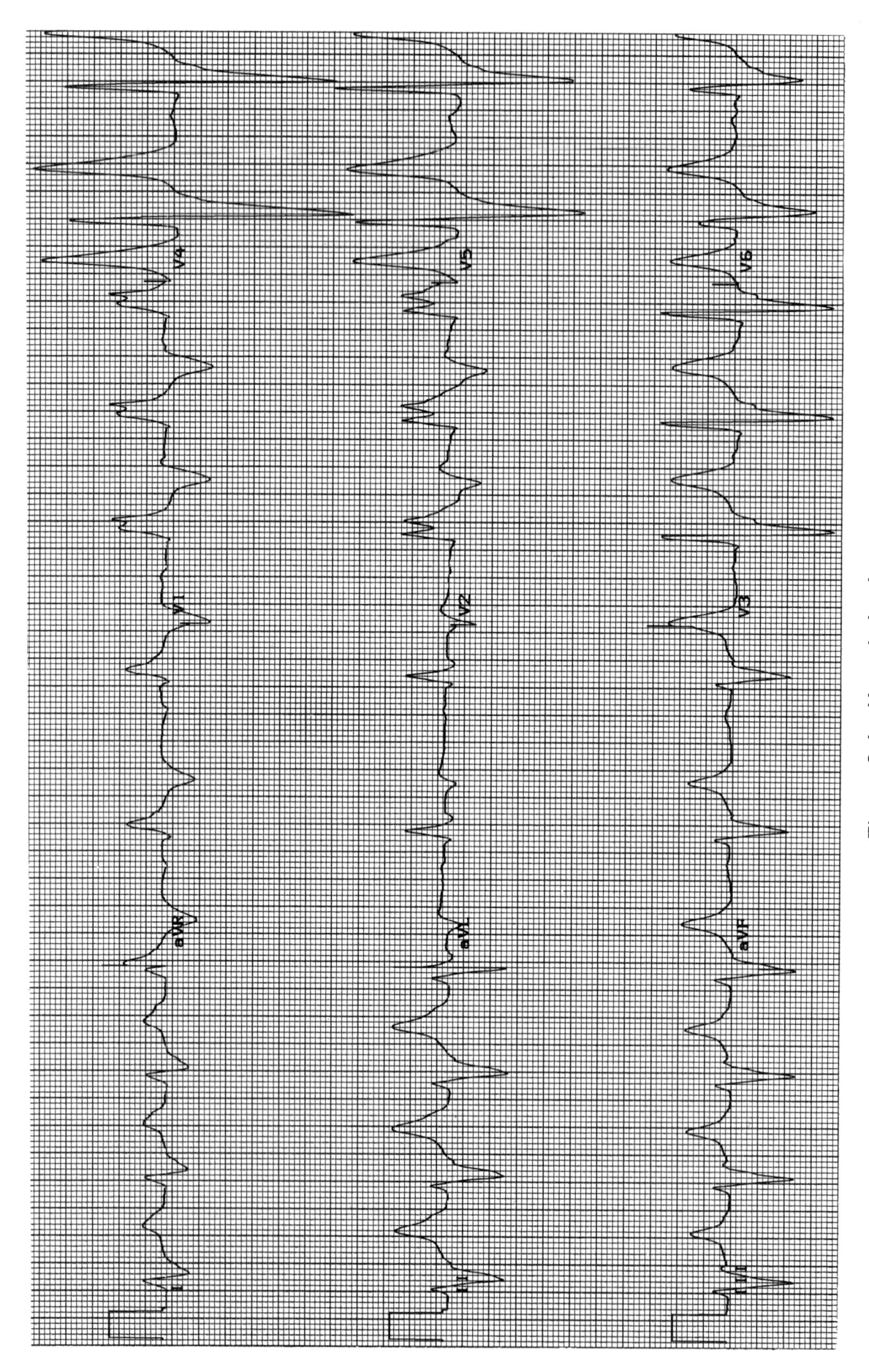

Figure 9 A. Hyperkalemia
Potassium level is 8.7 mEq/L.

Chapter 9 — Effects of Drugs and Electrolytes on the ECG

HYPOKALEMIA

Hypokalemic changes include a decrease in the amplitude of the T wave which may invert, an increase in U wave amplitude, prolongation of the QU interval, and depression of the ST segment. The U wave may be as large as or larger than the T wave. Recall the normal U wave is less than one-fourth the height of its T wave. When the amplitude of the T wave decreases and the U wave increases it is difficult to distinguish the U from the T. A QU interval may be mistaken for a prolonged QT interval.

The PR interval may be prolonged resulting in first degree AV heart block. An uncommon finding in advanced hypokalemia is an increase in the duration of the complex.

Hypokalemia causes ventricular arrhythmias most commonly in patients receiving digitalis; ventricular arrhythmias can be precipitated by hypokalemia alone.

Figure 9 B below is an example of hypokalemia:

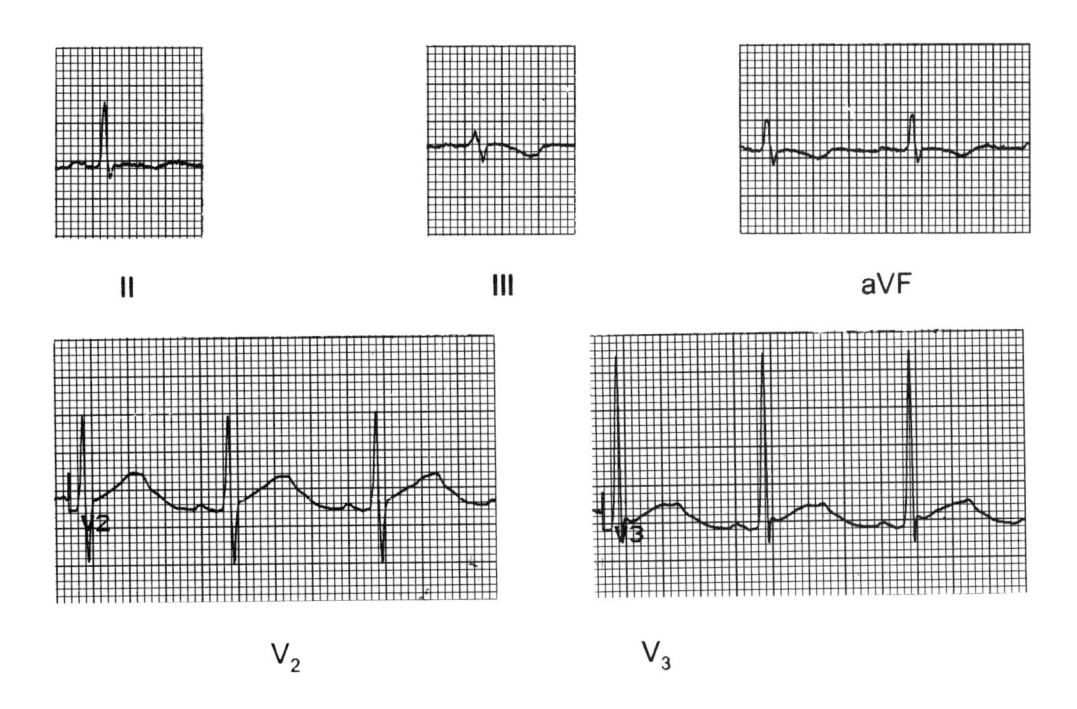

Figure 9 B. Potassium is 2.9 mEq/L. Note the inversion of the T wave in II, III, aVF and the notching of the T wave in V_2 and V_3. The notch is the U wave. The TU fusion gives the appearance of a prolonged QT interval.

Chapter 9 — Effects of Drugs and Electrolytes on the ECG

HYPERCALCEMIA

The normal serum calcium concentration is 8.6 to 10.3 mg/dl. Hypercalcemia decreases the QT interval by decreasing the ST segment which shortens or disappears. Cardiac arrhythmias are uncommon. The PR interval may be slightly increased resulting in first degree AV heart block.

Like hypokalemia, hypercalcemia may induce ventricular ectopics and potentiate the action of digitalis.

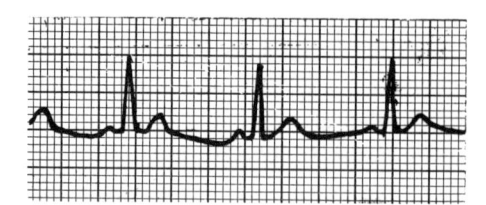

Figure 9 C. Hypercalcemia
Note the loss of the ST segment and the short QT interval.

HYPOCALCEMIA

The major ECG effect of hypocalcemia is prolongation of the QT interval due to an increase in the duration of the ST segment; the width of the T wave is unchanged. The P wave and the PR interval are not usually affected; cardiac arrhythmias are uncommon.

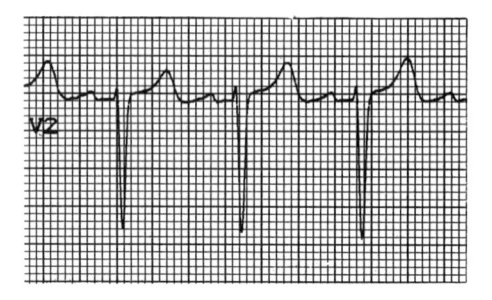

Figure 9 D. Hypocalcemia
Note the prolonged QT interval.

OTHER ELECTROLYTES

ECG changes of **hypomagnesemia** are less well established but may include tall peaked T waves, increased amplitude of the U wave, slight increase in the duration of the complex, ST segment depression, and QU prolongation.

Hypernatremia, hyponatremia, acidosis, and alkalosis alone do not cause any recognizable ECG changes.

Chapter 9 — Effects of Drugs and Electrolytes on the ECG

SUMMARY OF DRUG AND ELECTROLYTE ECG CHANGES

ECG Change	Drug and Electrolyte
P wave amplitude decreased	Hyperkalemia
P wave notched	Quinidine
PR interval increased	Hyperkalemia Hypokalemia Procainamide Quinidine
Complex duration increased	Hyperkalemia Norpace Procainamide Quinidine
ST segment depression	Digitalis Hypokalemia Quinidine
ST segment elevation	Hyperkalemia
T wave amplitude decreased	Digitalis Hypokalemia Procainamide
T wave amplitude increased	Hyperkalemia Quinidine
T wave flattened	Phenothiazines
T wave inversion	Hypokalemia Phenothiazines Quinidine
T wave notched/biphasic	Digitalis Quinidine Phenothiazines Procainamide
U wave amplitude increased	Digitalis Hypokalemia Hypomagnesemia Phenothiazines Procainamide Quinidine
QTI shortened	Digitalis Hypercalcemia
QTI prolonged	Hypocalcemia Norpace Phenothiazines Procainamide Quinidine

Therapeutic and toxic effects of various medications and electrolyte imbalances cause repolarization abnormalities which may not be recognized without the clinical information.

Chapter 9 — Effects of Drugs and Electrolytes on the ECG

NONSPECIFIC ST SEGMENT AND T WAVE CHANGES

Nonspecific ST segment and T wave changes are common 12 lead ECG interpretations. It means the ST segment and/or the T waves are not normal but the cause of these repolarization changes are unknown to the cardiologist interpreting the 12 lead ECG. There are many possible situations that effect repolarization. The clinician attending the patient is in a better position to assess the significance of this finding than the person reading the tracing who only has the 12 leads.

Fear, tension, stress, eating, drinking ice water, changes in body position, and hyperventilation, for example, can cause ST changes and/or T wave inversion. Gall bladder disease, acute pancreatitis, central nervous system disease, and endocrine disorders can also cause ST-T changes.

These nonspecific changes may be significant or they may be a normal variant. It is important that someone assess this ECG finding at the clinical level, taking care not to create iatrogenic heart disease.

Recall that ST segments are normally on the isoelectric line or no more than 1 millimeter above or below it.

T waves normally are in the same direction as the main part of the complex. An upright complex in lead II will have an upright T wave. The negative complex in aVR is accompanied by a negative T wave. Biphasic complexes in the frontal plane usually have a flat T wave.

The normal T wave in V_1 may be inverted, flat, biphasic, or upright. The T wave in the precordial leads usually is upright by V_2. The T normally remains upright to the left of V_2, i.e., V_3, V_4, V_5, and V_6.

Practice 12 lead ECGs #33, 57, and 68 on pages 103, 163, and 179 respectively, are examples of nonspecific ST-T wave changes.

Figure 9 E on the following page is an example of nonspecific ST-T wave changes.

Figure 9 F on page 274 is an example of nonspecific T wave changes.

Figure 9 E. Non-specific ST-T wave changes

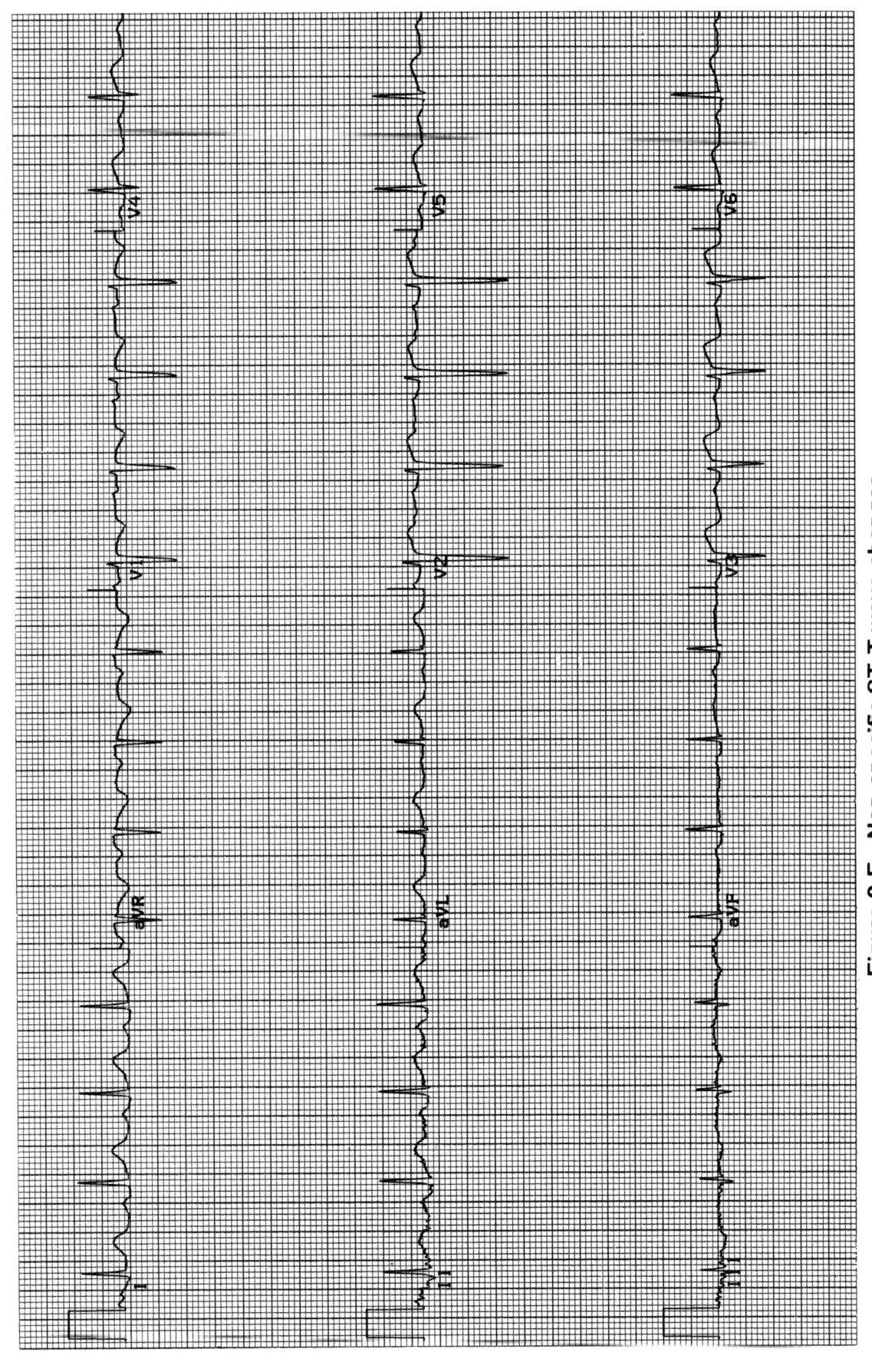

Note the inverted/flat T waves in III, aVF, and the slight elevation of the ST segments in V_3, V_4, and V_5.

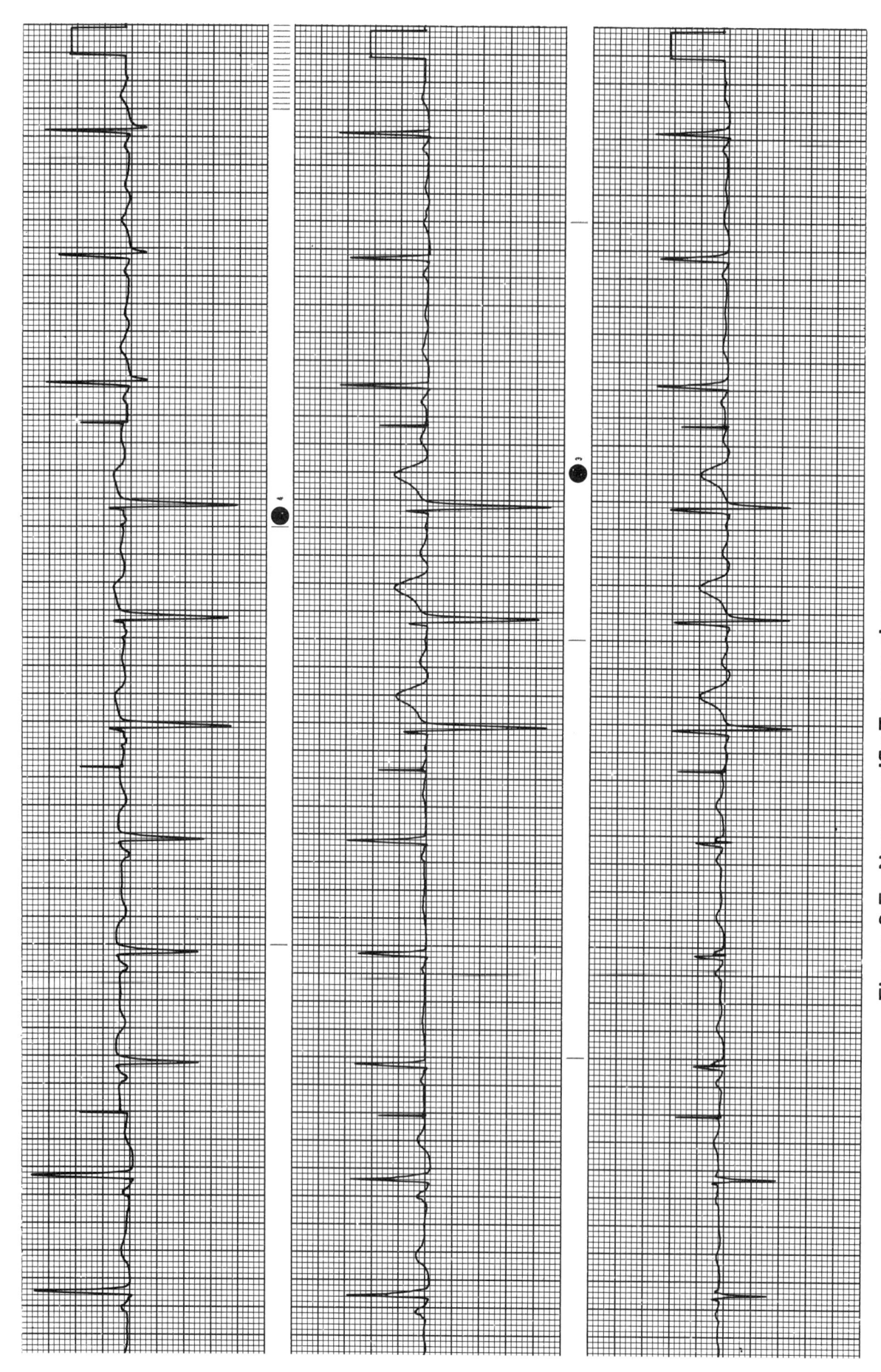

Figure 9 F. Non-specific T wave changes
Note the small T wave (compared to the complexes) in lead I, aVL, V$_5$, V$_6$.

CHAPTER 10
WOLFF-PARKINSON-WHITE (WPW) SYNDROME

Wolff, Parkinson, and White described this syndrome in 1930. The syndrome is also known as:

- **ventricular pre-excitation syndrome**
- **anonomalous atrioventricular excitation syndrome**
- **bundle of Kent syndrome**

The first two terms, ventricular pre-excitation syndrome and anomalous atrioventricular excitation syndrome mean the same thing. Recall the normal excitation via the AV node:

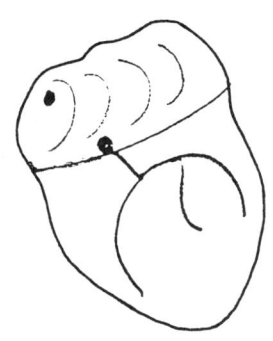

Normally the atria are stimulated and depolarize, and the AV node delays the conduction to the ventricles for a fraction of a second. This delay at the AV node allows the atria to depolarize, contact, and empty atrial blood into the ventricles which are still in diastole. This well-timed synchronization between the atria and ventricles accounts for approximately 15 percent of cardiac output in the normal individual.

1. **Ventricular pre-excitation** simply means that the ventricles are excited before they should be; in other words, the normal pathway with the AV node delaying the conduction between the atria and ventricles is bypassed.

2. **Anomalous atrioventricular excitation syndrome** indicates that the excitation between the atria and the ventricles is abnormal; the normal pathway with the AV node delaying the conduction between the atria and ventricles is bypassed.

3. **Bundle of Kent** is the name of the abnormal pathway which bypasses the normal pathway between the atria and the ventricles.

INCIDENCE OF WPW

This syndrome occurs in 0.15 percent of the population. The majority of those affected are asymptomatic and the syndrome is often identified on a routine ECG. The syndrome may be intermittent. Males are twice as likely to have WPW as females. People with hyperthyroidism also have a higher incidence; the reason for this is unknown.

Chapter 10 — Wolff-Parkinson-White (WPW) Syndrome

QUESTION: WPW syndrome is a prevalent nursing and medical problem.

A. True
B. False

ANSWER: B. False. It has been said that this syndrome is more fascinating than prevalent.

CAUSE OF WPW SYNDROME

WPW syndrome is caused by a faulty congenital development of the AV ring. Normally, the AV ring is a continuous sheet of fibrous tissue separating the atria and ventricles. With WPW, there is a congenital spilt in the ring which serves as an accessory pathway. This abnormal accessory pathway is called the bundle of Kent. The bundle of Kent can be on the right or the left side of the heart. Some people have more than one accessory pathway and their situation is more complex than this presentation.

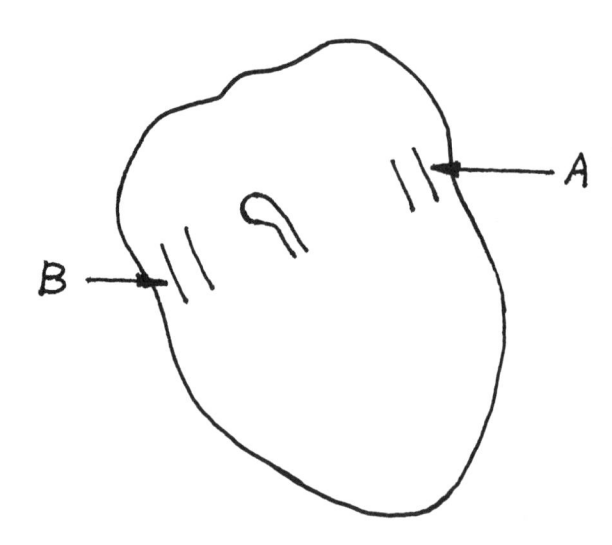

The atria are stimulated by the sinus node and depolarize. The electrical stimulation arrives at the AV node where it is delayed (normal), but it also arrives at the bundle of Kent. Notice there is no AV node between the atria and the ventricles via the bundle of Kent (A, B). Since there is no delay, depolarization is free to travel down the bundle of Kent and pre-excite the ventricles. So the

1. ventricles are pre-excited by this
2. anomalous atrioventricular accessory pathway which is called the
3. bundle of Kent

CLASSIFICATION: TYPES A AND B

WPW is conventionally classified into Type A and Type B using the morphology of the complex in the precordial leads. The morphology is explained in terms of the location of the bundle of Kent on the right or left side of the heart. Beware, however, it is not so clear cut in *real life.*

Chapter 10 — Wolff-Parkinson-White (WPW) Syndrome

TYPE A (left side accessory bundle of Kent)

In Type A, the bundle of Kent is located on the left side of the heart as depicted in the picture below. Pre-excitation of the left free wall of the ventricle is directed rightward. This premature activation in the left ventricle gives rise to the delta wave. The delta wave is directed anteriorly so that all precordial leads have complexes that are upright (positive, R waves).

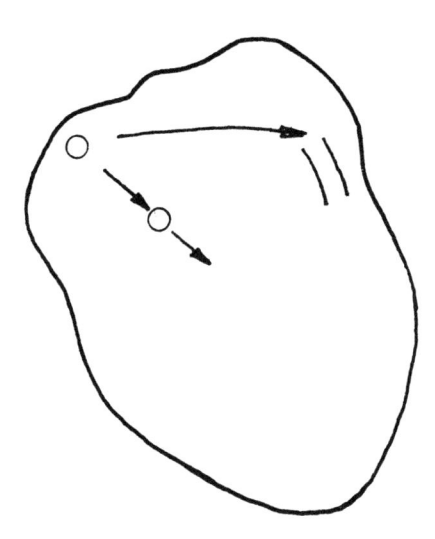

QUESTION: When all of the precordial leads have positive complexes it is referred to as *concordant pattern*.

A. True
B. False

ANSWER: A. True. When the precordial leads are all positive (or all negative) it is called concordant pattern.

The tall R waves in V_1 and V_2 simulate right ventricular hypertrophy, right bundle branch block, and posterior myocardial infarction.

The delta wave is often directed superiorly in the frontal plane in both Type A and Type B and this simulates inferior myocardial infarction. With a rapid ventricular rate both Type A and Type B can be mistaken for ventricular tachycardia.

In review, WPW TYPE A SIMULATES:

1. Right bundle branch block
2. Right ventricular hypertrophy
3. Posterior myocardial infarction
4. Inferior myocardial infarction
5. Ventricular tachycardia

Chapter 10 — Wolff-Parkinson-White Syndrome (WPW)

TYPE B (right side accessory bundle of Kent)

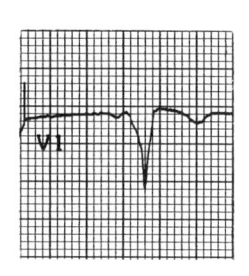

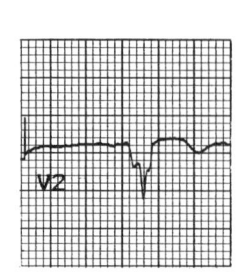

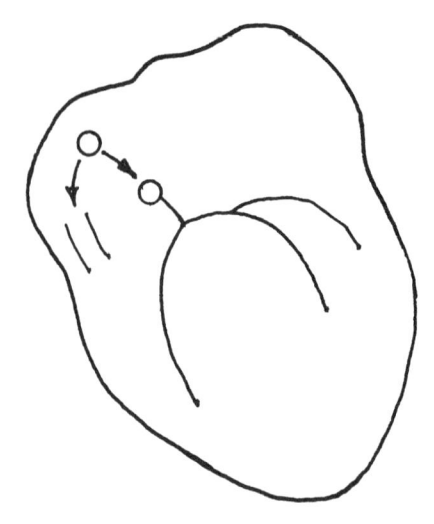

In Type B the bundle of Kent is located on the right side of the heart as depicted in the picture above. Pre-excitation of the right free wall of the ventricle is directed leftward. This premature activation in the right ventricle gives rise to the delta wave. The delta wave is directed away from the positive electrodes of V_1 and V_2 and a negative complex is inscribed in these leads. Then the wave is directed anteriorly so that the complexes usually are upright by V_3.

The QS pattern in V_1 and V_2 simulates left bundle branch block and anteroseptal myocardial infarction.

The delta wave is often directed superiorly in the frontal plane producing Q waves in II, III, aVF in both Type A and Type B; this simulates inferior myocardial infarction on the ECG.

With a rapid ventricular rate, both Type A and Type B can be mistaken for ventricular tachycardia.

In review, WPW TYPE B SIMULATES:

1. **Left bundle branch block**
2. **Anteroseptal myocardial infarction**
3. **Inferior myocardial infarction**
4. **Ventricular tachycardia**

Chapter 10 — Wolff-Parkinson-White (WPW) Syndrome

WPW ECG DIAGNOSTIC CRITERIA

Pre-excitation of the ventricles via the bundle of Kent results in the following ECG changes:

1. Slurring of the initial part of the complex — the delta wave. The delta wave is the result of early depolarization of the ventricles. See Figure 10 A below.

2. The PRI is shortened due to the delta wave.

3. The duration of the complex is prolonged due to the delta wave.

4. Secondary ST-T wave changes may be seen due to the altered repolarization. Secondary ST-T wave changes may or may not be present. If present they are usually seen in V_1, V_2 with Type A and V_5, V_6 with Type B.

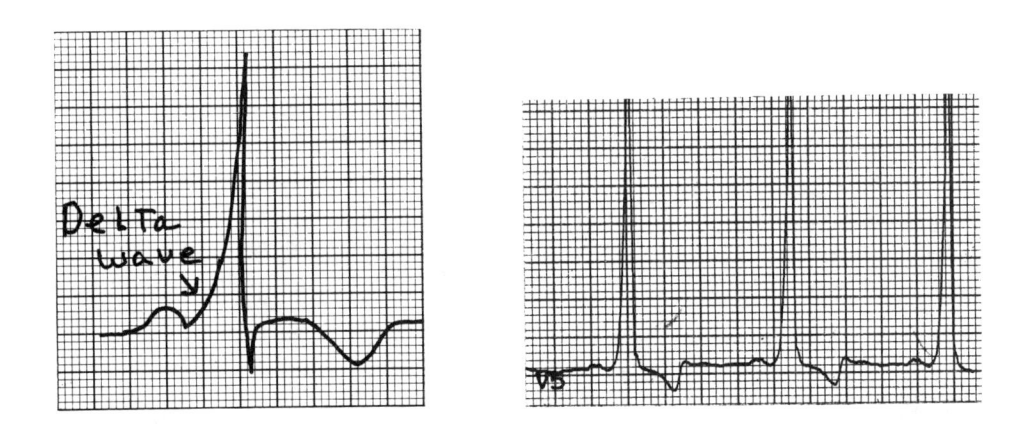

Figure 10 A WPW ECG Diagnostic Criteria

Figure 10 B and 10 C on pages 280 and 281 are examples of WPW Type A.
Figure 10 D and 10 E on pages 282 and 283 are examples of WPW Type B.

Figure 10 B. WPW Type A

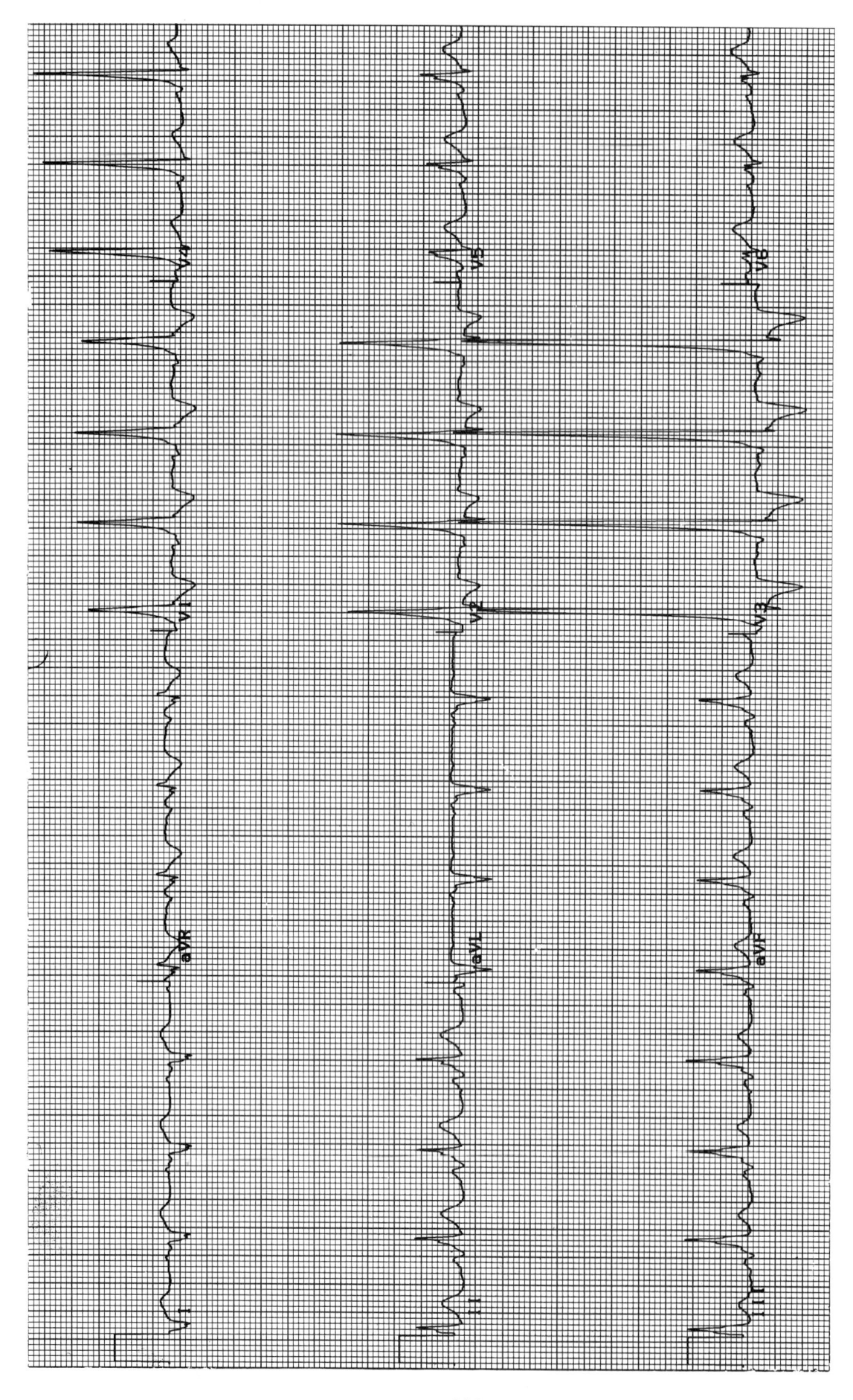

This is a young, thin, tall male which can account for the increased voltage in the precordial leads V_3 and V_4. Note the delta wave, short PR interval, wide complex, and secondary ST-T changes in V_1 through V_3.

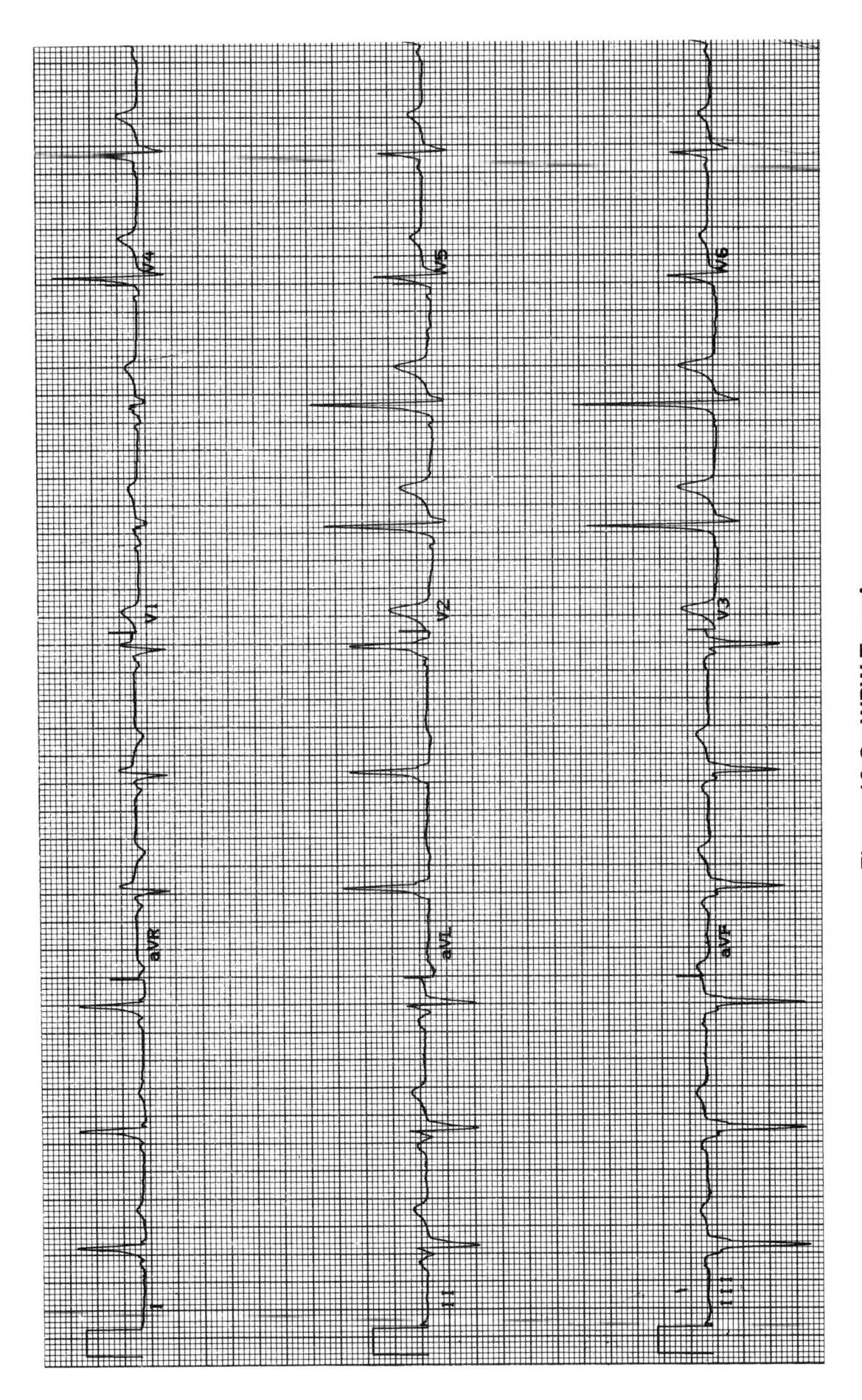

Figure 10 C. WPW Type A

Note the delta wave which results in a shortened PRi and widened complex. Q waves in III and aVF simulate inferior myocardial infarction.

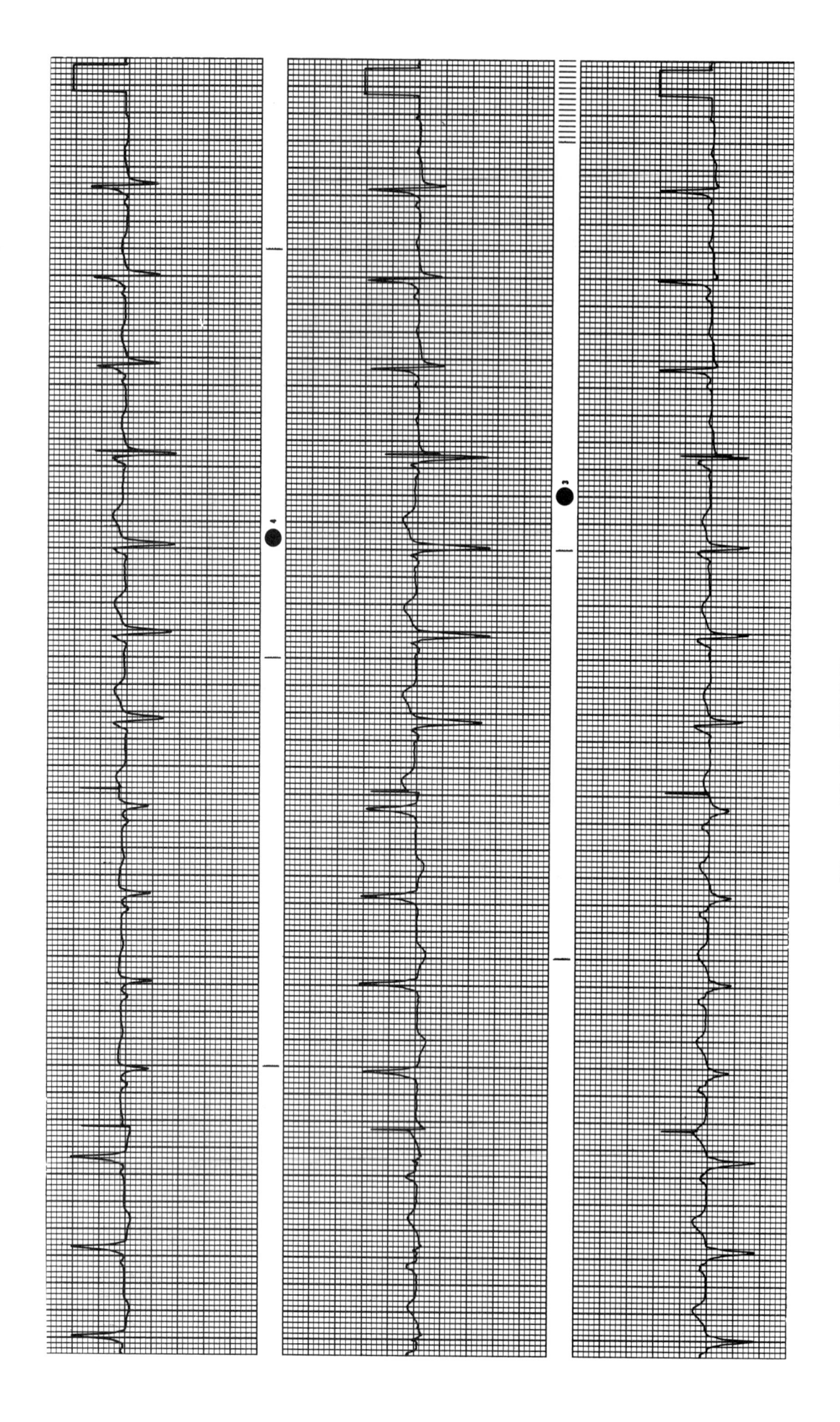

Figure 10 D. WPW Type B

Note the delta wave which results in a shortened PRi and widened complex. Q waves in II, aVF: a pseudoinferior myocardial infarction.

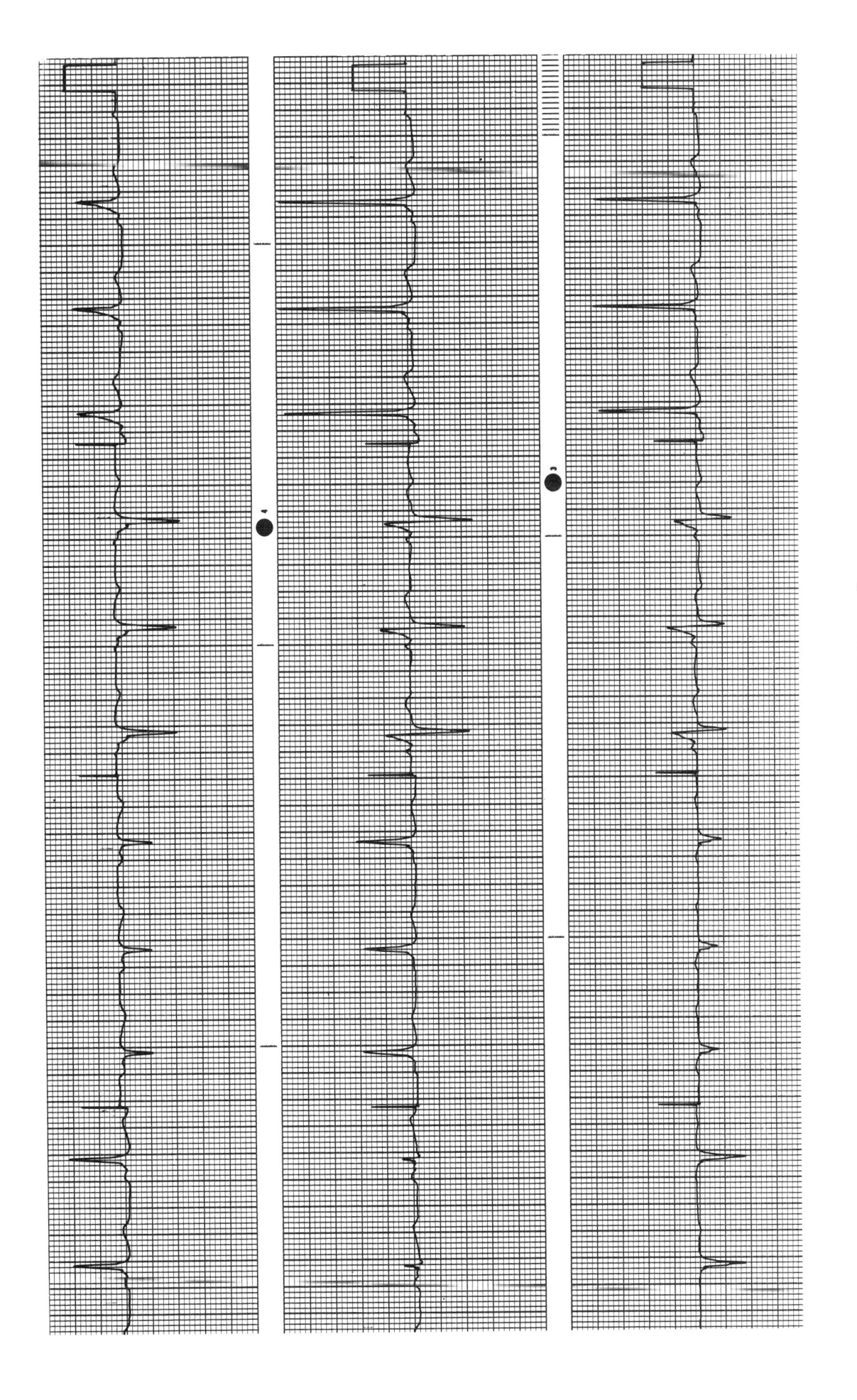

Figure 10 E. WPW Type B

Note the delta wave, short PRi, and prolonged complex. Also Q waves in II and aVF; a pseudoinferior myocardial infarction.

Chapter 10 — Wolff-Parkinson-White (WPW) Syndrome

CLINICAL SIGNIFICANCE

The WPW syndrome can cause a predisposition to atrial tachyarrhythmias due to reentry tachycardia as follows:

The conduction via the accessory bundle of Kent may be antegrade or retrograde.

Recall that antegrade means forward and retrograde means backwards.

RETROGRADE VERSUS ANTEGRADE AV NODE CONDUCTION

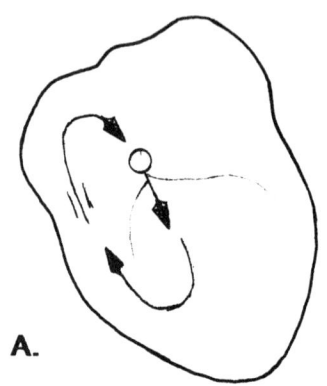

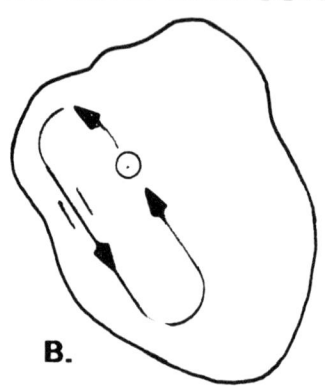

A. Antegrade through the AV Node

B. Retrograde through the AV Node

Picture A above shows antegrade conduction through the AV node with return to the atria via the bundle of Kent. A circus movement (reentrant tachycardia) may thus be initiated.

QUESTION: Would reentrant tachycardia with antegrade conduction through the AV node and a return to the atria via the bundle of Kent inscribe a normal complex or one with a delta wave?

A. Normal complex
B. Delta wave

ANSWER: A. A normal complex would be inscribed.

Please note that antegrade conduction through the AV node is also retrograde through the bundle of Kent. Likewise, retrograde conduction through the AV node is antegrade conduction through the bundle of Kent. It all depends on your frame of reference.

Picture B above shows the wave of depolarization entering the ventricle via the bundle of Kent and returning to the atria via the AV node (retrograde).

QUESTION: What kind of a complex would be inscribed with retrograde conduction through the AV node as depicted in picture B?

A. Normal
B. Abnormal

ANSWER: B. Abnormal

Chapter 10 — Wolff-Parkinson-White (WPW) Syndrome

When conduction occurs retrograde through the AV node a broad complex with a delta wave is inscribed. The tachycardia makes it difficult to see the delta wave. This is easily confused with ventricular tachycardia.

WPW type A and B can be mistaken for ventricular tachycardia:

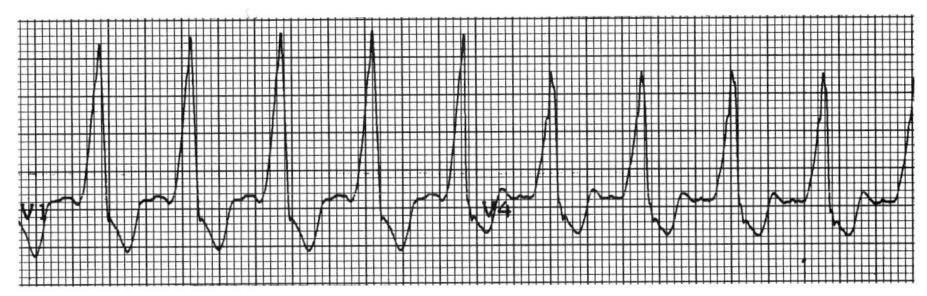

Figure 10 F

In Figure 10 F, the atrial impulses are conducted through the accessory bundle of Kent with a rapid ventricular response. This could easily be mistaken for ventricular tachycardia.

TREATMENT AND MEDICATION

WPW is considered an important clinical entity because of the frequent occurrences of tachyarrhythmias which compromise the patient. The tachycardia mechanism in WPW is a reentry phenomenon via the accessory and normal AV pathways as depicted in picture A and B on the previous page.

Chapter 10 — Wolff-Parkinson-White (WPW) Syndrome

Consider the effects of the following medications on the effective refractory period of the AV node and the bundle of Kent.

Medication	Effective Refractory Period — AV Node	Effective Refractory Period — Bundle of Kent
Amiodarone	Lengthen	Lengthen
Digitalis	Lengthen	Shorten
Lidocaine	No change	Lengthen
Procainamide	No change	Lengthen
Propranolol	Lengthen	No change
Quinidine	Shorten	Lengthen
Verapamil	Lengthen	Shorten

Note that digitalis and verapamil shorten the effective refractory period of the accessory pathway. The use of digitalis or verapamil on the patient with WPW may increase the conduction down the accessory pathway causing an increase in the ventricular rate and the possible development of ventricular fibrillation.

Note that lidocaine and procainamide lengthen the effective refractory period of the accessory pathway. If the tachycardia was traveling antegrade down the accessory pathway, lidocaine and procainamide would be effective in terminating the tachyarrhythmia.

Many patients with the WPW syndrome need long-term maintenance with medications such as propranolol, digitalis, and quinidine.

In a medical emergency situation, cardioversion applied immediately may convert the arrhythmia.

Patients with refractory tachyarrhythmias caused by WPW may benefit from an artificial pacemaker or surgical intervention.

CHAPTER 11
12 LEAD ECG REVIEW

It should be noted that the ECG must be interpreted in relation to the clinical condition of the patient and is no more than an aid to diagnosis, although considerable information can be derived from it.

This chapter reviews the ECG characteristics presented herein for:

- **Location of frontal plane axis**
- **Chamber enlargements**
- **Intraventricular conduction defects**
- **Myocardial ischemia, injury, and infarction**
- **Subendocardial infarctions**
- **Supraventricular aberrancy versus ventricular ectopy**
- **Effect of certain medications and electrolyte abnormalities**

FRONTAL PLANE AXIS

Normal axis is present when either:

1. Lead I and aVF both have positive complexes.
2. Lead I has a positive complex and aVF has an equiphasic complex.
3. Lead I has an equiphasic complex and aVF has a positive complex.

Clinically, it is not necessary to look for the exact degrees of a normal axis. Once you have ascertained the axis is normal, that's all you need to do. Degrees will be included herein just for the sake of practice.

I	aVF	Quadrant	Equiphasic	Axis
positive	negative	Left axis deviation	II	-30°
			aVR	-60°
negative	positive	Right axis deviation	II	+150°
			aVR	+120°
negative	negative	No man's land	III	-150°
			aVL	-120°

287

Chapter 11 — 12 Lead ECG Review

CHAMBER ENLARGEMENT

Right atrial enlargement

Peaked P in II, III, aVF, V_1
P amplitude > 2.5 mm II, III, aVF

Left atrial enlargement

Notched P in II, III, aVF
P duration > 0.11 seconds

Prominent negative P terminal in V_1

Biatrial enlargement

Peaked P wave in II, III, aVF
Tall P > 2.5 mm
Wide P > 0.11 seconds
Notched P in II, III, aVF
Abnormal P terminal in V_1

Right ventricular hypertrophy

Increased amplitude of r waves in V_1, V_2
Increased amplitude of the s wave in V_5, V_6
Secondary ST-T wave changes in V_1 and V_2
Increased VAT greater than 0.02 seconds in V_1, V_2
Right axis deviation

Chapter 11 — 12 Lead ECG Review

Left Ventricular Hypertrophy Estes Scoring System

CRITERIA		POINTS
Voltage		
S in V_1 or V_2: 25 mm or more		
R in V_5 or V_6: 25 mm or more	all or any one	3
R or S in any frontal plane lead: 20 mm or more		
Secondary ST-T changes		
Patient not on digitalis		3
Patient on digitalis		2
Abnormal P Terminal in V_1		3
Left axis deviation -30° or more		2
qRs interval: $\geq$ 0.09 seconds		1
VAT in V_5, V_6: 0.05 seconds or more		1

4 POINTS IS PROBABLE LVH

5 POINTS OR MORE STRONGLY INDICATES LVH

Chapter 11 — 12 Lead ECG Review

INTRAVENTRICULAR CONDUCTION DEFECTS

Right bundle branch block

rSR' (rabbit ears) V_1, V_2
s/S slurred V_5, V_6 (I, aVL)
Complex duration 0.12 seconds or greater
Secondary ST-T changes in the right precordial leads V_1, V_2

Left bundle branch block

QS or rS V_1, V_2
Loss of septal q wave V_5, V_6
Monophasic complex V_5, V_6
Complex duration 0.12 seconds or greater
Secondary ST-T changes in the left precordial leads V_5, V_6

Left anterior descending hemiblock (LADH)

Left axis deviation (-30° or more leftward)
Small r wave in lead II, III, or aVF
Small q wave in lead I or aVL

Left posterior hemiblock (LPH)

Right axis deviation (usually +110° or more rightward)
Small q wave in lead II, III, or aVF
Small r wave in lead I or aVL
No other evidence for right ventricular hypertrophy

Bifascicular block

RBBB + LADH
rSR' (rabbit ears) V_1, V_2
s/S slurred V_5, V_6 (I, aVL)
Complex duration 0.12 seconds or greater
Secondary ST-T changes in the right precordial leads V_1, V_2
Left axis deviation (-30° or more leftward)
Small r wave in lead II, III, or aVF
Small q wave in lead I or aVL

RBBB + LPH
rSR' (rabbit ears) V_1, V_2
s/S slurred V_5, V_6 (I, aVL)
Complex duration 0.12 seconds or greater
Secondary ST-T changes in the right precordial leads V_1, V_2
Right axis deviation (usually +110° or more rightward)
Small q wave in lead II, III, or aVF
Small r wave in lead I or aVL
No other evidence for right ventricular hypertrophy

Chapter 11 – 12 Lead ECG Review

Trifascicular block

    Bifascicular block plus some degree of AV heart block

TRANSMURAL MYOCARDIAL ISCHEMIA, INJURY, AND INFARCTION

Infarction = Pathological Q waves
Injury = Elevated ST segments
Ischemia = Inverted T waves

Age of Infarction

Recent/Acute = Q waves and elevated ST segments (normal or abnormal T waves)
Old = Q waves
Undetermined = Q waves, inverted T waves

Site of Infarction

Inferior = II, III, aVF
Lateral = I, aVL, V_5, V_6
Septum = V_1 (V_2)
Anterior = V_2, V_3, V_4
Posterior = V_1, V_2 (Tall R waves)

SUBENDOCARDIAL INFARCTION

ST segment depression } in the leads facing the infarcted wall as above
T wave inversion

Chapter 11 — 12 Lead ECG Review

SUPRAVENTRICULAR ABERRANCY	VENTRICULAR ECTOPY
Ashman's phenomena	Fusion beats
Triphasic complex V_1	Biphasic or predominantly positive complex in V_1 with taller left rabbit ear
Initial vector the same or similar	Opposite initial vector
P prime (P')	Absence of P prime
Noncompensatory pause	Compensatory pause
Ventricular rate greater than 170	Ventricular rate < 170
Slowed or terminated by vagal maneuvers	Unaffected by vagal maneuvers
	QS or rS in V_6
	Fat initial r greater than 0.03 seconds in V_1
Complex duration less than 0.14 seconds	Complex duration $\geq$ 0.14 seconds
	Concordant pattern
	Evidence of AV dissociation
	Left, right, or no man's land axis deviation

Chapter 11 — 12 Lead ECG Review

SUMMARY OF DRUG AND ELECTROLYTE ECG CHANGES

ECG Change	Drug and Electrolyte
P wave amplitude decreased	Hyperkalemia
P wave notched	Quinidine
PR interval increased	Hyperkalemia Hypokalemia Procainamide Quinidine
Complex duration increased	Hyperkalemia Norpace Procainamide Quinidine
ST segment depression	Digitalis Hypokalemia Quinidine
ST segment elevation	Hyperkalemia
T wave amplitude decreased	Digitalis Hypokalemia Procainamide
T wave amplitude increased	Hyperkalemia Quinidine
T wave flattened	Phenothiazines
T wave inversion	Hypokalemia Phenothiazines Quinidine
T wave notched/diphasic	Digitalis Quinidine Phenothiazines Procainamide
U wave amplitude increased	Digitalis Hypokalemia Phenothiazines Procainamide Quinidine
QTI shortened	Digitalis Hypercalcemia
QTI prolonged	Hypocalcemia Norpace Phenothiazines Procainamide Quinidine

Chapter 11 — 12 Lead ECG Review

WOLFF-PARKINSON-WHITE (WPW) SYNDROME

Delta wave
Short PRi
Duration of complex prolonged
Secondary ST-T changes

GLOSSARY

Aberrant: Deviating from the usual or normal course.

Absolute refractory period: Time during which the cardiac cells are incapable of responding to a stimulus, regardless of its strength. The absolute refractory period of the ventricles is from the beginning of the complex to the beginning of the T wave.

Acute reciprocal changes: Depressed ST segments in leads opposite an acute transmural myocardial infarction.

Anterior leads: V_2, V_3, V_4

Automaticity: Ability of myocardial cells to function as pacemakers and to spontaneously generate electrical impulses.

Baseline: The same as the isoelectric line.

Biphasic: Component of the ECG which is partly positive and partly negative; i.e., it is above and below the isoelectric line.

Cardiac output: The amount of blood ejected from the heart in one minute.
Cardiac Output = Stroke Volume X Heart Rate.

Cardioversion: Conversion of a pathological tachyarrhythmia to normal sinus rhythm, by use of electrical shock to the heart via electrodes placed on the chest wall.

Complex: The ECG waves due to ventricular depolarization. The waves of the complex are the q, r, and S. The complex consists of variations of these waves.

Circus movement: The same as reentrant tachycardia.

Concordant pattern: Presence of all positive or all negative complexes in all six of the precordial leads.

Conductivity: Ability of the cardiac cells to conduct electrical impulses.

Controlled atrial fibrillation: Ventricular rate less than 101 BPM.

Depolarization: Cardiac electrical stimulation which is normally followed by myocardial contraction.

Delta wave: Initial slurring of the complex seen in the WPW syndrome.

Dextrocardia: Having the heart on the right side of the body.

Diphasic: Another term for biphasic.

Dromotropic: Conduction velocity; may be positive (accelerated) or negative (slowed).

Ectopic: In reference to the heart, any pacemaker other than the sinus node.

Equiphasic: The same as biphasic except the wave is equally positive and negative.

Glossary

Excitability: The ability of the cardiac cell to respond to a given stimulation.

Frontal plane axis: The orientation of the heart's electrical activity in the frontal plane.

Fusion beats: Also known as Dressler and summation beats. There are two pacemakers spreading through the myocardium at the same time. These two impulses fuse and form a complex which is the fusion beat. The fusion beat on the ECG has some characteristics from each of the sources of its origin.

Galvanometer: An instrument for measuring small electrical currents.

Inferior leads: II, III, aVF.

Isoelectric line: The baseline of the ECG. When the ECG is isoelectric, no electrical activity is occurring in the heart and the stylus records a straight line.

Hypercalcemia: High serum calcium.

Hyperkalemia: High serum potassium.

Hypertrophy: An increase in the cardiac mass due to an increase in the size but not the number of cardiac cells.

Hypocalcemia: Low serum calcium.

Hypokalemia: Low serum potassium.

IVCD: Intraventricular conduction defect.

Iatrogenic: Abnormal condition induced by effects of the physician treating the patient. Implies that such effects could have been avoided by proper care on the part of the physician. Example: anxiety neurosis.

Left lateral leads: I, aVL, V_5, V_6.

Lidocaine reflex: The tendency to administer lidocaine for any wide, bizarre looking complex.

mm: millimeter.

Monophasic: A component of the ECG which is totally above or totally below the isoelectric line.

P' (P Prime): P wave caused by a PAC.

P mitrale: Left atrial enlargement.

P pulmonale: Right atrial enlargement.

P terminal: The negative terminal portion of the P wave. Normally, P terminal is equal to or less than the initial positive (upward) deflection of the P wave. An abnormal P terminal in lead V_1 is an ECG characteristic of P mitrale.

Glossary

P wave: The depolarizing electrical current recorded by the ECG when the atria are stimulated and depolarize.

PAC: Premature atrial contraction.

PAT: Paroxysmal atrial tachycardia.

PJC: Premature junctional contraction.

PVC: Premature ventricular contraction.

Physiological q waves: q Waves inscribed as the result of septal depolarization. Normally seen in V_5, V_6, I, aVL, may also be seen In II, III, aVF as a normal variant.

Posterior reciprocal changes: Tall R waves in V_1, V_2 as the result of posterior myocardial infarction.

Primary ST-T wave abnormalities: ECG changes that reflect an actual change in ventricular repolarization and not caused secondarily by changes in the complex which are due to altered depolarization.

Purkinje fibers: Specialized conducting cells at the distal end of the bundle branches which spread the electrical stimulus through the ventricular myocardium.

Q wave: When the initial deflection of the complex is negative it is called a q wave (q if less than 5 mm in depth; Q if the depth is 5 mm or more).

qRs complex: The depolarizing electrical current recorded by the ECG when the ventricles are stimulated and depolarize.

QT interval: Beginning of the complex to the end of the T wave.

R wave: The first positive deflection of the complex. If the deflection is less than 5 mm it is an r wave; if the deflection is 5 mm or more it is an R wave.

Reciprocal changes: Unfortunately, the term reciprocal has two meanings in 12 lead ECG interpretation. The terms *acute reciprocal changes* and *posterior reciprocal changes* are used in this book to help differentiate the two terms.

Refractory: Resistant to ordinary treatment.

Relative refractory period: A stronger than normal stimulus is capable of exciting the cardiac cell. The relative refractory period of the ventricles is from the beginning of the T wave to almost the end of the T wave.

Repolarization: After depolarization, the return of the heart muscle cells to their resting state.

Right ventricular leads: V_1 and V_2.

Septal leads: V_1 and sometimes V_2.

Glossary

Septal q waves: The same as physiological q waves.

Sick sinus syndrome: Caused by dysfunction of the sinus node - usually manifested as bradycardia, or bradycardia with episodes of tachycardia.

Stroke Volume: The amount of blood the heart ejects with each systole.

Subendocardial infarction: Necrosis that involves only the inner half of the total thickness of the ventricular wall. The only ECG change may be the presence of deep, symmetrically inverted T waves without any pathological Q waves.

Torades de pointes: A French term for ventricular tachycardia, which means "twisting of the points." The vector of the complexes appear to rotate cyclically, pointing downward for several beats and then twisting and pointing upward in the same lead.

Transition: In the precordial leads, the lead in which the amplitude of the R wave becomes as great or greater than the S wave. Transition normally occurs in V_3 but may occur in V_2 or V_4 as a normal variant.

Transmural myocardial infarction: Necrosis affecting the entire thickness of the ventricular wall.

Triphasic: Component of the ECG which is above, below, above the isoelectric line, i.e., or below, above, below the isoelectric line.

Uncontrolled atrial fibrillation: Ventricular rate greater than 100 BPM.

Vector: A force with direction and magnitude. In electrocardiography, direction is the most important parameter; an arrow represents the direction of the flow of electrical current in the heart.

BIBLIOGRAPHY

Chou, Te-Chuan. (1986). <u>Electrocardiography in Clinical Practice</u>. Second Edition. New York: Grune and Stratton Inc.

Goldberger, A.L., and Goldberger, E. (1986). <u>Clinical Electrocardiography: A Simplified Approach</u>. Third Edition. St Louis, Missouri: The C.V. Mosby Company.

Khan, G.M., (1988). <u>Manual of Cardiac Drug Therapy</u>. Second Edition. Philadelphia: W.B. Saunders.

Marriott, H.J.L. (1988). <u>Practical Electrocardiography</u>. Eighth Edition. Baltimore: Williams and Wilkins.

Norman, A.E. (1989). <u>Rapid ECG Interpretation: A Self-Teaching Manual</u>. New York: Macmillan Publishing Company.

Thomas, C.L. (Ed.) (1989). <u>Taber's Cyclopedic Medical Dictionary.</u> Sixteenth Edition. Philadelphia: F.A. Davis Company.

Wong, E.T., Zappaterreno, G. (Eds.), (1991). <u>Laboratories and Pathology Mini Handbook: A Guide to Using the Laboratory Effectively</u>. Los Angeles: Los Angeles County+University of Southern California Medical Center.